Healthcare Code Sets, Clinical Terminologies, and Classification Systems

FOURTH EDITION

KATHY GIANNANGELO

MA, RHIA, CCS, CPHIMS, FAHIMA

VOLUME EDITOR

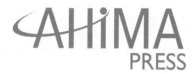

AHIMA STAFF
Chelsea Brotherton, MA, Production Development Editor
Colton Gigot, MA, Production Development Editor
Megan Grennan, Managing Editor
James Pinnick, Senior Director, Publications
Caitlin Wilson, Project Editor

Cover image: © gremlin, iStockphoto

American Health Information Management Association
233 North Michigan Avenue, 21st Floor
Chicago, Illinois 60601-5809
ahima.org

Contents

Part I

Healthcare Code Sets and Classifications Commonly Used for Administrative and Statistical Reporting

Part II

Other Terminologies and Classification Systems

Part III

HIT Data Standards and Interoperability

Part IV

Application of Terminologies and Classification Systems in Healthcare

Detailed Contents

Part I

Healthcare Code Sets and Classifications Commonly Used for Administrative and Statistical Reporting — *5*

2   Current Procedural Terminology (CPT)

Andrei Besleaga, RHIT

3   Healthcare Common Procedure Coding System (HCPCS)   87

June Bronnert, MHI, RHIA, CCS, CCS-P

4   National Drug Codes (NDCs)   109

Gary L. Saner

5   Current Dental Terminology (CDT)

Mark W. Jurkovich, DDS, MBA, MHI

Part II

Other Terminologies and Classification Systems

6   SNOMED Clinical Terms (SNOMED CT)

Mary H. Stanfill, MBI, RHIA, CCS, CCS-P, FAHIMA

11   International Classification of Functioning, Disability, and Health   299

Heather R. Porter, PhD, CTRS

12   Terminologies Used in Nursing Practice   329

Susan Matney, PhD, RNC-OB, FAAN, FACMI

13   Other Terminology and Classification Systems   *353*

Kathy Giannangelo, RHIA, CCS, CPHIMS, FAHIMA

Part III

HIT Data Standards and Interoperability 387

14 Healthcare Data Governance and Data Set Standards 389

Mary H. Stanfill, MBI, RHIA, CCS, CCS-P, FAHIMA

15 Data Interchange Standards 425

Jay Lyle, PhD

Part IV

Application of Terminologies and Classification Systems in Healthcare

16   Centralized Locations and Tools for Multiple Terminologies: Servers, Services, Databases, and Registries

Susan A. Matney, PhD, RNC-OB, FAAN, FACMI

17   Data Mapping of Clinical Terminologies, Classifications, and Ontologies

James R. Campbell, MD

About the Editor and Authors

KATHY GIANNANGELO, MA, RHIA, CCS, CPHIMS, FAHIMA, has a comprehensive background in the field of clinical terminologies, classification, and data standards with more than forty years of experience in the health information management field. She is president of Kathy Giannangelo Consulting, LLC. Her consulting work involves clinical terminology feasibility assessments, adoption methodology appraisals, and implementation support. Previous positions include map lead for SNOMED International, where she provided expertise, support, and consensus for the development, review, and maintenance of mappings between SNOMED CT and other code systems. As a coding specialist for the National Committee for Quality Assurance, her work focused on the analysis of quality measures and assignment of various vocabulary standards to value sets used in the measure criteria.

For six years, she taught a graduate-level course on clinical vocabularies and classification systems. Other previously held positions include director of content management for Apelon, Inc., where she oversaw the terminologies found within the Core Content suite and helped clients define terminology requirements, create or extend structured terminologies, or integrate terminology components into their products. As a medical informaticist with Language and Computing (L&C), her role was to support the ontology, modeling, sales, and product development activities related to the creation and implementation of natural language processing applications where clinical terminology and classification systems are utilized. Prior to L&C, she was director, practice leadership, with the American Health Information Management Association (AHIMA) in Chicago. Kathy has also served as senior nosologist for a health information services company and worked in various HIM roles, including vice president of product development, education specialist, director of medical records, quality assurance coordinator, and research team manager for the Centers for Disease Control and Prevention.

Contributing Authors

Andrei Besleaga, RHIT, is an experienced health information management (HIM) professional serving as a healthcare coding analyst at the American Medical Association (AMA) since 2016. He is one of the contributing staff writers for the AMA's *CPT Assistant* newsletter. Andrei completed his associate of applied science degree in HIM, followed by a bachelor of science degree in pre-medical biology with a concentration on cellular and molecular biology, and obtained his registered health information technician (RHIT) certification in 2009. Before joining the AMA, Andrei served in various roles for both nonprofit and for-profit organizations, including Kaiser Permanente Health Plan and Lincoln Financial Group. He is also an active partner in Elsevier's eLearning projects and a current member of the American Health Information Management Association. In his spare time, Andrei enjoys traveling, road trips, playing the piano, and spending time with his chocolate Labrador, Wrigley.

June Bronnert, MSHI, RHIA, CCS, CCS-P, is the director of terminology mapping at Intelligent Medical Objects Inc. (IMO), where she provides health information management (HIM) subject matter expertise while overseeing daily operations of code mappings for IMO's terminology solutions.

Prior to joining IMO, she held various positions including professional practice director at the American Health Information Management Association (AHIMA), where she provided professional expertise to develop AHIMA products and services aimed at furthering the art and science of HIM. She was responsible for content development and technical reviews of AHIMA's products and resources.

Mrs. Bronnert's experience includes positions ranging from coding professional and coding supervisor to director at various facilities, including the Department of Veterans Affairs (VA). She was a member of the National Coding Council at the VA, where she provided coding educational programs.

Mrs. Bronnert was also an adjunct educator for the Cincinnati State RHIT program and University of Cincinnati RHIA program for numerous years while being active in her state and local HIM association. She obtained her master's degree in health informatics from Northeastern University and her HIM degree from Indiana University.

James Campbell, MD, FACP, FACMI, is a physician board certified in primary care internal medicine and a professor of medicine at the University of Nebraska Medical Center. He retired from clinical practice in 2017 after 45 years of caring for patients. Dr. Campbell earned a bachelor of science degree in physics from the University of Rochester in 1968 with training in computer science. He became convinced of the future of the electronic health record (EHR) in 1979 and recognized the sentinel role of well-formed terminologies and ontologies in achieving that vision. He implemented his first EHR, a problem-oriented enhancement of COSTAR®, in 1982. Dr Campbell has worked with standards organizations since 1995, including SNOMED International, LOINC, and HL7. He is a consultant terminologist certified by SNOMED. Dr. Campbell has developed terminology extensions, deployed those in EHRs that he has used for patient care, and researched and published widely on the use of terminology for advanced decision support and data analytics.

Christopher Chute, MD, DrPH, is a Bloomberg Distinguished Professor of health informatics and professor of medicine, public health, and nursing at Johns Hopkins University; he is chief research information officer for Johns Hopkins Medicine. He received his undergraduate and medical training at Brown University, internal medicine residency at Dartmouth, and doctoral training in epidemiology and biostatistics at Harvard. He is board certified in internal medicine and clinical informatics and an elected Fellow of the American College of Physicians, the American College of Epidemiology, HL7, the America Medical Informatics Association, and the American College of Medical Informatics (ACMI), as well as a Founding Fellow of the International Academy of Health Sciences Informatics. He is currently president of ACMI through 2018.

Dr. Chute's career has focused on how we can represent clinical information to support analyses and inferencing, including comparative effectiveness analyses, decision support, best evidence discovery, and translational research. He has had a deep interest in semantic consistency, harmonized information models, and ontology. His current research focuses on translating basic science information to clinical practice and how we classify dysfunctional phenotypes (disease). He became founding chair of biomedical informatics at Mayo Clinic in 1988 and retired from Mayo in 2014, where he remains an emeritus professor of biomedical informatics. He is presently PI on a spectrum of high-profile informatics grants from NIH spanning translational science. He has been active on many HIT standards efforts and chaired ISO Technical Committee 215 on Health Informatics and the World Health Organization International Classification of Disease Revision (ICD-11).

Michael B. First, MD, is a professor of clinical psychiatry at Columbia University and a research psychiatrist in the Division of Behavioral Health Sciences and Policy Research, Diagnosis and Assessment Unit at the New York State Psychiatric Institute. He maintains a schematherapy and psychopharmacology practice in Manhattan. Dr. First is a nationally and internationally recognized expert on psychiatric diagnostic and assessment issues and conducts expert forensic psychiatric evaluations in both criminal and civil matters.

Dr. First is the co-chair of the DSM-5 text revision, an editorial and coding consultant for the DSM-5, the chief technical and editorial consultant on the World Health Organization's ICD-11 revision project, and an external consultant to the National Institute of Mental Health's Research Domain Criteria (RDoC) project. Dr. First was the editor of the DSM-IV-TR and the editor of text and criteria for the DSM-IV and the American Psychiatric Association's *Handbook on Psychiatric Measures*. He has co-authored and co-edited a number of books, including the fourth edition of the two-volume psychiatry textbook *A Research Agenda for DSM-V* as well as *DSM-5 Handbook for Differential Diagnosis, Structured Clinical Interview for DSM-5 (SCID-5)*, and *Learning DSM-5 by Case Example*. He has trained thousands of clinicians and researchers in diagnostic assessment and differential diagnosis.

Mark Jurkovich, DDS, MBA, MHI, is a graduate of the University of Minnesota School of Dentistry. He also has master's degrees in business and health informatics. He has utilized Current Dental Terminology (CDT) codes as a clinician and has served on the CDT Code Maintenance Committee. He serves on advisory groups for various interested parties that have voting privileges on the Code Maintenance Committee. He continues his work in terminologies by serving as the co-lead for the SNOMED International Dental Clinician Resource Group and chairing the ANSI SNODENT Maintenance Committee. He also serves as vice chair of the Standards Committee of Dental Informatics and has a strong interest and involvement in health information exchange and how terminologies directly assist in enhancing that information transfer. He has spoken nationally and internationally on code use in dentistry.

Jay Lyle, PhD, is a clinical data standards architect for JP Systems. He serves as the current terminology project manager for the Federal Health Information Model and as a consultant to the Veterans Health Administration for standards implementation. He is also a founding partner of the US affiliate of the Global e-Health Collaborative, an organization focused on developing collaborative solutions to complex health data issues.

After teaching composition and literature in high school and college, he worked in systems integration as a business architect and project manager before focusing his efforts on data standards, which he has been designing and helping to implement for over 10 years. Dr. Lyle serves as co-chair of the Patient Care Work Group for the Health Level Seven International standards development organization. He holds a PhD in Renaissance literature from the University of Virginia and an MBA from Emory University's Goizueta Business School.

Susan Matney, PHD, RNC-OB, FAAN, FACMI, FHIMSS, is a medical informaticist with Intermountain Healthcare. She has more than 20 years of experience in informatics and 30 years in nursing. In 2002, she took the terminology Logical Observation Identifiers Names and Codes (LOINC) to the American Nurses Association to be recognized as a terminology for use in nursing. She represents nursing at national and international conferences and organizations, including SNOMED CT, Health Level Seven (HL7), LOINC, and the Federal Health Information Model Terminology team. She is chair of the LOINC Nursing Subcommittee, past chair of the SNOMED CT Nursing Special Interest Group, and current member of the HL7 Terminology Authority.

Terri Meredith, RPh, MSCIS, is a medical editor with responsibilities that include the National Library of Medicine's RxNorm database. Prior to her work at the National Library of Medicine, she was the director of clinical vocabularies at Cerner Corporation. She has over 20 years of experience with drug vocabularies such as RxNorm, SNOMED, the UK's Dictionary of Drugs and Medical Devices, and Australia's NeHTA drug database. She works with both national and international standards organizations, including the National Council for Prescription Drug Programs and Health Level Seven International, to promote interoperability in drug vocabularies.

Brooke N. Palkie, EdD, RHIA, is a tenured associate professor for the Department of Health Informatics and Information Management at the College of St. Scholastica with a teaching focus on classifications, vocabularies, and clinical data standards as well as assessing healthcare quality and corporate compliance. Dr. Palkie is an AHIMA-approved ICD-10-CM/PCS trainer and has been involved with several ICD-10 educational training programs and grant-funded projects. She also serves as a coauthor on the AHIMA Press publication *Basic ICD-10-CM and ICD-10-PCS*

Coding. Prior to her higher education career, Dr. Palkie worked in management roles both within the hospital setting and for the State of Minnesota. Dr. Palkie graduated from the College of St. Scholastica with a bachelor's and master's degree in health information management and received her EdD from Capella University with a focus on educational leadership.

Heather Porter, PhD, CTRS, is an associate professor in the Rehabilitation Sciences Department, Recreational Therapy Program at Temple University in Philadelphia, PA. She has a dual bachelor of science in recreational therapy and sport/recreation management, a master of science in counseling psychology with a certificate in marriage and family counseling, and a PhD in health studies (recreational therapy and public health). She has a strong clinical background in inpatient and outpatient physical rehabilitation and is an avid proponent of the International Classification of Functioning, Disability and Health (ICF). She was the author of the first book about the ICF other than the ICF book itself, which was spotlighted in the ICF Clearinghouse newsletter (a CDC publication). She served as the chair for the American Therapeutic Recreation Association's World Health Organization ICF team for three years and has been a member of the team since its inception in 2004. She contributed to the development of the lower limb amputation ICF Core Set, gives ICF presentations to local and national audiences, and developed a graduate-level ICF academic course. She serves as the editor for Idyll Arbor's Recreational Therapy Practice series, which focuses on the infusion of the ICF into recreational therapy practice, and is the director of the ICF and evidence-based recreational therapy research lab at Temple University. She has published numerous journal articles and book chapters, created and maintains the Recreational Therapy Wise Owls website (www.rtwiseowls.com) to promote evidence-based practice, provides evidence-based research consultation to recreational therapy academic programs, and has received several teaching awards.

Gary L. Saner is senior manager of information solutions in the life sciences group at Reed Technology and Information Services Inc. and an experienced leader in establishing regulatory solutions for the life sciences industry. He monitors regulations, forms solution concepts for industry needs, and facilitates system development and client implementation.

Mr. Saner has over 35 years of experience in the areas of software development, process management, and data administration, with the last 15 years focused on the life sciences industry. With an understanding of regulations, business requirements, and systems, he has helped shape and implement successful solutions at Reed Tech for US drug labeling submission, XML publishing, EU XEVMPD medicinal product information, and US medical device unique device identification (UDI).

Within the life sciences community, Mr. Saner is a recognized subject matter expert on Structured Product Labeling (SPL), FDA electronic Drug Registration and Listing (eDRL), and medical device UDI compliance. He is an active member of industry's SPL Leadership Team and SPL Process Team and serves as co-chair of the SPL Technical Team. He is involved with other industry groups including the EMA SPOR Task Force, IRISS IDMP, DIA, and RAPS; he also serves on the advisory board of the Medical Devices Group.

Mary H. Stanfill, MBI, RHIA, CCS, CCS-P, FAHIMA, is vice president of health information management (HIM) consulting services for United Audit Systems, Inc. (UASI), based in Cincinnati, OH. Mary has over 30 years of experience within the HIM profession. She served as the vice president of HIM Practice Resources for the American Health Information Management Association from 2006 to 2011 before joining UASI in 2011. Throughout her career, she has been directly involved in clinical documentation requirements for classification systems, mapping and map validation for clinical terminologies and classification systems, and compliance with healthcare data standards and reporting specific data sets. For six years, she taught a graduate-level course on managing clinical classifications and terminologies.

Ms. Stanfill has published over 35 articles in industry journals and presented over 45 presentations nationally and internationally on various healthcare classification and clinical terminology topics. She has also designed and delivered numerous educational courses and programs, both online and in person.

Ms. Stanfill holds a bachelor of science degree in HIM from Mercy College of Detroit and a master of science degree in biomedical informatics from the Oregon Health Sciences University School of Medicine in Portland, Oregon. She also holds a mini-MBA from Northwestern University in Chicago, Illinois, and completed the SNOMED CT master's course from the College of American Pathologists in 2006.

Daniel Vreeman, PT, DPT, MS, FACMI, is an associate research professor and the Regenstrief-McDonald Scholar in Data Standards at the Indiana University School of Medicine and a research scientist at the Regenstrief Institute, Inc. As director, LOINC and health data standards, at the Regenstrief Center for Biomedical Informatics, he leads the development of LOINC, a freely available international standard for identifying health measurements, observations, and documents. Dr. Vreeman's primary research focus is on the role of standardized clinical vocabularies and standards to support electronic health information exchange. He provides leadership to the terminology services that underpin the Indiana Network for Patient Care, the nation's largest interorganizational clinical data repository with more than 10 billion clinical data elements. He is the author of the book *LOINC Essentials: A step-by-step guide for getting your local codes mapped to LOINC*. Dr. Vreeman also teaches medical informatics at Indiana University. More information on Dr. Vreeman's research and professional interests can be found at: https://danielvreeman.com.

Foreword

John D. Halamka, MD, MS

In 2019, academia, industry, and government are turning their attention to machine learning to improve healthcare quality, safety, and workflow. But training artificial intelligence tools requires curated data. Data must be codified and normalized, otherwise even the most powerful tools will suffer from "garbage in, garbage out" dysfunction.

As healthcare embraces the next generation of decision support, metadata about the underlying data is more important than ever. We cannot move the industry forward to enhance interoperability, empower patients, or evolve EHRs into highly usable decision support tools without coding.

Healthcare Code Sets, Clinical Terminologies, and Classification Systems is a key resource for this transformation. It provides all the resources needed for health information professionals to ensure the data used in the next generation of tools is organized, comparable, and consistent.

ICD-10, SNOMED-CT, and other vocabularies are now required as part of the US Core Data for Interoperability (USCDI), and these coding systems are soon to be part of new CMS and ONC regulations accelerating interoperability among providers, payers, and patients.

Think of this textbook as a roadmap to help you navigate the next phase of healthcare innovation. Machine learning, application programming interfaces, mobile technologies, cloud services, and telemedicine are all empowered by the coding systems described in this volume.

John D. Halamka, MD, MS, is a professor of medicine at Harvard Medical School, chief information officer of Beth Israel Deaconess Medical Center, chairman of the New England Healthcare Exchange Network (NEHEN), co-chair of the national HIT Standards Committee, co-chair of the Massachusetts HIT Advisory Committee, and a practicing emergency physician.

Online Resources

For Instructors

Instructor materials for this book are provided only to approved educators. Materials include test bank, Check Your Understanding and review question answer keys, PowerPoint slides, and other useful reminders and resources. Please visit http://www.ahima.org/publications/educators.aspx for further instruction. If you have any questions regarding the instructor materials, please contact AHIMA Customer Relations at (800) 335-5535 or submit a customer support request at https://my.ahima.org/messages.

For Students

This textbook includes a student workbook featuring application exercises, a Check Your Understanding answer key, and additional chapter review content.

Acknowledgments

The volume editor would like to thank

Keith W. Boone
Fred Horowitz, DMD
Emily A. Kuhl, PhD
William E. Narrow, MD, MPH
Stuart J. Nelson, MD, FACMI
Theresa A. Rihanek, RHIA, CCS
Rita A. Scichilone, MHSA, RHIA, CCS, CCS-P
Amy Sheide, MPH, RN
Bedirhan Üstün, MD
Judith J. Warren, PhD, RN, BC, FAAN, FACMI
Ann Zeisset, RHIT, CCS, CCS-P

for their contributions to the textbook.
AHIMA Press would like to acknowledge Kimberly Huey, MJ, CHC, CPC, CCS-P, PCS, CPCO, COC, for her review of this edition.

Introduction

Kathy Giannangelo, MA, RHIA, CCS, CPHIMS, FAHIMA

The coding of healthcare encounters has been one of the core functions of health information management (HIM) almost since the beginning of the profession. In fact, many consider the function of identifying and organizing clinical data to be the essence of the profession (Sheehy 1991). Given this observation, what better way is there to name and arrange medical content than through terminologies, classifications, and code sets?

This core function has been considered in a number of American Health Information Management Association (AHIMA) projects. For example, AHIMA's Coding Futures Task Force studied the likely futures of HIM professionals in the domain of coding practice. The group determined that HIM professionals must be educationally prepared to go well beyond the assignment of diagnostic and procedural codes and into broader areas of formalization that will ensure a leading position in the development of algorithmic translation, concept representation, and mapping among clinical nomenclatures and reimbursement methods (Johns 2000). This was further reinforced in market research conducted to determine specific job skills, job competencies and role specialties needed to align with the healthcare industry's future needs. One of the key findings of that study was that survey participants in both clinical and nonclinical segments identified skills and capabilities in data standards, classifications, and terminologies as a priority (Vault Consulting 2017).

While HIM professionals have a long history with a select group of terminologies, classifications, and code sets, such as the Health Insurance Portability and Accountability Act (HIPAA) standard healthcare code sets, they also need to become cognizant of and knowledgeable about many others. As a landmark Institute of Medicine report concluded, "No single terminology has the depth and breadth to represent the broad spectrum of medical knowledge; thus, a core group of well-integrated, nonredundant clinical terminologies will be needed to serve as the backbone of clinical information and patient safety systems" (IOM 2004). In addition, multiple systems were recommended for reporting structured data elements under the Promoting Interoperability Program developed by the Centers for Medicare and Medicaid Services (CMS). Thus, standard code sets, clinical terminologies, and classification systems are a key element for interoperable electronic health records (EHRs).

In 2018, National Library of Medicine staff collaborated with the National Committee for Vital and Health Statistics Subcommittee on Standards to produce an environmental scan on health terminologies. The report again reinforced their importance and application in today's electronic environment by indicating "terminologies provide structured domain knowledge and are increasingly being used as the foundation of healthcare information systems" (NCVHS 2018).

The current landscape of standards and implementation specifications is published by the Office of the National Coordinator for Health Information Technology (ONC) through the Interoperability Standards Advisory. Section I of the guide lists the standards available to address clinical health information interoperability needs. Among those noted, some of which are well known by HIM professionals and others not so much, are:

- International Classification of Diseases, Tenth Revision, Clinical Modification (ICD-10-CM)
- ICD-10, Procedure Coding System (ICD-10-PCS)
- Current Procedural Terminology, Fourth Edition (CPT) (also known as HCPCS Level I)
- Code on Dental Procedures and Nomenclature (CDT)
- National Drug Codes (NDCs)
- Healthcare Common Procedure Coding System (HCPCS Level II)
- RxNorm
- Logical Observation Identifiers Names and Codes (LOINC)
- SNOMED Clinical Terms (SNOMED CT)
  (ONC 2018)

In addition to expanding knowledge of clinical terminologies and classifications, HIM professionals must understand their tie to data governance along with health information technology (HIT) data set and data interchange standards. Data sets are needed to create and populate forms and templates, to enhance database management, and to help build a data warehouse for use in executive and clinical decision support. Moreover, data interchange standards are necessary for the capture, exchange, and use of data for various purposes.

Having uniform data sets and standards for the electronic exchange of health record information results in the ability to send and receive medical and administrative data in an understandable and usable manner. Some standards, such as the Uniform Hospital Discharge Data Set, have been in existence since the late 1960s. Others, often referred to using their acronyms, such as *CDA, FHIR, DICOM,* or *USCDI,* exist because of their connection to electronic systems interoperability.

The HIM professional's role in terminologies and classifications as well as data governance and data standards is essential to unified clinical information and administrative systems. However, this alone will not result in interoperability. In 2006, a joint effort between the American Medical Informatics Association (AMIA) and AHIMA produced a report addressing the role of terminologies and classifications in forming the information content in EHRs. AMIA and AHIMA state:

A robust universe of health-related terminologies and classifications identifying the clinical data is required, and simply having a list of relevant words is not the same as representing all the relevant data in a computable form. Thus, while coherent systems of terminologies and classifications are essential, they are not sufficient, especially in the context of data and information representation. The process of data or information representation begins with information models, not just the terms and codes alone (AMIA and AHIMA Terminology and Classification Policy Task Force 2006).

Contained in the pages that follow is educational material covering the above topics. Part I, Healthcare Code Sets and Classifications Commonly Used for Administrative and Statistical Reporting, and Part II, Other Terminologies and Classification Systems, supply detail on the various code sets, clinical terminologies, and classification systems either currently in use or having the potential for use in an EHR. This information combined with that found in Part III, HIT Data Standards and Interoperability, and Part IV, Application of Terminologies and Classification Systems in Healthcare, translates into a comprehensive textbook for HIM professionals. This resource will expand your knowledge of code sets, clinical terminologies, and classification systems; explain their connection to data governance, data sets, and data interchange standards; identify implementation issues surrounding their use in an electronic environment; and describe the connection between terminology and semantic interoperability.

References

American Medical Informatics Association (AMIA) and American Health Information Management Association (AHIMA) Terminology and Classification Policy Task Force. 2006. Healthcare terminologies and classifications: An action agenda for the United States. White paper. *Perspectives in Health Information Management*. http://bok.ahima.org/PdfView?oid=71880.

Institute of Medicine (IOM), Committee on Data Standards for Patient Safety. 2004. Patient Safety: Achieving a New Standard for Care. Washington, DC: National Academies Press.

Johns, M. 2000. Crystal ball for coding. *Journal of AHIMA* 71(1):26–33.

National Committee for Vital and Health Statistics (NCVHS), Subcommittee on Standards. 2018. Health terminologies and vocabularies environmental scan. https://ncvhs.hhs.gov/wp-content/uploads/2018/10/Report-Health-Terminologies-and-Vocabularies-Environmental-Scan.pdf.

Office of the National Coordinator for Health Information Technology (ONC). 2018. Interoperability Standards Advisory, 2018. https://www.healthit.gov/isa/.

Sheehy, Kathryn H. 1991. Coding and classification systems: Implications for the profession. White paper. *Journal of the American Medical Record Association* 62:44–49.

Vault Consulting, LLC. 2017. American Health Information Management Association: Health information management skills, education, and credential research. White paper. http://bok.ahima.org/PdfView?oid=302482.

Part I

Healthcare Code Sets
and Classifications
Commonly Used for
Administrative
and Statistical Reporting

1

International Classification of Diseases (ICD) and the US Modifications

Dr. Brooke Palkie, EdD, RHIA

LEARNING OBJECTIVES

- Describe the purpose and function of the International Classification of Diseases
- Identify the developer, revision process, and guidelines for ICD-10, ICD-10-CM, and ICD-10-PCS
- Summarize the differences between WHO's International Classification of Diseases and ICD-10-CM and ICD-10-PCS
- Demonstrate understanding of the ICD-10-CM process for the US
- Compare the different classification systems
- Explain the structure of ICD-10-CM and ICD-10-PCS
- Examine the relationships ICD-10-CM and ICD-10-PCS have with other classifications, terminologies, and code sets

KEY TERMS

- Centers for Medicare and Medicaid Services (CMS)
- Classification of diseases
- Clinical Data Abstraction Center (CDAC)
- *Coding Clinic*
- Cooperating Parties
- Coordination and Maintenance Committee (C&M Committee)

- Department of Health and Human Services (HHS)
- Encoder
- Hierarchical Condition Category (HCC) risk adjustment model
- International Classification of Diseases (ICD)
- Morbidity
- Mortality
- Mortality Reference Group (MRG)
- National Center for Health Statistics (NCHS)
- Prospective Payment System (PPS)
- Update and Revision Committee (URC)
- World Health Organization (WHO)

Introduction to ICD

This chapter discusses the International Classification of Diseases (ICD), specifically the Tenth Revision (ICD-10), ICD-10 Clinical Modification (ICD-10-CM), and ICD-10 Procedure Coding System (ICD-10-PCS). Each classification is discussed in terms of how it was developed, its purpose, its content, its principles and guidelines, and the process for revision and updates. This chapter also reviews how ICD relates to other terminologies, classification systems, code sets, tools available to access, and adoption and use.

International Classification of Diseases

The **World Health Organization (WHO)** in Geneva, Switzerland is responsible for the development and publication of the **International Classification of Diseases (ICD)**. A **classification of diseases** can be defined as a "system of categories to which morbid entities are assigned according to established criteria" (WHO 2016). The purpose of ICD is to permit the systematic recording, analysis, interpretation, and comparison of **mortality** and **morbidity** data collected in different countries. Mortality data identifies the causes of death and morbidity data the causes of disease. The classification system then is used to translate diagnoses, diseases, and other health problems from words into codes. This translation permits easy reporting, storage, retrieval, and analysis of data (WHO 2016).

ICD was developed in the early 20th century as a way to collect data from governments on the causes of death worldwide. As revisions were developed, it became increasingly evident that classifications needed to be considered from a broader perspective. The classification of sickness and injury is closely linked with the classification of causes of death. Today, many countries use ICD-10 to record both mortality and morbidity data. Having an international coding system provides a way in which data can be collected, analyzed, interpreted, and compared.

WHO publishes the International Classification of Diseases as a standardized diagnostic tool for epidemiology, management of health, and other clinical purposes. The intent of the classification is to monitor the incidence and prevalence of diseases and other health problems (WHO 2018a). The overall concept of monitoring is to analyze the health of a population. Population groups can then be compared and assessed within regional, state, national, and international levels. According to WHO, ICD is the foundation for all clinical and research purposes due to its hierarchical structure. This allows for easy storage and retrieval, analysis, sharing, and comparing of health information. Today, the use of ICD-10 codes for reimbursement is a vital part of healthcare operations in most types of facilities. The ICD-10 provides defined codes for the purposes of:

- Classifying morbidity and mortality information for statistical purposes
- Indexing hospital records by disease and operations
- Reporting diagnoses and procedures for reimbursement
- Storing and retrieving data
- Determining patterns of care among healthcare providers
- Analyzing payments for health services
- Performing epidemiological studies, clinical trials, and clinical research
- Measuring quality, safety, and efficacy of care
- Designing payment systems
- Setting health policy
- Monitoring resource utilization
- Implementing operational and strategic plans
- Designing healthcare delivery systems
- Improving clinical, financial, and administrative performance
- Preventing and detecting healthcare fraud and abuse
- Tracking public health and risks

ICD has become the international standard diagnostic classification for all general epidemiological and many health management purposes.

International Statistical Classification of Diseases and Related Health Problems, Tenth Revision (ICD-10)

Development of the tenth revision of ICD began in 1983. Volume 1, Tabular List, was first published in 1992, followed by volume 2, Instruction Manual, in 1993, and volume 3, Alphabetic Index, in 1994. This edition was a major revision from the previous ICD-9 version.

Developer

ICD-10 is a collaborative product among WHO and 10 international centers, although WHO holds the copyright. The Forty-third World Health Assembly endorsed ICD-10 in May 1990, and the system came into use by WHO Member States in 1994. The US implemented ICD-10 in January 1999.

Purpose

Many countries around the world have implemented ICD-10 for reporting mortality statistics. The US is bound by international treaty to report mortality data to WHO using ICD-10 codes. ICD-10 has been used in the US as a mortality classification for the coding of death certificates since 1999. A morbidity classification contains substantially more detail than is required in a mortality classification. Some of these countries use ICD-10 to report morbidity data; others have chosen to modify ICD-10 for that same purpose. WHO has authorized for the development of modifications of ICD-10 under specific requirements. In the US, this clinical modification of ICD includes ICD-10-CM. Clinically modified systems have also been implemented in Australia (ICD-10-AM), Canada (ICD-10-CA), Germany (ICD-10-GM), and Thailand (ICD-10-TM), amongst others. The necessary clinical modifications of ICD-10, ICD-10-CM, and ICD-10-PCS were needed prior to the US implementation on October 1, 2015.

Content

ICD-10 is a statistical classification, hierarchical in structure. It provides many more categories for disease and other health-related conditions than previous revisions through its alphanumeric coding scheme. In addition, it includes chapter rearrangements compared to ICD-9, additions and revisions, and extensive changes to the mental and behavioral disorders (chapter V), the injury, poisoning, and certain other consequences of external causes (chapter XIX), and the external causes of morbidity and mortality (chapter XX). It also includes additional categories for post-procedural disorders.

General Structure

Although the collaborating centers discussed a different structure and evaluated other models after the ninth revision, the tenth revision maintains the long-established arrangement for morbidity and mortality statistics. This variable-axis classification places diseases, disorders, injuries, and other reasons for a patient to receive healthcare services into chapters according to what is most appropriate for general epidemiological purposes. This method influences the way diseases are grouped in ICD-10. The five ways are:

- Epidemic diseases
- Constitutional or general diseases
- Local diseases arranged by site (the body system chapters)
- Development diseases
- Injuries

Four of the five groupings are considered "special." The exception is local diseases arranged by site. The special groups bring together disorders that, for epidemiological study, make sense to be placed together rather than classified mainly by anatomical site. In other words, the conditions are assigned principally to one of the four special-group chapters, which have priority over the body system chapters. In order to assign codes and interpret statistics properly, it is important to keep this in mind.

Structural Components

ICD-10 is divided into three volumes, consists of twenty-two chapters (including a placeholder chapter for codes for new diseases of uncertain etiology), and uses alphanumeric codes, described in the following subsections.

THE VOLUMES

Volume 1, Tabular List, contains an alphanumeric listing of ICD-10 codes arranged by chapter. It also includes notes and other coding instructions. Volume 2, Instruction Manual, contains background information, instructional materials on how to use volumes 1 and 3, and rules and guidelines for mortality and morbidity coding. Volume 3, Alphabetic Index, is the alphabetic index to the diseases, disorders, injuries, and other conditions found in volume 1. Volume 1 also contains instructions on how to use the index. The Instruction Manual is available online at WHO's ICD website.

THE CHAPTERS

ICD-10 includes separate chapters for diseases of the nervous system (VI), diseases of the eye and adnexa (VII), and diseases of the ear and mastoid process (VIII). Moreover, ICD-10 does not separate the codes that explain the external causes of injury and poisoning and the factors influencing health status and contact with health services from the core classification.

Since the ICD-10 codes begin with an alphabetic character, many of the chapters begin with a new letter. It is important to keep in mind that some chapters use more than one letter and some chapters share a letter. For example,

Chapter II, Neoplasms (C00–D48)

Chapter III, Diseases of the blood and blood-forming organs and certain disorders involving the immune mechanism (D50–D89)

Chapter XIX, Injury, poisoning and certain other consequences of external causes (S00–T98)

The order and content of the ICD-10 chapters for diseases of the skin and subcutaneous tissue (XII) and diseases of the musculoskeletal system and connective tissue (XIII) follow the chapter on diseases of the digestive system. Next are chapters for diseases of the genitourinary system (XIV), pregnancy, childbirth, and the puerperium (XV), certain conditions originating in the perinatal period (XVI), and congenital malformations, deformations, and chromosomal abnormalities (XVII). Disorders involving the immune mechanism are included with diseases of the blood and blood-forming organs (III).

Category restructuring and code reorganization have occurred in a number of ICD-10 chapters, which has resulted in different classification of certain diseases and disorders. For example, Streptococcal sore throat and its inclusion terms, found in the infectious and parasitic disease chapter of ICD-9, are reclassified in ICD-10 to Chapter X, Diseases of the Respiratory System.

THE CODES

To serve a wider variety of needs for reporting mortality and healthcare data, the tenth revision has implemented a completely alphanumeric coding scheme. The first character is a letter. All the letters of the alphabet are used. The letter *U* has been set aside by WHO for the provisional assignment of new diseases of uncertain etiology or emergency use (U00–U49) or for resistance to antimicrobial and antineoplastic drugs (U82–U85). For example, category U04 has been assigned to severe acute respiratory syndrome (SARS). When this condition is better understood, a code (or codes) will be created to classify this condition to the appropriate ICD-10 chapter.

The code letter is followed by two numbers. Each code must have the first three characters, followed by a decimal point, followed by additional characters if needed.

C19   Malignant neoplasm of rectosigmoid junction

I50.0   Congestive heart failure

S02.1   Fracture of base of skull

Features

Some of the other features of ICD-10 are:

- *Exclusion notes:* These notes have been expanded at the beginning of each chapter to clarify the hierarchy of the chapters. As explained previously, the special-group chapters have priority over the organ or system chapters. In addition, the chapters for pregnancy, childbirth, and the puerperium (XV) and certain conditions originating in the perinatal period (XVI) take precedence over the other special-group chapters.

- *Blocks:* After the appropriate Includes and Excludes notes, chapters are further subdivided into blocks of three-character categories. To explain the chapter structure, the beginning of each chapter contains a listing of blocks and, where applicable, the asterisk (manifestation) categories.

- *Notes:* The notes in the Tabular List apply to both mortality and morbidity use. Rules specific to one or the other are found in volume 2.

- *Drug-induced conditions:* What began with the ninth revision regarding the identification of drug-induced conditions has been expanded in the tenth revision.

- *Mental and Behavioral Disorders (Chapter V); Injury, Poisoning, and Certain Other Consequences of External Causes (Chapter XIX); and External Causes of Morbidity and Mortality (Chapter XX):* These chapters are significantly revised in ICD-10.

- *Disorders of the immune system:* The categories for disorders of the immune system have been expanded and are placed with diseases of blood and blood-forming organs rather than with endocrine, nutritional, and metabolic diseases.

- *Diseases of the eye and adnexa and diseases of the ear and mastoid process:* Sense organs have been separated from nervous system disorders, creating two new chapters for diseases of the eye and adnexa and for disorders of the ear and mastoid process.

- *Injuries:* Injuries are grouped by body part and not by categories of injury; thus, all injuries of the head and neck are grouped together, rather than all fractures or all open wounds. Figure 1.1 compares injury codes in ICD-10 with those in ICD-9.

- *Postprocedural disorders:* ICD-10 contains new categories placed toward the end of each body system chapter for postprocedural complications.

- *Etiology and manifestation:* The asterisk codes (manifestations) are found in specific three-character categories, resulting in less confusion on their appropriate use in conjunction with the dagger codes (etiology).

FIGURE 1.1. Differences in injury codes in ICD-9 and ICD-10

```
ICD-9-CM
    – Fractures (800–829)
    – Dislocations (830–839)
    – Sprains and strains (840–848)
ICD-10-CM
    – Injuries to the head (S00–S09)
    – Injuries to the neck (S10–S19)
    – Injuries to the thorax (S20–S29)
```

Conventions Used in ICD-10

Like its predecessors, ICD-10 contains conventions that must be understood and used, where necessary, in order to properly use the classification and assign accurate codes. Following is a summary of those found in the Tabular List and Alphabetic Index.

INSTRUCTIONAL TERMS AND NOTES

Terms or notes providing information or instructions are found either at the beginning of a chapter or a block or after a three-, four-, or five-character code. Their position is important in that the terms or notes that appear at the beginning of a chapter apply to all the categories in the chapter. The same rule applies to terms or notes found at the block or code level. Following are some examples of the various types of instructional notes and terms found in ICD-10:

- Inclusion and exclusion terms at category level

  K31 Other diseases of stomach and duodenum

  Includes: functional disorders of stomach

  Excludes: diverticulum of duodenum (K57.0–K57.1)

                   gastrointestinal haemorrhage (K92.0–K92.2)

- Includes notes and exclusion notes at chapter level

  Chapter V Mental and behavioral disorders (F00–F99)

  Includes: disorders of psychological development

  Excludes: symptoms, signs and abnormal clinical and laboratory findings, not elsewhere classified (R00–R99)

- Use additional code at category level

  N34   Urethritis and urethral syndrome

        Use additional code (B95–B98), if desired, to identify infectious agent.

PUNCTUATION MARKS

ICD-10 uses the following punctuation marks for the purposes stated:

- Parentheses ( ) enclose supplementary words, a code contained in an excludes note, a code range for a block, or a dagger or asterisk code in the Tabular List. Parentheses are used in the Alphabetic Index to enclose nonessential modifiers, cross-referenced terms, or morphology codes.

- Square brackets [] are used to enclose a note or pages and direct the user elsewhere. They also are used to enclose synonyms, alternative words, and explanatory phrases.
- Colons : indicate that one of the modifying terms after the main term (that is, the condition listed above the colon) is required before the code can be assigned.
- Braces { } are used to identify incomplete terms. The terms may precede or follow the brace. One or more of the terms after the brace complete or qualify the terms before the brace.
- A dash is used in both the ICD-10 Index and the Tabular List. The Index uses the dash to show the level of indentation. In the Tabular List, a dash preceded by a decimal point (.–) indicates an incomplete code.

Examples:

K63.1   Perforation of intestine (nontraumatic)

B20   Human immunodeficiency virus [HIV] disease resulting in infectious and parasitic diseases

C48   Malignant neoplasm of retroperitoneum and peritoneum
    Excludes: Kaposi's sarcoma (C46.1)
                     mesothelioma (C45.–)

ABBREVIATIONS

The abbreviation *NEC* stands for not elsewhere classified. A residual category, subdivision, or subclassification provides a location for "other" types of specified conditions that have not been classified elsewhere.

The abbreviation *NOS* stands for not otherwise specified. The unspecified, or NOS, codes are available for use when documentation of the condition identified by the provider is not specific to the defined axis.

Examples:

L98.4   Non-pressure chronic ulcer of skin, not elsewhere classified
    Chronic ulcer of skin NOS
    Tropical ulcer NOS
    Ulcer of skin NOS
    Excludes: decubitus [pressure] ulcer and pressure area (L89.–)
                     gangrene (R02)
                     skin infections (L00-L08)

specific infections classified to A00-B99

ulcer of lower limb NEC (L97)

varicose ulcer (I83.0, I83.2)

R07.89 Other chest pain

Anterior chest-wall pain NOS

RELATIONAL TERMS

ICD-10 contains the following types of relational terms:

- *And:* When the term *and* is contained in code titles, it should be interpreted to mean and/or.
- *With, with mention of, associated with, in:* These terms join together conditions. The combination must be present to assign the code; however, an indication of a cause-and-effect relationship is unnecessary.
- *Without, not associated with:* These terms indicate that the two conditions should not be present together. When both conditions are present, a different code should be selected.
- *Due to, resulting in:* The cause-and-effect relationship should be clear from the documentation. In some cases, however, ICD-10 presumes a cause-and-effect relationship.

Examples:

C41.3	Malignant neoplasm of ribs, sternum and clavicle
E50.5	Vitamin A deficiency with night blindness
H33.3	Retinal breaks without detachment
J15.2	Pneumonia due to staphylococcus

DAGGER (ETIOLOGY) AND ASTERISK (MANIFESTATION)

A dual-classification system is available for the identification of the etiology or underlying cause and the manifestation of certain disease. In ICD-10, the dagger symbol (†) indicates the underlying disease and the asterisk symbol (*) is for the manifestation.

LEAD TERMS

The Alphabetic Index to Diseases and Nature of Injury, the Table of Neoplasms, the External Causes of Injury Index, and the Table of Drugs and Chemicals are organized in ICD-10 by lead terms describing the disease condition, other reason for an encounter with the healthcare provider, or the underlying cause or means of an injury.

MODIFIERS OR QUALIFIERS

Descriptors, essential and nonessential modifiers that further specify the lead term, may be listed as subterms or in parentheses.

CROSS-REFERENCES

The Alphabetic Index contains the following cross-references: *see* and *see also*. The *see* cross-reference requires the coder to check another term in the index; the *see also* cross-reference provides the option to review a different term in the index if the specificity is not found with the original indexed term.

Examples:

Perinephritis (*see also* Infection, kidney) N15.9
–purulent (*see also* Abscess, kidney) N15.1

Paget's disease
–with infiltrating duct carcinoma – *see* Neoplasm, breast, malignant (M8541/3)

Principles and Guidelines

The guidelines for mortality and morbidity coding are located in the fourth section of volume 2, Instructional Manual. These rules have been adopted by the WHO to provide guidance on selecting the underlying cause of death and the main and secondary conditions analysis for morbidity data.

When reporting the underlying cause of death to the WHO, the rules specified in section 4 must be applied consistently for meaningful statistics to be obtained from these data. Included are standard definitions on "underlying cause of death," "live birth," "maternal death," and many others.

As one can see from the major section headings listed below (including the 4.1 subsection example), a coder assigning ICD-10 codes has many guidelines to understand and apply for appropriate reporting.

Process for Revision and Updates

The WHO established the **Update and Revision Committee (URC)** in 2000 to recommend mortality and morbidity changes to ICD-10. The URC manages the update process and recommends changes to the Heads of WHO Collaborating Centres each year. Before ICD-10, updates were not made between revisions. Because health classifications provide a common language for clinicians and administrators and must allow for the addition of new disease processes, the need for updates was recognized. An additional group, the **Mortality Reference Group (MRG)** was established to make recommendations regarding mortality to the URC. An update cycle was established. The Tabular List is updated every three years with major changes, and annually for minor changes. The Index is updated annually with changes that do not impact the structure of the Tabular List.

The URC assesses the need for updating the ICD and develops detailed proposals for annual meetings. It fosters reference groups for specific areas of interest and addresses issues brought forward by reference groups. The Committee may identify where major revision is required and how such a revision could be undertaken. Once a revision is approved by the Network, the URC Committee may undertake or direct the revision work. The Official Updates to the published volumes of ICD-10 are available as annual lists of changes. The lists indicate the source of recommendation and implementation date. These updates are approved annually at the October meeting of Heads of WHO Collaborating Centres for the Family of International Classifications (WHO 2018b). Each version of updates is available on WHO's ICD website.

ICD-10-CM and ICD-10-PCS

The uses of coded data go well beyond the purposes for which coding systems were originally designed or even contemplated in the 1970s. ICD was used primarily in the hospital inpatient setting for indexing purposes at the time the clinical modification of ICD-9 (ICD-9-CM) was implemented in the US. Used in many more healthcare settings, ICD-9-CM became a key component of several American healthcare reimbursement systems. Many reimbursement systems that are not based on a prospective payment methodology also require complete, accurate, and detailed coding in order to negotiate or calculate appropriate reimbursement rates, determine coverage, and establish medical necessity. However, ICD-9-CM had become inadequate for meeting the needs of noninpatient hospital settings or serving the many other purposes for which ICD data is used.

On January 16, 2009, the **Department of Health and Human Services (HHS)** published 45 CFR Part 162—HIPAA Administrative Simplification: Modifications to Medical Data Code Set Standards to Adopt ICD-10-CM and ICD-10-PCS in the *Federal Register*. This final rule adopted ICD-10-CM (and ICD-10-PCS) to replace ICD-9-CM in HIPAA transactions, effective October 1, 2013. The implementation of ICD-10 was delayed from October 1, 2013 to October 1, 2014 by final rule CMS-0040-F issued on August 24, 2012, and delayed a second time with the passage of H.R. 4302, Protecting Access to Medicare Act of 2014 until no earlier than October 1, 2015. On October 1, 2015, ICD-10-CM replaced ICD-9-CM volumes 1 and 2 (for diagnosis reporting), and ICD-10-PCS replaced ICD-9-CM volume 3 (for procedure coding).

In a separate final regulation, HHS adopted the updated X12 standard, Version 5010, and the National Council for Prescription Drug Programs standard, Version D.0, for electronic transactions, such as healthcare claims. Version 5010 is essential to use of the ICD-10 codes. Replacement of ICD-9-CM was an absolute necessity because the code set was more than 30 years old and had become obsolete. It no longer met the needs for accurate and complete data in the healthcare setting.

Being aware of the transition from ICD-9-CM to ICD-10-CM and ICD-10-PCS is essential as data previously coded in ICD-9-CM may need to be utilized for research, quality management, and other assessment purposes. For this reason, the **Centers for Medicare and Medicaid Services (CMS)** created a crosswalk between the ICD-9-CM and ICD-10-CM and ICD-10-PCS classification systems.

International Classification of Diseases, Tenth Revision, Clinical Modification (ICD-10-CM)

In 1994, the **National Center for Health Statistics (NCHS)** awarded a contract to the Center for Health Policy Studies (CHPS) to conduct a comprehensive evaluation of ICD-10 to determine whether it was a significant improvement over ICD-9-CM and should be implemented in the US. A technical advisory panel concluded that modifications were needed.

All modifications to ICD-10 must conform to WHO conventions. WHO authorized development of the modification of ICD-10 for use in the US. Per the agreement with WHO, NCHS was required to conform with system conventions and code structure. Moreover, any changes to code titles could not alter the meaning.

ICD-10-CM is in the public domain. In general, the classification will allow greater specificity in code assignment.

Developer

NCHS, the federal agency responsible for the use of ICD-10 in the US, developed a clinical modification of the classification for morbidity purposes called *International Classification of Diseases, Tenth Revision, Clinical Modification (ICD-10-CM)*.

ICD-10-CM represents a significant improvement over both ICD-9-CM and ICD-10. It incorporates much greater specificity and clinical detail, which will result in major improvements in the quality and usefulness of the data for all the current uses of the coding system. Moreover, information relevant to ambulatory and managed care encounters has been added.

Purpose

ICD-10-CM is used to report diseases and conditions of patients treated in the US healthcare system. When **prospective payment systems (PPSs)** came into existence, the concerns for data quality, coding education, and medical record documentation received new emphasis. The consequences of inaccurate claims data in a fee-for-service environment had not been nearly as critical. ICD-10-CM identifies the diagnosis for the PPSs and has a direct impact on payment.

Many reimbursement systems that are not based on a prospective payment methodology also require complete, accurate, and detailed coding in order to negotiate or calculate appropriate reimbursement rates, determine coverage, and establish medical necessity. For example, the **Hierarchical Condition Category (HCC) risk adjustment model** is mandated by CMS. The CMS-HCC model's purpose is to promote fair payments, reward efficiency, and encourage excellent care for the chronically ill (Hess and Frosch 2017). Risk adjustment is a method used to adjust bidding and payment based on the health status and demographic characteristics of an enrollee (CMS 2014). It is a method to adjust for observable differences between patients. HCC is a payment model that was implemented by Medicare in 2004 to adjust payments for the health expenditure risk of their enrollees (Pope et al. 2004). Uses of the CMS-HCC risk model are included within Medicare Advantage, Medicare Shared Savings Program (MSSP), Accountable Care Organizations, Comprehensive Primary Care Plus (CPC+), and Quality Payment Program (QPP)/Medicare Access and CHIP (Children's Health Insurance Program) Reauthorizations Act of 2015 (MACRA).

The CMS risk adjustment model measures medical conditions that include HCC categories that are correlated to diagnosis codes (CMS 2011). HCC codes are mapped to diagnoses that are supported by provider documentation. ICD-10-CM guidelines provide the standards used to support correct diagnostic coding. In essence, documentation impacts whether a diagnosis is considered an HCC or not. Conditions that are mapped to an HCC include high-risk chronic conditions and some acute high-risk conditions such as acute myocardial infarction (AMI) or acute renal failure, for example. Providers must show evidence with documentation that the patient's conditions were monitored, evaluated, assessed, and treated.

Risk adjustment occurs both to compare effectiveness and to remove variances in order to improve the delivery of high-value care. The risk adjustment model is "an actuarial tool used to predict health care costs based on the relative actuarial risk of enrollees in risk adjustment covered plans" (45 CFR 153.20). The risk score is developed via the Risk Adjustment Factor (RAF) score. The RAF score is set for each patient and includes the demographic elements (age, sex, and dual eligibility status) and incremental increases based on the HCC diagnoses submitted on claims (CMS 2017). Face-to-face encounters with qualified practitioners are used to determine the RAF score. HCC coding in the current year sets the RAF and subsequent funding for the next year. The focus is on the estimated expenditure risk for Medicare beneficiaries (Premera 2015).

The risk score includes chronic conditions that remain from year to year (for example, COPD, diabetes, CHF, and the like). Risk adjustment scores are higher for patients with chronic conditions and lower for healthier patients (Omachi et al. 2013). A risk adjustment system (RAS) executes the risk adjustment model and calculates the risk score. The risk score is normalized to the average of the population.

In order to validate submitted diagnoses, audits that compare health record documentation to the submitted diagnoses are conducted annually on selected plans. This again brings to light the importance of good clinical documentation.

Content

ICD-10-CM consists of the Alphabetic Index, an alphabetical list of terms and their corresponding codes, and the Tabular Lists, a structured list of codes divided into chapters based on body system or condition. The Alphabetic Index consists of the following parts: the Index of Diseases and Injury, the Index of External Causes of Injury, the Table of Neoplasms, and the Table of Drugs and Chemicals. The process to locate a code is to first identify a term within the Alphabetic Index and then verify the code and code description in the Tabular List.

Structure

ICD-10-CM has a hierarchical structure in which all codes with the same first three characters have common traits and each character beyond three characters adds greater specificity. ICD-10-CM also incorporates guidance through conventions and published guidelines. Moreover, ICD-10-CM uses notes and instructions. When a note appears under a three-character code, it applies to all codes within that category. However, instructions under a specific code apply only to that single code.

ICD-10-CM contains 21 chapters and its code composition is alphanumeric; letters I and O and numbers 1 and 0 should not be confused because the first character is always a letter. Letters are not case-sensitive. A chapter may encompass more than one letter, and more than one chapter may share a letter.

In ICD-10-CM, all letters are used except the letter U. Each code must be at least three characters, and the first three characters indicate the category. All codes in ICD-10-CM have full titles; thus, referral back to a common fourth or fifth character is unnecessary. For example, the full title of C4A.12 is merkel cell carcinoma of left eyelid, including canthus. There is no need to refer back to C4A.1, merkel cell carcinoma of eyelid, including canthus or C4A, merkel cell carcinoma to know the description of C4A.12. The fourth, fifth, or sixth characters provide additional specificity. A sixth character has been added in some chapters for further specificity. These additional characters provide the etiology, anatomic site, or severity of conditions. (See table 1.1 for examples of ICD-10-CM code composition.)

Seventh characters have been added in some chapters of ICD-10-CM, primarily in the obstetrics, injury, and external cause chapters. Seventh characters are added to the end of the code in the seventh position to add additional information when applicable. Table 1.2 lists general seventh-character extensions for the injury and external cause chapters and specific ones for fractures.

A placeholder x is used in some codes to allow for future expansion and to enable the use of a seventh character when the code contains fewer than seven characters.

ICD-10-CM diagnosis codes consist of three to seven characters. A decimal point is used after the third character when other characters are present. The structure is three characters to the left of the decimal point and up to four additional characters to the right. A three-character category may represent a single-disease entity (generally based on frequency or severity) or a group of closely related conditions. An example of a category is D51, Vitamin B_{12} deficiency anemia. Most, but not all, three-character categories have been subdivided. An example of a complete three-character code is P90, Convulsions of newborn. Up to four characters may follow the decimal to further describe such things as etiology, anatomic site, and severity. However, not every code will have four characters after the decimal. When the first three characters after the decimal are insufficient to describe the condition, a seventh character may appear after the three characters to the right of the decimal. Figure 1.2 shows the format of ICD-10-CM.

TABLE 1.1. Examples of ICD-10-CM code composition

ICD-10-CM Codes	Diagnoses
B20	Human immunodeficiency virus [HIV] disease
J20.0	Acute bronchitis due to Mycoplasma pneumoniae
D57.80	Other sickle-cell disorders without crisis
C50.311	Malignant neoplasm of lower-inner quadrant of right female breast
S59.222A	Salter-Harris Type II physeal fracture of lower end of radius, left arm, initial encounter for closed fracture

Source: CMS 2018.

TABLE 1.2. Use of seventh character extensions in ICD-10-CM

Injury and External Cause Chapters	Seventh Character	Definition
	A	Initial encounter
	D	Subsequent encounter
	S	Sequela
Fracture		
	A	Initial encounter for closed fracture
	B	Initial encounter for open fracture
	D	Subsequent encounter for fracture with routine healing
	G	Subsequent encounter for fracture with delayed healing
	K	Subsequent encounter for fracture with nonunion
	P	Subsequent encounter for fracture with malunion
	S	Sequelae

FIGURE 1.2. Format of ICD-10-CM

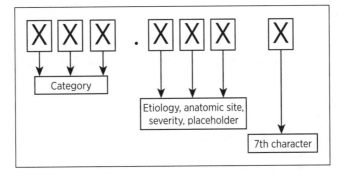

Alphabetic Index

The Alphabetic Index has two major sections, the Index to Diseases and Injuries and the Index to External Causes. In addition, there is a Neoplasm Table and a Table of Drugs and Chemicals. ICD-10-CM uses a dash (-) at the end of an entry to indicate that additional characters are required and will be found during the verification process in the Tabular List. In practice, all codes should be verified in the Tabular List. Characteristics of each of the sections are displayed in table 1.3. Figure 1.3 displays an example of the Alphabetic Index.

TABLE 1.3. Major sections of ICD-10-CM, Alphabetic Index

Section	Characteristics
Index to Diseases and Injuries	Includes terminology for all the codes appearing in the Tabular List of ICD-10-CM except external causes. The Alphabetic Index employs three levels of indentations: Main terms Subterms Carryover lines
External Cause of Injuries Index	Classifies environmental events, circumstances, and other conditions as the cause of injury and other adverse effects.
Table of Neoplasms	Provides codes for neoplasms by anatomical site, and then for each site there are six possible codes according to whether the neoplasm in question is malignant primary, malignant secondary, in situ, benign, of uncertain behavior, or of unspecified behavior.
Table of Drugs and Chemicals	Reports substances to identify poisoning states, toxic effects, underdosing, and external causes of adverse effects. The table lists the drug or chemical and columns to identify circumstances such as accidental, self-harm, assault, undetermined, adverse effect, or underdosing.

FIGURE 1.3. Sample of the Alphabetic Index to Diseases of ICD-10-CM

Prematurity NEC (less than 37 completed weeks) —*see* Preterm, newborn
- extreme (less than 28 completed weeks) —*see* Immaturity, extreme
Premenstrual
- dysphoric disorder (PMDD) F32.81
- tension (syndrome) N94.3
Premolarization, cuspids K00.2
Prenatal
- care, normal pregnancy —*see* Pregnancy, normal
- screening of mother —*see also* Encounter, antenatal screening Z36.9
- teeth K00.6
Preparatory care for subsequent treatment NEC
- for dialysis Z49.01
- peritoneal Z49.02
Prepartum —*see* condition
Preponderance, left or right ventricular I51.7
Prepuce —*see* condition
PRES (posterior reversible encephalopathy syndrome) I67.83
Presbycardia R54
Presbycusis, presbyacusia H91.1-
Presbyesophagus K22.8
Presbyophrenia F03
Presbyopia H52.4

Tabular List

The Tabular List of Diseases and Injuries contains the codes in alphanumeric order. All codes should be verified in the Tabular List. ICD-10-CM contains the following 21 chapters:

1	Certain infectious and parasitic diseases (A00–B99)
2	Neoplasms (C00–D49)
3	Diseases of the blood and blood-forming organs and certain disorders involving the immune mechanism (D50–D89)
4	Endocrine, nutritional and metabolic diseases (E00–E89)
5	Mental, Behavioral and Neurodevelopmental disorders (F01–F99)
6	Diseases of the nervous system (G00–G99)
7	Diseases of the eye and adnexa (H00–H59)
8	Diseases of the ear and mastoid process (H60–H95)
9	Diseases of the circulatory system (I00–I99)
10	Diseases of the respiratory system (J00–J99)
11	Diseases of the digestive system (K00–K95)
12	Diseases of the skin and subcutaneous tissue (L00–L99)
13	Diseases of the musculoskeletal system and connective tissue (M00–M99)
14	Diseases of the genitourinary system (N00–N99)
15	Pregnancy, childbirth and the puerperium (O00–O9A)
16	Certain conditions originating in the perinatal period (P00–P96)
17	Congenital malformations, deformations and chromosomal abnormalities (Q00–Q99)
18	Symptoms, signs and abnormal clinical and laboratory findings, not elsewhere classified (R00–R99)
19	Injury, poisoning and certain other consequences of external causes (S00–T88)
20	External causes of morbidity (V00–Y99)
21	Factors influencing health status and contact with health services (Z00–Z99)

Each chapter is divided into blocks, categories, subcategories, and, when appropriate, fifth-, sixth-, or seventh-character subclassifications. Table 1.4 illustrates the subdivisions.

The codes in the Tabular List must be assigned to the highest level of specificity.

The newest revision of the Tabular List, Index, guidelines, and mappings for ICD-10-CM are available at NCHS's ICD-10-CM website.

Organization

Following are some of the organizational components of ICD-10-CM (some of which were mentioned in the ICD-10 section of this chapter):

TABLE 1.4. ICD-10-CM subdivisions

Format	Description	Example
Blocks	Blocks are groups of three-character categories that represent a single disease entity or a group of similar or closely related conditions.	DORSOPATHIES (M40–M54)
Categories	Each three-character category represents a single disease entity or a group of similar or closely related conditions.	M40 Kyphosis and lordosis
Subcategories	The fourth- or fifth-character subcategories provide more specificity or information regarding the etiology (cause of a disease or illness), site (location), or manifestation (display of characteristic signs, symptoms, or secondary processes of a disease or illness).	M40.0 Postural kyphosis M48.4 Fatigue fracture of vertebra M48.8 Other specified spondylopathies
Subclassifications	Codes may be three, four, five, six, or seven characters. Subclassifications provide additional information about the encounter type (initial, subsequent, or sequelae).	M40.03 Postural kyphosis, cervicothoracic region M48.42XA Fatigue fracture of vertebra, cervical region, initial encounter for fracture M48.8x3 Other specified spondylopathies, cervicothoracic region

- Excludes notes at the beginning of each chapter have been expanded to provide guidance on the hierarchy of chapters and to clarify priority of code assignment (Excludes1 and Excludes2). Examples from diseases of genitourinary system (N00–N99) include:

  - Excludes certain conditions originating in perinatal period (P04–P96)
  - Excludes complications of pregnancy, childbirth, and puerperium (O00–O9A)

- Combination codes have been created, such as arteriosclerotic heart disease with angina, poisonings, and external causes. In some cases, this resolves sequencing issues. For example, pathological fractures are distinguished by underlying cause.
- The concept of laterality (right–left) has been added. With regard to laterality, affected codes are in neoplasm and injury chapters as well as others.
- With regard to obstetric codes, the axis of classification indicating episode of care has been eliminated. The last character in the code will now report the patient's trimester. Because certain obstetric conditions or complications occur at only one point in the obstetric period, not all codes will include all three trimesters, and some codes will not include a character to describe the trimester at all.
- Information relevant to ambulatory and managed care encounters has been added.

- The codes for postoperative complications have been expanded and a distinction has been made between intraoperative complications and postprocedural disorders.
- Alcohol and drug abuse codes have been expanded to include information about abuse and dependence at the fourth-character level, and information about intoxication, withdrawal, mood disorders, psychotic disorders, and other specified or unspecified disorders at the fifth-character level. A sixth character further specifies manifestations.
- ICD-10-CM includes other code expansions that provide greater specificity (for example, diabetes, epilepsy, radiation-related skin conditions, and family history).
- With regard to diabetes, controlled versus uncontrolled is not considered in the classification. To identify uncontrolled, it is now captured as diabetes mellitus with hyperglycemia or diabetes mellitus with hypoglycemia when the physician specifies the meaning of uncontrolled as hyperglycemia or hypoglycemia.
- The time frames in some codes have changed. For example, the time frame for abortion versus fetal death in the chapter on pregnancy, childbirth, and the puerperium has been changed from 22 to 20 weeks.
- In the chapter on the circulatory system, there are no longer subdivisions describing the initial and subsequent episodes of care. Guidelines do exist however on sequencing new and old AMIs.

As stated above, some codes include a seventh character. Table 1.2 shows how some of these seventh characters are used. Table 1.5 shows the level of detail in a few selected ICD-10-CM codes.

TABLE 1.5. Level of detail in selected ICD-10-CM codes

Concept	Code	Description
Laterality	C50.512	Malignant neoplasm of lower-outer quadrant of left female breast
Combination Codes	K71.51	Toxic liver disease with chronic active hepatitis with ascites
Expansion of Injury Codes	S00.411A	Abrasion of right ear, initial encounter
Postoperative Complications	K91.61	Intraoperative hemorrhage and hematoma of digestive system organ or structure complicating a digestive system procedure
Expansion of diabetes mellitus codes	E11.311	Type 2 diabetes mellitus with unspecified diabetic retinopathy with macular edema
Expansion of alcohol/drug abuse codes	F10.180	Alcohol abuse with alcohol-induced anxiety disorder
Expansion of decubitus ulcer codes	L89.112	Pressure ulcer of right upper back, stage 2

Principles, Conventions, and Guidelines

Within the Department of Health and Human Services (HHS) are the Centers for Medicare and Medicaid Services (CMS) and the National Center for Health Statistics (NCHS). They have the responsibility for developing and maintaining the *ICD-10-PCS Official Guidelines for Coding and Reporting* and *ICD-10-CM Official Guidelines for Coding and Reporting*, respectively. The guidelines should be used as a companion document to the official version of ICD-10-CM.

In addition to CMS and NCHS, the American Hospital Association (AHA) and the American Health Information Management Association (AHIMA) form the **Cooperating Parties**. The Official Guidelines have been approved by these four organizations. Published by HHS, the guidelines also appear in the ***Coding Clinic***, an AHA publication (AHA 2018).

The purpose of the guidelines is to assist users in coding and reporting in situations where ICD-10-CM does not provide direction (although coding and sequencing instructions in ICD-10-CM take precedence over any guidelines). For example, one of the guidelines expands on what is included in ICD-10-CM regarding the requirement for the use of a placeholder character "X" at certain codes to allow for future expansion. The seventh character must always be in the seventh character position in the data field. Where a seventh character exists, the X must be used in order for the code to be considered a valid code.

Another example is the ICD-10-CM guideline that clarifies the meaning of "with." According to the *ICD-10-CM Official Guidelines for Coding and Reporting*:

> The word "with" or "in" should be interpreted to mean "associated with" or "due to" when it appears in a code title, the Alphabetic Index (either under a main term or subterm), or an instructional note in the Tabular List. The classification presumes a causal relationship between the two conditions linked by these terms in the Alphabetic Index or Tabular List. These conditions should be coded as related even in the absence of provider documentation explicitly linking them, unless the documentation clearly states the conditions are unrelated or when another guideline exists that specifically requires a documented linkage between two conditions (e.g., sepsis guideline for "acute organ dysfunction that is not clearly associated with the sepsis").
>
> For conditions not specifically linked by these relational terms in the classification or when a guideline requires that a linkage between two conditions be explicitly documented, provider documentation must link the conditions in order to code them as related.
>
> The word "with" in the Alphabetic Index is sequenced immediately following the main term, not in alphabetical order. (NCHS 2018)

The conventions, general guidelines, and chapter-specific guidelines apply to the proper use of ICD-10-CM, regardless of the healthcare setting. A joint effort among the attending physician, clinical documentation specialist (CDI) staff, and coder is essential to achieve complete and

TABLE 1.6. Table of Contents of the *ICD-10-CM Official Guidelines for Coding and Reporting*

Section	Title	Content and Uses
I	Conventions, general coding guidelines, and chapter-specific guidelines	Used by all regardless of setting Contains three parts ICD-10-CM conventions General coding guidelines Chapter-specific guidelines
II	Selection of principal diagnosis	Used by those covered by the Uniform Hospital Discharge Data Set (UHDDS) guidelines. This includes all inpatient and nonoutpatient settings (acute care, short term, long term care, and psychiatric hospitals; home health agencies; rehab facilities; nursing homes, etc.). Provides information on sequencing and reporting.
III	Reporting additional diagnoses	Used by those covered by the Uniform Hospital Discharge Data Set (UHDDS) guidelines. This includes all inpatient and nonoutpatient settings (acute care, short term, long term care, and psychiatric hospitals; home health agencies; rehab facilities; nursing homes, etc.). Provides information on abnormal findings, general rules, previous conditions, and uncertain diagnosis.
IV	Diagnostic coding and reporting guidelines for outpatient services	Used by hospital-based outpatient services and provider-based office visits.
Appendix I	Present on Admission (POA) Reporting Guidelines	Used as a supplement to the Guidelines to facilitate assignment of POA indicators.

Source: NCHS 2018.

accurate documentation, code assignment, and diagnosis and procedure coding. The importance of consistent, complete documentation in the health record cannot be overemphasized. Without such documentation, the application of all coding guidelines is a difficult, if not impossible, task.

It should be pointed out that the guidelines for coding and reporting are not exhaustive. The Cooperating Parties review the guidelines on an ongoing basis and develop new ones as needed. Users of ICD-10-CM should be aware that only guidelines approved by the Cooperating Parties are official. Revision of the guidelines and new guidelines are published by HHS after the Cooperating Parties have approved them. The *Official Guidelines for Coding and Reporting* currently are divided into four sections, as shown in table 1.6. The *ICD-10-CM Official Guidelines for Coding and Reporting* are available on the NCHS website.

Process for Revision and Updates

The HIPAA Administrative Simplification: Modification to Medical Data Code Set Standards to Adopt ICD-10-CM and ICD-10-PCS: Proposed Rule established that an ICD-10-CM/PCS

Coordination and Maintenance Committee (C&M Committee) be formed to follow the same procedures that had been used by the ICD-9-CM Coordination and Maintenance Committee to consider new codes and revisions to existing codes. Moreover, AHA's *Coding Clinic* will continue to provide advice on coding.

The changes and updates to ICD-10-CM and ICD-10-PCS are managed by the C&M Committee, a federal committee co-chaired by representatives from NCHS and CMS. ICD-10-CM is expected to undergo biannual updates in the US to remain current.

NCHS is responsible for maintaining the diagnosis classification and CMS is responsible for maintaining the procedure classification (ICD-10-PCS). AHIMA and the AHA give advice and assistance, as do health information management (HIM) practitioners, physicians, and other users of ICD-10-CM. C&M Committee meetings are open to the public, and the discussion topics are available on their websites.

ICD-10-Procedure Coding System (ICD-10-PCS)

CMS is the federal agency responsible for the use of ICD-10-PCS in the US. A major strength of the system is its detailed structure, which enables users to recognize and report more precisely the procedures that were performed.

Developer

In 1990, the US Health Care Financing Administration (HCFA) (now known as CMS) funded a pilot project to produce a preliminary design to replace volume 3 of ICD-9-CM. In 1995, CMS awarded 3M Health Information Systems a three-year contract to complete development of the ICD-10-Procedure Coding System (ICD-10-PCS). The system underwent an informal test in October 1996, which was followed by a formal test conducted by CMS. **Clinical Data Abstraction Centers (CDACs)** were trained on the use of ICD-10-PCS and found it to be an improvement in that it provided greater specificity in coding for use in research, statistical analysis, and administrative areas.

Purpose

ICD-10-PCS has a multi-axial, seven-character, alphanumeric code structure that provides a unique code for all substantially different procedures and allows new procedures to be easily incorporated as new codes.

Procedures in ICD-10-PCS are divided into sections that relate to the general type of procedure. The first character of the procedure code always specifies the section or type of procedure. The second through seventh characters have a standard meaning within each section but may

TABLE 1.7. Essential characteristics of ICD-10-PCS

Characteristics	Explanation
Completeness	There should be a unique code for all substantially different procedures.
Expandability	As new procedures are developed, the structure of ICD-10-PCS should allow them to be easily incorporated as unique codes.
Multi-axial	The structure should be a multi-axial structure, with each code character having the same meaning within a specific procedure section and across procedure sections.
Standard Terminology	It should include definitions of the terminology used. Although the meaning of specific words can vary in common usage, ICD-10-PCS should not include multiple meanings for the same term, and each term must be assigned a specific meaning.

Source: CMS 2016.

have a different meaning across sections. In ICD-10-PCS, the term *procedure* is used to refer to the complete specification of the seven characters. All terminology in ICD-10-PCS is defined precisely, with a specific meaning attached to all terms used in the system.

Although the coding system requires coders to have a greater knowledge of anatomy and physiology and complete documentation of a procedure to be available prior to coding, ICD-10-PCS provides complete and accurate descriptions of the procedures performed. All procedures on a particular body part, by a particular approach, or by another characteristic can be easily retrieved using ICD-10-PCS data. The codes provide very specific information about each particular procedure.

Development of ICD-10-PCS was based on four major objectives. These essential characteristics are shown in table 1.7.

Content

ICD-10-PCS has a seven-character alphanumeric code structure. Each character has many different possible values. The digits 0–9 and the letters A–H, J–N, and P–Z are used. The letters O and I are not used in order to avoid confusion with the digits 0 and 1. The letters and numbers are intermingled throughout the code.

Because of the format of the codes into seven characters that have distinct definitions, it is literally possible to code each procedure with a distinct code that identifies components of the procedure, such as the specific body part value and the specific approach.

Procedures are divided into sections that relate to the general type of procedure (medical and surgical, imaging, obstetrics, nuclear medicine, and so on). The first character of the procedure code always specifies the section (see table 1.8 for the sections).

TABLE 1.8. Sections of ICD-10-PCS

Section	Title
0	Medical and Surgical
1	Obstetrics
2	Placement
3	Administration
4	Measurement and Monitoring
5	Extracorporeal or Systemic Assistance and Performance
6	Extracorporeal or Systemic Therapies
7	Osteopathic
8	Other Procedures
9	Chiropractic
B	Imaging
C	Nuclear Medicine
D	Radiation Therapy
F	Physical Rehabilitation and Diagnostic Audiology
G	Mental Health
H	Substance Abuse Treatment
X	New Technology

Source: CMS 2018

ICD-10-PCS Manual

The ICD-10-PCS online manual is divided into parts, including:

- ICD-10-PCS Tables
- Index
- Definitions
- Body Part Key
- Device Key
- Substance Key
- Device Aggregation Table

The Index allows codes to be located by an alphabetic lookup; however, only the first three or four characters are usually provided. Occasionally, all characters are provided in the Index.

FIGURE 1.4. Sample of ICD-10-PCS tabular grid

0DB

Section	**0**	Medical and Surgical
Body System	**D**	Gastrointestinal System
Operation	**B**	Excision: Cutting out or off, without replacement, a portion of a body part

Body Part	Approach	Device	Qualifier
1 Esophagus, Upper **2** Esophagus, Middle **3** Esophagus, Lower **4** Esophagogastric Junction **5** Esophagus **7** Stomach, Pylorus **8** Small Intestine **9** Duodenum **A** Jejunum **B** Ileum **C** Ileocecal Valve **E** Large Intestine **F** Large Intestine, Right **H** Cecum **J** Appendix **K** Ascending Colon **P** Rectum	**0** Open **3** Percutaneous **4** Percutaneous Endoscopic **7** Via Natural or Artificial Opening **8** Via Natural or Artificial Opening Endoscopic	**Z** No Device	**X** Diagnostic **Z** No Qualifier
6 Stomach	**0** Open **3** Percutaneous **4** Percutaneous Endoscopic **7** Via Natural or Artificial Opening **8** Via Natural or Artificial Opening Endoscopic	**Z** No Device	**3** Vertical **X** Diagnostic **Z** No Qualifier
G Large Intestine, Left **L** Transverse Colon **M** Descending Colon **N** Sigmoid Colon	**0** Open **3** Percutaneous **4** Percutaneous Endoscopic **7** Via Natural or Artificial Opening **8** Via Natural or Artificial Opening Endoscopic	**Z** No Device	**X** Diagnostic **Z** No Qualifier
G Large Intestine, Left **L** Transverse Colon **M** Descending Colon **N** Sigmoid Colon	**F** Via Natural or Artificial Opening With Percutaneous Endoscopic Assistance	**Z** No Device	**Z** No Qualifier
Q Anus	**0** Open **3** Percutaneous **4** Percutaneous Endoscopic **7** Via Natural or Artificial Opening **8** Via Natural or Artificial Opening Endoscopic **X** External	**Z** No Device	**X** Diagnostic **Z** No Qualifier
R Anal Sphincter **U** Omentum **V** Mesentery **W** Peritoneum	**0** Open **3** Percutaneous **4** Percutaneous Endoscopic	**Z** No Device	**X** Diagnostic **Z** No Qualifier

Source: CMS 2018.

The Index entry will refer to a specific location in the table. Reference to the table is always required to obtain the complete code because the codes are "built" from the tables in ICD-10-PCS.

Each page of the ICD-10-PCS tables is arranged in a grid that specifies the valid combinations of character values for the code. The upper portion of the grid contains a description of the first three characters of the procedure code. These characters were obtained in the Index. An example of one of these grids is provided in figure 1.4. The third character is also considered the axis since all characters following the axis are selected based on the correct row use of the table.

Medical and Surgical Procedures

The medical and surgical procedures section is used frequently in the hospital inpatient setting, so the following demonstrates the meanings of the seven characters in this section (see figure 1.5). It is important to remember, however, that the characters have a slightly different meaning in each section, but that they are well defined in the coding system.

In the medical and surgical procedures section, the first character specifying the section is 0. The second character indicates the body system (for example, the Endocrine system). Table 1.9 lists the Medical and Surgical section (0) body systems.

The third character indicates the root operation, which specifies the objective of the procedure (for example, Control). ICD-10-PCS has done an exemplary job of defining these terms in the classification's guidelines. It also has included examples of each term for clarification. Table 1.10 provides the list of root operations with their respective definitions.

The term *anastomosis* is not a root operation because it is a means of joining and is an integral part of another procedure such as a bypass or a resection; therefore, it can never stand alone. Incision is not a root operation because it is a means of opening and is always an integral part of another procedure. Repair is only coded when none of the other operations apply and is therefore the NEC option for the root operation character. It is used when none of the other root operations apply to the procedure.

The body part is specified in the fourth character and indicates the specific part of the body system on which the procedure was performed (for example, stomach).

FIGURE 1.5. Meaning of characters for medical and surgical procedures

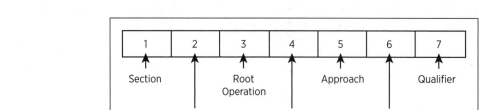

TABLE 1.9. ICD-10-PCS Medical and Surgical section (0) body systems

Character	Title
0	Central Nervous System and Cranial Nerves
1	Peripheral Nervous Systems
2	Heart and Great Vessels
3	Upper Arteries
4	Lower Arteries
5	Upper Veins
6	Lower Veins
7	Lymphatic and Hemic Systems
8	Eye
9	Ear, Nose, Sinus
B	Respiratory System
C	Mouth and Throat
D	Gastrointestinal System
F	Hepatobiliary System and Pancreas
G	Endocrine System
H	Skin and Breast
J	Subcutaneous Tissue and Fascia
K	Muscles
L	Tendons
M	Bursae and Ligaments
N	Head and Facial Bones
P	Upper Bones
Q	Lower Bones
R	Upper Joints
S	Lower Joints
T	Urinary System
U	Female Reproductive System
V	Male Reproductive System
W	Anatomical Regions, General
X	Anatomical Regions, Upper Extremities
Y	Anatomical Regions, Lower Extremities

Source: CMS 2018.

TABLE 1.10. Root operations with their respective definitions

Operation	Definition, Explanation, Examples	
Alteration	Definition	Modifying the natural anatomic structure of a body part without affecting function of the body part.
	Explanation	Principal purpose is to improve appearance.
	Examples	Face-lift, breast augmentation.
Bypass	Definition	Altering the route of passage of the contents of a tubular body part.
	Explanation	Rerouting contents of a body part to a downstream area of the normal route, to a similar route and body part, or to an abnormal route and dissimilar body part. Includes one or more anastomoses, with or without the use of a device.
	Examples	Coronary artery bypass, colostomy formation.
Change	Definition	Taking out or off a device from a body part and putting back an identical or similar device in or on the same body part without cutting or puncturing the skin or a mucous membrane.
	Explanation	All CHANGE procedures are coded using the approach EXTERNAL.
	Examples	Urinary catheter change, gastrostomy tube change.
Control	Definition	Stopping, or attempting to stop, postprocedural bleeding.
	Explanation	The site of the bleeding is coded as an anatomical region and not to a specific body part.
	Examples	Control of postprostatectomy hemorrhage, control of retroperitoneal hemorrhage.
Creation	Definition	Putting in or on biological or synthetic material to form a new body part that to the extent possible replicates the anatomic structure or function of an absent body part.
	Explanation	Used for gender reassignment surgery and corrective procedures in individuals with congenital anomalies.
	Examples	Creation of vagina in a male, creation of right and left atrioventricular valve from common atrioventricular valve.
Destruction	Definition	Physical eradication of all or a portion of a body part by the direct use of energy, force, or a destructive agent.
	Explanation	None of the body part is physically taken out.
	Examples	Fulguration of rectal polyp, cautery of skin lesion.
Detachment	Definition	Cutting off all or a portion of the upper or lower extremities.
	Explanation	The body part value is the site of the detachment, with a qualifier if applicable to further specify the level where the extremity was detached.
	Examples	Below-knee amputation, disarticulation of shoulder.

TABLE 1.10. Continued

Operation	Definition, Explanation, Examples	
Dilation	Definition	Expanding an orifice or the lumen of a tubular body part.
	Explanation	The orifice can be a natural orifice, or an artificially created orifice. Accomplished by stretching a tubular body part using intraluminal pressure or by cutting part of the orifice or wall of the tubular body part.
	Examples	Percutaneous transluminal angioplasty, internal urethrotomy.
Division	Definition	Cutting into a body part without draining fluids and/or gases from the body part in order to separate or transect a body part.
	Explanation	All or a portion of the body part is separated into two or more portions.
	Examples	Spinal cordotomy, osteotomy.
Drainage	Definition	Taking or letting out fluids and/or gases from a body part.
	Explanation	The qualifier DIAGNOSTIC is used to identify drainage procedures that are biopsies.
	Examples	Thoracentesis, incision and drainage.
Excision	Definition	Cutting out or off, without replacement, a portion of a body part.
	Explanation	The qualifier DIAGNOSTIC is used to identify excision procedures that are biopsies.
	Examples	Partial nephrectomy, liver biopsy.
Extirpation	Definition	Taking or cutting out solid matter from a body part.
	Explanation	The solid matter may be an abnormal byproduct of a biological function or a foreign body. The solid matter is imbedded in a body part or is in the lumen of a tubular body part. The solid matter may or may not have been previously broken into pieces.
	Examples	Thrombectomy, choledocholithotomy.
Extraction	Definition	Pulling or stripping out or off all or a portion of a body part by the use of force.
	Explanation	The qualifier DIAGNOSTIC is used to identify extraction procedures that are biopsies.
	Examples	Dilation and curettage, vein stripping.
Fragmentation	Definition	Breaking solid matter in a body part into pieces.
	Explanation	The solid matter may be an abnormal byproduct of a biological function or a foreign body. Physical force (e.g., manual, ultrasonic) applied directly or indirectly is used to break the solid matter into pieces. The pieces of solid matter are not taken out.
	Examples	Extracorporeal shockwave lithotripsy, transurethral lithotripsy.

(continued)

TABLE 1.10. Continued

Operation	Definition, Explanation, Examples	
Fusion	Definition	Joining together portions of an articular body part rendering the articular body part immobile.
	Explanation	The body part is joined together by fixation device, bone graft, or other means.
	Examples	Spinal fusion, ankle arthrodesis.
Insertion	Definition	Putting in a non-biological device that monitors, assists, performs, or prevents a physiological function but does not physically take the place of a body part.
	Explanation	N/A
	Examples	Insertion of radioactive implant, insertion of central venous catheter.
Inspection	Definition	Visually and/or manually exploring a body part.
	Explanation	Visual exploration may be performed with or without optical instrumentation. Manual exploration may be performed directly or through intervening body layers.
	Examples	Diagnostic arthroscopy, exploratory laparotomy.
Map	Definition	Locating the route of passage of electrical impulses and/or locating functional areas in a body part.
	Explanation	Applicable only to the cardiac conduction mechanism and the central nervous system.
	Examples	Cardiac mapping, cortical mapping.
Occlusion	Definition	Completely closing an orifice or the lumen of a tubular body part.
	Explanation	The orifice can be a natural orifice or an artificially created orifice.
	Examples	Fallopian tube ligation, ligation of inferior vena cava.
Reattachment	Definition	Putting back in or on all or a portion of a separated body part to its normal location or other suitable location.
	Explanation	Vascular circulation and nervous pathways may or may not be reestablished.
	Examples	Reattachment of hand, reattachment of avulsed kidney.
Release	Definition	Freeing a body part from an abnormal physical constraint by cutting or by use of force.
	Explanation	Some of the restraining tissue may be taken out, but none of the body part is taken out.
	Examples	Adhesiolysis, carpal tunnel release.

TABLE 1.10. Continued

Operation	Definition, Explanation, Examples	
Removal	Definition	Taking out or off a device from a body part.
	Explanation	If the device is taken out and a similar device is put in without cutting or puncturing the skin or mucous membrane, the procedure is coded to the root operation CHANGE. Otherwise, the procedure for taking out the device is coded to the root operation REMOVAL.
	Examples	Drainage tube removal, cardiac pacemaker removal.
Repair	Definition	Restoring, to the extent possible, a body part to its normal anatomic structure and function.
	Explanation	Used only when the method to accomplish the repair is not one of the other root operations.
	Examples	Colostomy takedown, suture of laceration.
Replacement	Definition	Putting in or on biological or synthetic material that physically takes the place and/or function of all or a portion of a body part.
	Explanation	The body part may have been previously taken out or replaced, or may be taken out, physically eradicated, or rendered nonfunctional during the Replacement procedure. A Removal procedure is coded for taking out the device used in a previous replacement procedure.
	Examples	Total hip replacement, bone graft, free skin graft.
Reposition	Definition	Moving to its normal location or other suitable location all or a portion of a body part.
	Explanation	The body part is moved to a new location from an abnormal location, or from a normal location where it is not functioning correctly. The body part may or may not be cut out or off to be moved to the new location.
	Examples	Reposition of undescended testicle, fracture reduction.
Resection	Definition	Cutting out or off, without replacement, all of a body part.
	Explanation	N/A
	Examples	Total nephrectomy, total lobectomy of lung.
Restriction	Definition	Partially closing an orifice or the lumen of a tubular body part.
	Explanation	The orifice can be a natural orifice, or an artificially created orifice.
	Examples	Esophagogastric fundoplication, cervical cerclage.
Revision	Definition	Correcting, to the extent possible, a portion of a malfunctioning device or the position of a displaced device.
	Explanation	Revision can include correcting a malfunctioning or displaced device by taking out or putting in components of the device such as a screw or pin.
	Examples	Adjustment of position of pacemaker lead, recementing of hip prosthesis.

(continued)

TABLE 1.10. Continued

Operation	Definition, Explanation, Examples	
Supplement	Definition	Putting in or on biological or synthetic material that physically reinforces and/or augments the function of a portion of a body part.
	Explanation	The biological material is non-living, or the biological material is living and from the same individual. The body part may have been previously replaced, and the SUPPLEMENT procedure is performed to physically reinforce and/or augment the function of the replaced body part.
	Examples	Herniorrhaphy using mesh, free nerve graft, mitral valve ring annuloplasty, put a new acetabular liner in a previous hip replacement.
Transfer	Definition	Moving, without taking out, all or a portion of a body part to another location to take over the function of all or a portion of a body part.
	Explanation	The body part transferred remains connected to its vascular and nervous supply.
	Examples	Tendon transfer, skin pedicle flap transfer.
Transplantation	Definition	Putting in or on all or a portion of a living body part taken from another individual or animal to physically take the place and/or function of all or a portion of a similar body part.
	Explanation	The native body part may or may not be taken out, and the transplanted body part may take over all or a portion of its function.
	Examples	Kidney transplant, heart transplant.

Source: CMS 2018.

The fifth character indicates the approach or the technique of the procedure. Table 1.11 provides the surgical approaches.

The device is specified in the sixth character and is only used to specify devices that remain after the procedure is completed. Materials incidental to procedures, such as clips and sutures, are not considered devices. If no device is applicable, the letter *Z* is used.

There are four general types of devices:

- Biological or synthetic material that takes the place of all or a portion of a body part (such as skin grafts and joint prosthesis)
- Biological or synthetic material that assists or prevents a physiological function (such as an intrauterine device [IUD])
- Therapeutic material that is not absorbed by, eliminated by, or incorporated into a body part (such as radioactive implants)
- Mechanical or electronic appliances used to assist, monitor, take the place of, or prevent a physiological function (such as a cardiac pacemaker or orthopedic pins)

TABLE 1.11. Surgical approach

Approach Value	Approach Definition
Open	Cutting through the skin or mucous membrane and any other body layers necessary to expose the site of the procedure.
Percutaneous	Entry, by puncture or minor incision, of instrumentation through the skin or mucous membrane and/or any other body layers necessary to reach the site of the procedure.
Percutaneous Endoscopic	Entry, by puncture or minor incision, of instrumentation through the skin or mucous membrane and/or any other body layers necessary to reach and visualize the site of the procedure.
Via Natural or Artificial Opening	Entry of instrumentation through a natural or artificial external opening to reach the site of the procedure.
Via Natural or Artificial Opening Endoscopic	Entry of instrumentation through a natural or artificial external opening to reach and visualize the site of the procedure.
Via Natural or Artificial Opening With Percutaneous Endoscopic Assistance	Entry of instrumentation through a natural or artificial external opening and entry, by puncture or minor incision, of instrumentation through the skin or mucous membrane and any other body layers necessary to aid in the performance of the procedure.
External	Procedures performed directly on the skin or mucous membrane and procedures performed indirectly by the application of external force through the skin or mucous membrane.

Source: CMS 2018.

The seventh character is for the qualifier. The qualifier has a unique meaning for some individual procedures and adds an additional attribute of the procedure performed. It could have narrow application such as being used to identify the second site included in a bypass or to identify that a biopsy is a diagnostic procedure (diagnostic excision, i.e., biopsy).

Principles and Guidelines

CMS publishes the ICD-10-PCS guidelines. In addition, the four Cooperating Parties approve them, including any updates. The guidelines complement the conventions and instructions found within ICD-10-PCS. However, the instructions in ICD-10-PCS take precedence over any guidelines.

For example, one of the guidelines explains the purpose of the Alphabetic Index, which is to locate the appropriate table that contains all information necessary to construct a procedure code. The PCS table is consulted to find the most appropriate valid code. However, it is not necessary to consult the Index first before proceeding to the tables to complete the code. A valid code may be chosen directly from the tables. Additional guidance on the PCS table states valid codes include all combinations of choices in characters four through seven contained in the same row of the table. In the example below, 0JHT3VZ is a valid code, and 0JHW3VZ is *not* a valid code.

Section: 0 Medical and Surgical

Body System: J Subcutaneous Tissue and Fascia

Operation: H Insertion: Putting in a nonbiological appliance that monitors, assists, performs, or prevents a physiological function but does not physically take the place of a body part

Body Part	Approach	Device	Qualifier
S Subcutaneous Tissue and Fascia, Head and Neck V Subcutaneous Tissue and Fascia, Upper Extremity W Subcutaneous Tissue and Fascia, Lower Extremity	0 Open 3 Percutaneous	1 Radioactive Element 3 Infusion Device Y Other Device	Z No Qualifier
T Subcutaneous Tissue and Fascia, Trunk	0 Open 3 Percutaneous	1 Radioactive Element 3 Infusion Device V Infusion Device, Pump Y Other Device	Z No Qualifier

Another example from the ICD-10-PCS guidelines is the statement that all seven characters must be specified for the code to be valid. If the documentation is incomplete for coding purposes, the physician should be queried for the necessary information.

TABLE 1.12. General principles followed in the development of ICD-10-PCS

Guideline	Explanation
Diagnostic information is not included in procedure description	The disease or disorder is not specified in procedures.
Not otherwise specified (NOS) options are restricted	Many NOS options are provided in ICD-9-CM, but these options are restricted in ICD-10-PCS. A minimal level of specificity is required for components in the procedure.
Limited use of not elsewhere classified (NEC) option	All possible components of a procedure are specified in ICD-10-PCS. Thus, in general, there is no need for a NEC option, although ICD-10-PCS does use this in very limited situations when necessary. For example, because new devices are being developed, there is a NEC option for devices until the new device can be explicitly added to the coding system.
Level of specificity	Based on the combinations of the seven alphanumeric characters, all possible procedures were defined. A code was created for any procedure that could be performed.

Source: CMS 2016.

Several general principles were followed in the development of ICD-10-PCS (see table 1.12). The full set of *ICD-10-PCS Official Guidelines for Coding and Reporting* are available at the CMS ICD-10 website.

Process for Revision and Updates

CMS has updated ICD-10-PCS each year since it was published. The process for revisions and updates is the same as that described earlier in this chapter for ICD-10-CM. CMS is responsible for maintaining the procedure classification (ICD-10-PCS).

Relationship with Other Clinical Terminologies, Classification Systems, and Code Sets

Clinical terminologies are a set of standardized terms that provide a means for organizing information and defining semantics of information in a consistent way. Although clinical classifications utilize terminologies, they do serve different functions. While classifications such as ICD-10-CM and ICD-10-PCS represent a broader characterization of information, such as a diagnosis, terminologies represent specific documentation elements and other data, such as lab values. Terminologies support information capture within the electronic health record (EHR) at the point of documentation. It is therefore necessary to have specifications that identify particular terminologies and classifications, such as in the HIPAA transaction standards mentioned earlier. The intent is to create standardization for interoperability between electronic health systems. Interoperability is the "extent to which systems and devices can exchange data and interpret that shared data" (HIMSS 2018). For example, SNOMED Clinical Terms (SNOMED CT) was adopted as a federal information technology interoperability standard to define diagnosis and problem lists (IHTSDO 2018). In terms of data standardization, mapping is the function that reuses data captured for one purpose to be used for another. Mapping is discussed in detail in chapter 17. Mapping is necessary because a wide variety of classifications and terminologies are available for use in the healthcare setting and no single system can meet all the needs independently. Thus, different maps are created for different purposes. For example, a map created for reimbursement purposes (SNOMED CT to ICD-10-CM mapping) would be different from public health tracking (LOINC to Current Procedural Terminology [CPT] mapping).

The following are some examples of relationships that ICD-10-CM and ICD-10-PCS have with other clinical terminologies, classification systems, and code sets.

ICD-11 Revision for Mortality and Morbidity Statistics

The WHO released the International Classification of Diseases 2018 Revision for Mortality and Morbidity Statistics (ICD-11-MMS) in June 2018, 18 years after the launch of ICD-10. It has been hailed as a vast improvement and was released in a completely electronic format that should improve the agility and longevity of this revision. It has, however, been built with traditional use cases of earlier revisions in mind to ensure consistency. ICD-11-MMS also complements the chapter structure of the current version (ICD-10) but will include additional detail, such as anatomy, substances, infectious agents, or place of injury. In correlation with its electronic format, ICD-11-MMS provides a set of rules and explanations for use, required reporting formats, and necessary metadata (WHO 2018a).

The Alphabetic Index includes a list of 120,000 clinical terms. ICD-11-MMS also includes basic coding reporting guidelines, similar to ICD-10. ICD-11-MMS codes always have a letter in the second position and the first character relates to the chapter number or letter. This is a noted change from ICD-10, along with code ranges within a single chapter always having the same character in the first position. ICD-11-MMS codes remain alphanumeric and range from 1A00.00–ZZ9Z.ZZ. One additional notable change in the general features includes ICD-11 categories that include both a short and long description. Short descriptions identify things that are always true about the condition and the long descriptions provide additional information about a condition without a length restriction. For detailed content regarding ICD-11-MMS, see Chapter 7 of this text.

SNOMED CT

Although ICD-10-CM, ICD-10-PCS, and SNOMED CT are similar in terms of representing diagnoses and procedures, several differences in purpose and structure exist. SNOMED CT is considered a reference terminology rather than a classification such as ICD-10-CM or ICD-10-PCS. SNOMED CT includes unique codes for more than 300,000 concepts including procedures (Stearns and Fuller 2014). The analogy of input systems and output systems is often used to describe classifications and terminologies in terms of the value of health information contained within an EHR. Classification systems represent the output system, as they are not designed for robust clinical care documentation (Bowman 2005). Reference terminologies, on the other hand, are considered input systems. This is because they are common sources of high-level specificity of clinical information for patient care (Bowman 2005). Clinical classifications lack the granularity of individual clinical concepts and relationships while reference terminologies fail to meet the needs of reimbursement and statistical analysis due to their immense size and complex hierarchies (Bowman 2005). However, when linked together through the process of mapping, information for multiple purposes can be obtained. In fact, for the purposes of health information exchange, EHR standards require the incorporation of specific classifications and terminologies for standardization of protected health information (PHI) electronic transmission. SNOMED CT is discussed in detail in chapter 6.

DSM-5

The *Diagnostic and Statistical Manual of Mental Disorders*, Fifth Edition (DSM-5) contains the diagnosis criteria to guide healthcare professionals in the diagnosis of mental disorders. The intent is to provide a resource containing common language for the providers. According to the American Psychiatric Association (APA), the DSM-5 and ICD-10-CM should be looked at as companion documents (APA 2018). As mentioned, the DSM-5 contains the criteria for diagnosing mental disorders while ICD-10-CM contains the codes needed for reimbursement and statistical monitoring purposes of the diagnoses. Although compatible, certain variations do exist. This is particularly true now that the DSM-5 utilizes spectrum disorders. This will require providers to document with specificity in order to get to the correct ICD-10-CM code. The APA will continue to work closely with CMS and NCHS to ensure the compatibility of the two systems. See Chapter 9 DSM-5 for further information.

CPT and HCPCS

ICD-10-CM and ICD-10-PCS systems are used to capture diagnoses and procedures within the inpatient or acute settings. ICD-10-CM is also used for diagnosis capture within the outpatient or ambulatory settings. In connection with ICD-10-CM for diagnosis reporting, the Healthcare Common Procedure Coding System (HCPCS) is used to capture outpatient procedures and services. HCPCS is divided into two levels. Level I includes the CPT codes, and Level II includes products, supplies, and other services not included within CPT. The purpose of CPT is "to provide a uniform language that accurately describes medical, surgical and diagnostic services, and thereby serves as an effective means for reliable nationwide communication among physicians, patients, and third parties" (AMA 2018). CPT and HCPCS include the procedure codes set for physician services, physical and occupational therapy services, radiological procedures, clinical laboratory tests, other medical diagnostic procedures, hearing and vision services, and transportation services including ambulance (AMA 2018). The diagnosis and outpatient services must correlate on the claim submissions to receive payment for reimbursement. Chapter 2, Current Procedural Terminology (CPT), and chapter 3, Healthcare Common Procedure Coding System (HCPCS), provide specific content on each system.

Tools to Access and Use

Several tools are available to access and use toward accurate clinical documentation and code capture of ICD-10-CM and ICD-10-PCS. These examples include both free and cost-associated electronic resources and tools for use in the successful application of ICD-10-CM and ICD-10-PCS:

- The Index, Tables, and Tabular of ICD-10-CM can be located and downloaded from the NCHS website. (See [NCHS 2018] in the reference list at the end of this book). This site also includes the forward and backward mappings between ICD-9-CM and ICD-10-CM and the *ICD-10-CM Official Guidelines for Coding and Reporting*. Also available are the POA Exempt Codes and the full Tabular Code Descriptions.

- The Index and Table sections of ICD-10-PCS can be obtained from the CMS website. (See [CMS 2018] in the reference list at the end of this book). This site also has the forward and backward mappings between ICD-9-CM and ICD-10-PCS and the *ICD-10-PCS Official Guidelines for Coding and Reporting*. Also available are additional tutorials and, although no longer updated, the ICD-10-PCS Reference Manual.

- Electronic browsers, such as ICD10Data.com found at https://www.icd10data.com/ICD10CM/Codes, provide a free reference website designed for the fast lookup of all current ICD-10-CM and ICD-10-PCS codes. Another example is a free one-year access to SuperCoder Smart Assistant at https://www.supercoder.com/icd-10-codes-lookup. This advanced online code search allows free ICD-10-CM code lookup. The Healthcare Cost and Utilization Project (HCUP) is a family of healthcare databases and related software tools and products made available for free by a Federal-State-Industry Partnership sponsored by the Agency for Healthcare Research and Quality (AHRQ). The HCUP at https://hcup-us.ahrq.gov/datainnovations/icd10_resources.jsp summarizes key issues for researchers using HCUP and other administrative databases that include ICD-10-CM/PCS coding. The contents include general ICD-10-CM/PCS information, ICD-10-CM/PCS databases and related data elements, and ICD-10-CM/PCS data analysis.

- Vendor offerings also provide several tools and resources for a fee. These include mappings between code sets, documentation improvement guides, and integrated coding tools for the EHR, mobile digital devices, and other electronic devices. The intent is to provide utility and quick functionality with point-of-care assistance for documentation and accurate code capture.

- To assist organizations in the successful implementation of ICD-10-CM and ICD-10-PCS, encoders have been provided in the marketplace. An **encoder** is a specialty software that converts information (documentation) to code format (AHIMA 2017). The intent is to assist the coder within an EHR in standardization and speed in the correct code selection process.

Adoption and Use Case

The CMS regulation published on August 17, 2000 to implement the Health Insurance Portability and Accountability Act (HIPAA) names the following code set standards:

- International Classification of Diseases, 10th revision, Clinical Modification (ICD-10-CM)
- International Classification of Diseases, 10th revision, Procedure Coding System (ICD-10-PCS)

The HIPAA Transactions and Code Set Standards are the rules to standardize the electronic exchange of PHI in order to carry out heathcare financial or administrative activities (CMS 2017). ICD-10-CM is the current *diagnosis* coding system and ICD-10-PCS is the current *procedure* coding system. The compliance date for ICD-10-CM for diagnoses and ICD-10-PCS for inpatient hospital procedures was set on October 1, 2015 (45 CFR 162.1002). Electronic transactions are now required for health plan claim submissions in order to increase efficiency and improve the quality accuracy of information while reducing overall costs (CMS 2017). In addition to the transaction standards, the Affordable Care Act also implemented provisions regarding the use of transactions. Together, the two are referred to as Administration Simplification due to the combined effort to simplify the business of healthcare through technology (CMS 2017).

Quality measure developers have adopted administrative data as a way to express healthcare performance data used in the measures. ICD is one of the code systems that identify the administrative data. For example, the AHRQ Inpatient Quality Indicators (IQIs) are measures of hospital quality and safety that use administrative data found in the typical discharge record (AHRQ n.d.). The IQI technical specifications include ICD-10-CM/PCS codes. Contained within the various E-measures are data elements, such as principal diagnosis code, that are defined by ICD and are required measurements for the national quality inpatient measures.

Use Case One: Calculating Performance Measurement

A hospital submits an electronic claim, which includes diagnoses coded with ICD-10-CM.

A 54-year-old female was treated as an inpatient for an acute non-ST anterior wall myocardial infarction. She also has atrial fibrillation. After five days she was discharged from the hospital. Two weeks later the same patient presented to the emergency department and was diagnosed with an acute inferior wall myocardial infarction. She is still being monitored following her initial heart attack two weeks earlier and continues to have atrial fibrillation. She will be transferred to a larger facility for cardiac catheterization and possible further intervention.

The following codes are assigned for this stay:

I22.1   Subsequent ST elevation (STEMI) myocardial infarction of inferior wall

I21.4   Non-ST elevation (NSTEMI) myocardial infarction

I48.91   Unspecified atrial fibrillation

Following the *ICD-10-CM Official Coding Guidelines for Coding and Reporting*, the subsequent AMI is sequenced as the principal diagnosis, followed by the initial AMI because the subsequent AMI was within four weeks of the initial AMI, as specified by the guidelines. The atrial fibrillation was treated and also listed. There were no procedures since the patient is being transferred to receive cardiac catheterization and intervention. Using these diagnoses, the Medicare Severity Diagnosis Related Group (MS-DRG) is calculated. This data is then used for reporting the diagnoses on the electronic claim submission to the payer for reimbursement and for reporting administrative data.

The payer uses the codes to determine the readmission rate following an AMI hospitalization, one of the outcome measures monitored by the payer to assess hospital performance. (Barta et al. 2016)

Use Case Two: Billing Inpatient Hospital Services

To be compliant with HIPAA, hospital inpatient services are coded using ICD-10-CM and ICD-10-PCS.

Hospital inpatient admission: The patient, gravida II, para 1, was admitted at approximately 33 weeks gestation with mild contractions. She was contracting every 7–8 minutes. An ultrasound showed twins of approximately 4 pounds each. The patient was given magnesium sulfate to stop the contractions, but she contracted through the drug. After developing a fever with suspected chorioamnionitis, a low cervical cesarean section was performed. The umbilical cord was wrapped tightly around the neck of twin 1.

The following codes are assigned for this case on the mother's record:

O60.14X0	Preterm labor third trimester with preterm delivery third trimester
O30.003	Twin pregnancy, unspecified number of placenta and unspecified number of amniotic sacs, third trimester
O41.1230	Chorioamnionitis, third trimester
O69.1XX1	Labor and delivery complicated by cord around neck, with compression, fetus 1
Z37.2	Twins, both liveborn
Z3A.33	Weeks of gestation of pregnancy, 33 weeks
10D00Z1	Extraction, products of conception, open, low cervical

Diagnosis code O60.14X0, preterm delivery at 33 weeks, is sequenced as the principal diagnosis. ICD-10-CM Coding Guideline I.15.b.4 states that if the reason for the admission/encounter was unrelated to the condition resulting in the cesarean delivery, the condition related to the reason for the admission/encounter should be selected as the principal diagnosis. In this case, the reason for the admission was the preterm labor that could not be stopped. The third trimester of pregnancy is defined as 28 weeks 0 days until delivery. A note appears prior to O60.1 stating that a seventh character is to be assigned to each code under subcategory O60.1. The seventh character

0 is for single gestations and multiple gestations where the fetus is unspecified. Code O30.003 indicates the twin gestation with the sixth character indicating the third trimester. The code for the chorioamnionitis complication is O41.1230 with the sixth character indicating the third trimester and the seventh character indicating an unspecified fetus. A note appears under O41 stating that a seventh character is to be assigned to each code under category O41. Seventh character 0 is for single gestations and multiple gestations where the fetus is unspecified. The code for the complication of cord around the neck of twin 1 is O60.1xx1 with the seventh character indicating that it is fetus 1 that is affected by the complication. A note appears under O69 stating that a seventh character is to be assigned to each code under category O69. The characters 1 through 9 are for cases of multiple gestations to identify the fetus for which the code applies. This code also requires the use of a character X in the fifth and sixth character positions in order for the code to be a valid code. ICD-10-CM Coding Guideline I.A.5 states that if a code that requires a seventh character is not six characters, a placeholder X must be used to fill in the empty characters. The correct outcome of delivery code is Z37.2 indicating that both twins were liveborn. In the Tabular at the beginning of Chapter 15, the following note appears: "Use additional code from category Z3A, Weeks of gestation, to identify specific week of pregnancy." Code Z3A.33 specifies that this is 33 weeks.

The cesarean section is coded to 10D00Z1 with the seventh character indicating a low cervical cesarean section.

The ICD-10-CM and ICD-10-PCS codes are submitted on an electronic claim to the payer for processing and payment (Barta et al. 2016).

CHECK YOUR UNDERSTANDING

1. What is the classification system that the US clinically modified from the WHO's *International Classification of Diseases, Tenth Revision*, and what is the intent of classification for use in the US?

2. What is the new revision of ICD released from WHO, and how is it related to the previous revision?

3. Define the format of an ICD-10-CM code. What are the first three characters identified as? What are the fourth, fifth, and sixth characters identified as? What is the seventh character identified as? Define the minimum and maximum characters of an ICD-10-CM code and explain how a coder would know what character to code to.

4. Define the format of an ICD-10-PCS code. What does each of the ICD-10-PCS characters stand for under the Medical Surgical Section? Define the minimum and maximum characters of an ICD-10-PCS code.

5. Define the process for revision and updates for ICD-10, ICD-10-CM, and ICD-10-PCS.

REVIEW

1. Fracture codes in ICD-10-CM have seventh characters for which of the following circumstances?

   a. Initial versus subsequent encounter
   b. Routine versus delayed healing
   c. Open versus closed fracture
   d. All of the above

2. Which group approves the *Official Guidelines for Coding and Reporting?*

   a. WHO, CMS
   b. NCHS, CHPS
   c. Coordination and Maintenance Committee
   d. Cooperating Parties

3. What agency is responsible for the use of ICD-10 in the US?

4. What agencies are responsible for maintaining the changes and updates to ICD-10-CM and ICD-10-PCS?

5. In the medical and surgical section of ICD-10-PCS, what does the fifth character represent?

   a. Root operation
   b. Device
   c. Qualifier
   d. Approach

6. The root operation in ICD-10-PCS specifies the

   a. Objective of the procedure.
   b. Body system involved.
   c. Body part involved.
   d. Technique used.

7. Which section(s) of the *ICD-10-CM Official Guidelines for Coding and Reporting* are followed for the coding of hospital inpatients?

   a. Section I
   b. Section I, II
   c. Section I, II, III, IV
   d. Section I, II, III

8. Which of the following is considered a valid root operation in ICD-10-PCS?

   a. Incision
   b. Anastomosis
   c. Resection
   d. Modification

9. Fill in the blank: The (.–) at the end of an entry in the ICD-10-CM Index means _____. Give an example of how this is used.

10. The *ICD-10-CM Official Guidelines for Coding and Reporting* are developed and maintained by the

   a. Centers for Medicare and Medicaid Services (CMS).
   b. National Center for Health Statistics (NCHS).
   c. American Hospital Association (AHA).
   d. World Health Organization (WHO).

References

45 CFR 162.1002: Administrative requirements. 2014 (Aug. 4).

45 CFR 153.20: Standards related to reinsurance, risk corridors, and risk adjustment under the Affordable Care Act: Subpart A – General provisions. 2017 (October 1).

Agency for Healthcare Research and Quality (AHRQ). n.d. "Inpatient Quality Indicators Overview. http://www.qualityindicators.ahrq.gov/modules/iqi_overview.aspx.

American Health Information Management Association (AHIMA). 2017. *Pocket Glossary of Health Information Management and Technology*, 5th ed. Chicago: AHIMA.

American Hospital Association (AHA). 2018. Central Office. http://www.ahacentraloffice.org.

American Medical Association (AMA). 2018. CPT Purpose and Mission. https://www.ama-assn.org/practice-management/cpt-purpose-mission.

American Psychiatric Association (APA). 2018. DSM-5: Frequently Asked Questions. https://www.psychiatry.org/psychiatrists/practice/dsm/feedback-and-questions/frequently-asked-questions.

Barta, A., K. DeVault, and M. Endicott. 2016. *ICD-10-CM and ICD-10-PCS Coder Training Manual*. Chicago, IL: AHIMA.

Bowman, S. E. 2005. Coordinating SNOMED-CT and ICD-10: Getting the most out of electronic health record systems. *Journal of AHIMA* 76(7):60–61.

Centers for Medicare and Medicaid Services (CMS). 2018. 2019 ICD-10-PCS. http://www.cms.hhs.gov/ICD10/.

Centers for Medicare and Medicaid Services (CMS). 2017. Transaction Overview. https://www.cms.gov/Regulations-and-Guidance/Administrative-Simplification/Transactions/TransactionsOverview.html.

Centers for Medicare and Medicaid Services (CMS). 2016. ICD-10-PCS Reference Manual. https://www.cms.gov/Medicare/Coding/ICD10/2016-ICD-10-PCS-and-GEMs.html.

Centers for Medicare and Medicaid Services (CMS). 2014. Medicare Managed Care Manual: Chapter 7–Risk Adjustment; Transmittal for Chapter 7; 20-Purpose of Risk Adjustment. https://www.cms.gov/regulations-and-guidance/guidance/manuals/downloads/mc86c07.pdf.

Centers for Medicare and Medicaid Services (CMS). 2011. Evaluation of the CMS-HCC Risk Adjustment Model. https://www.cms.gov/Medicare/Health-Plans/MedicareAdvtgSpecRateStats/downloads/evaluation_risk_adj_model_2011.pdf.

Hess, P. C. and K. Frosch. 2017. Outpatient CDI: A solution for navigating risk adjustment. *Journal of AHIMA* 88(7): 22–27.

HIMSS. 2018. Interoperability Toolkit – Interoperability 101. https://www.himss.org/library/interoperability-standards/toolkit.

International Health Terminology Standards Development Organisation. 2018. About SNOMED CT. http://www.ihtsdo.org/snomed-ct/what-is-snomed-ct.

National Center for Health Statistics. 2018. ICD-10-CM. ICD-10-CM Official Guidelines for Coding and Reporting FY 2019. https://www.cdc.gov/nchs/icd/icd10cm.htm.

Omachi, T. A., S. E. Gregorich, M. D. Eisner, R. A. Penaloza, I. V. Tolstykh, E. H. Yelin, C. Irarren, et al. 2013. Risk adjustment for health care financing in chronic disease: What are we missing by failing to account for disease severity? *Medical Care* 51(8):740–747.

Pope, G. C., J. Kautter, R. P. Ellis, A. S. Ash, J. Z. Ayanian, L. I. Lezzoni, M. J. Ingber, et al. 2004. Risk adjustment of Medicare capitation payments using the CMS-HCC model. *Health Care Financing Review* 25(4):119–141.

Premera. 2015. Medicare Advantage–Risk Adjustment Coding. https://www.premera.com/documents/033050.pdf.

Stearns, M. and J. C. Fuller. 2014. What's the difference? SNOMED CT and ICD systems are suited for different purposes. *Journal of AHIMA* 85(11):70–72.

World Health Organization (WHO). 2018a. ICD-11 Reference Guide. https://icd.who.int/browse11/content/refguide.ICD11_en/html/index.html#1.2.0StructureandtaxonomyofICD|structure-and-taxonomy-of-the-icd-classification-system|c1-2.

World Health Organization (WHO). 2018b. The WHO Update and Revision Committee. http://www.who.int/classifications/committees/updating/en/.

World Health Organization (WHO). 2016. ICD-10 International Statistical Classification of Diseases and Related Health Problems 10th Revision Volume 2 Instruction Manual. http://www.who.int/classifications/en/.

Resources

Bowman, S. 2008. Why ICD-10 is worth the trouble. *Journal of AHIMA* 79(3):24–29.

Centers for Medicare and Medicaid Services (CMS). 2018. ICD-10-PCS Official Guidelines for Coding and Reporting 2019. http://www.cms.hhs.gov/ICD10/.

Federal Register. Vol. 73. No. 164. Monday, September 3, 2018. http://www.access.gpo.gov/su_docs/fedreg/a080822c.html.

Giannangelo, K. 2004. The regulatory journey to destination 10: Understanding the process for adoption of ICD-10-CM and ICD-10-PCS. AHIMA Web Extra. http://library.ahima.org/xpedio/groups/public/documents/ahima/bok1_023199.hcsp?dDocName=bok1_023199.

H.R. 4302, Protecting Access to Medicare Act of 2014. http://www.gpo.gov/fdsys/pkg/BILLS-113hr4302enr/pdf/BILLS-113hr4302enr.pdf.

National Center for Health Statistics. 2018. http://www.cdc.gov/nchs.

National Center for Health Statistics. 2018. ICD-10-CM and guidelines http://www.cdc.gov/nchs/icd/icd10cm.htm.

Schraffenberger, L.A., and B. N. Palkie. 2019. *Basic ICD-10-CM and ICD-10-PCS Coding*. Chicago: AHIMA.

World Health Organization. 2018. History of the development of the ICD. http://www.who.int/classifications/en/.

World Health Organization. 2016. *International Statistical Classification of Diseases and Related Health Problems, Tenth Revision*. Geneva: WHO.

World Health Organization. 2008. The WHO Update and Revision Committee. http://www.who.int/classifications/en/.

2

Current Procedural Terminology (CPT)

Andrei Besleaga, RHIT

LEARNING OBJECTIVES

- Describe the development and purpose of CPT
- Explain the types of CPT codes
- Differentiate the component parts of CPT
- Review the process for updating CPT
- Examine the relationship CPT has with other classifications, terminologies, and code sets
- Compare tools available to access and use
- Demonstrate how CPT is used in an electronic environment

KEY TERMS

- Counseling
- CPT Editorial Panel
- Current Procedural Terminology (CPT)
- Evaluation and management (E/M) codes
- Modifiers
- Semicolon
- Separate procedure
- Surgical package

Introduction to Current Procedural Terminology (CPT)

This chapter discusses the American Medical Association's (AMA) **Current Procedural Terminology (CPT)**, a comprehensive terminology describing diagnostic and therapeutic procedures and medical and surgical services. The chapter focuses on the content of CPT, the process for updating the terminology, and principles of its application.

Developer

The AMA developed CPT to describe medical services and procedures performed by physicians and other healthcare providers. As a procedural terminology, CPT contains no diagnosis codes. One of the most widely used terminologies in healthcare, CPT was first introduced in 1966 and has subsequently been published in four editions. In 1983, the Centers for Medicare and Medicaid Services (CMS) adopted CPT as the standard for physician and hospital outpatient service coding. With implementation of the Health Insurance Portability and Accountability Act (HIPAA) code set standards, CPT in combination with the Healthcare Common Procedure Coding System (HCPCS) became the only acceptable system for reporting services in these settings. These services include, but are not limited to:

- Physician services
- Physical and occupational therapy services
- Radiologic procedures
- Clinical laboratory tests
- Other medical diagnostic procedures
- Hearing and vision services
- Transportation services including ambulance

In addition, CPT codes are reported with ICD-10-CM diagnosis codes to obtain reimbursement for physician services regardless of the setting, hospital outpatient and freestanding ambulatory surgery centers, and other appropriate outpatient settings.

Purpose

The purpose of CPT is "to provide a uniform language that accurately describes medical, surgical, and diagnostic services, and thereby serves as an effective means for reliable nationwide communication among physicians and other healthcare providers, patients, and third parties" (AMA 2018). CPT is used to report physician services, many nonphysician services, and surgical services performed in hospital outpatient departments and ambulatory surgery centers.

Increasingly, CPT is used for healthcare trending and planning, benchmarking, and measurement of quality of care.

Content

CPT is part of a larger coding system called the Healthcare Common Procedure Coding System (HCPCS), which contains both CPT codes (HCPCS Level I) and HCPCS National Codes (HCPCS Level II), which are administered by CMS. HCPCS codes are required for reporting physician services and hospital outpatient services (see chapter 3).

CPT is composed of three types of codes: category I, category II, and category III. Notably, a new subsection dedicated to proprietary laboratory analyses (PLA) was added in 2016. These codes can be provided either by a single ("sole-source") laboratory or licensed or marketed to multiple providing laboratories (cleared, or approved, by the FDA). They include advanced diagnostic laboratory tests (ADLTs) and clinical diagnostic laboratory tests (CDLTs) as defined under the Protecting Access to Medicare Act (PAMA) of 2014.

Category I Codes

Category I codes are five-digit numeric codes. For a procedure or service to receive a category I CPT code, it must:

- Have FDA clearance or approval for all devices and drugs necessary to provide the service
- Be performed by many healthcare professionals across the country
- Meet the literature and documentation requirement demonstrating clinical efficacy
- Be consistent with current medical practice
- Not be a fragmentation of another procedure or reportable by current CPT codes

Thus, new technologies or procedures of unproven efficacy would not receive CPT category I codes. An example of a current category I code is 27830, *Closed treatment of proximal tibiofibular joint dislocation; without anesthesia.*

Category II Codes

Introduced in 2004, category II codes are five-character alphanumeric codes with an *F* in the fifth position. These codes are supplemental tracking codes that can be used for performance measurement. They are reported in addition to standard evaluation and management (E/M) codes, not in place of them.

Category II codes are intended to facilitate data collection on quality of care by coding certain services that support performance measurements and have been agreed upon as contributing to quality patient care. The use of category II codes is completely optional. They are used only in conjunction with category I codes and cannot be reported alone.

The category II codes are grouped into the following sections:

Composite codes	0001F-0015F
Patient management	0500F-0584F
Patient history	1000F-1505F
Physical examination	2000F-2060F
Diagnostic/screening processes or results	3006F-3776F
Therapeutic, preventive or other interventions	4000F-4563F
Follow-up or other outcomes	5005F-5250F
Patient safety	6005F-6150F
Structural measures	7010F-7025F
Nonmeasure code listing	9001F-9007F

Examples of category II codes are:

0557F	Plan of care to manage anginal symptoms documented (CAD)
1000F	Tobacco use assessed (CAD, CAP, COPD, PV) (DM)
3014F	Screening mammography results documented and reviewed (PV)
4012F	Warfarin therapy prescribed (NMA-No Measure Associated)

For Physician Quality Reporting System (PQRS) quality measures, CPT category II codes are used to report quality measures on a claim for measurement calculation.

Figure 2.1 is an example of a performance measure that has incorporated category II codes into its criteria.

Category III Codes

Introduced into CPT in 2002, category III codes are five-character temporary alphanumeric codes with a T in the fifth position. These codes are used to describe emerging technologies that do not yet qualify for CPT category I codes. Some category III codes may become category I codes when the procedure satisfies the criteria for inclusion as a category I code outlined above. Medicare, Medicaid, and many private insurance companies accept category III codes for reimbursement purposes.

Category III status does not imply clinical efficacy, safety, or applicability to clinical practice. The category III codes do not conform to the usual requirements for category I codes, but rather provide a means of tracking for research purposes or evaluation of frequency. Where a category

FIGURE 2.1. Measure #6 (NQF 0067): Coronary Artery Disease (CAD): Antiplatelet therapy

DESCRIPTION:
Percentage of patients aged 18 years and older with a diagnosis of coronary artery disease (CAD) seen within a 12 month period who were prescribed aspirin or clopidogrel.

INSTRUCTIONS: This measure is to be reported a minimum of **once per reporting period** for patients with CAD seen during the reporting period. This measure may be reported by clinicians who perform the quality actions described in the measure for the primary management of patients with CAD based on the services provided and the measure-specific denominator coding.

Measure Reporting:
The listed denominator criteria is used to identify the intended patient population. The numerator options included in this specification are used to submit the quality actions allowed by the measure. The quality-data codes listed do not need to be submitted for registry-based submissions; however, these codes may be submitted for those registries that utilize claims data.

DENOMINATOR:
All patients aged 18 years and older with a diagnosis of coronary artery disease seen within a 12 month period.

Denominator Criteria (Eligible Cases):
Patients aged ≥18 years on date of encounter.

AND

Diagnosis for coronary artery disease (ICD-10-CM): I20.0, I20.1, I20.8, I20.9, I21.01, I21.02, I21.09, I21.11, I21.19, I21.21, I21.29, I21.3, I21.4, I22.0, I22.1, I22.2, I22.8, I22.9, I24.0, I24.1, I24.8, I24.9, I25.10, I25.110, I25.111, I25.118, I25.119, I25.2, I25.5, I25.6, I25.700, I25.701, I25.708, I25.709, I25.710, I25.711, I25.718, I25.719, I25.720, I25.721, I25.728, I25.729, I25.730, I25.731, I25.738, I25.739, I25.750, I25.751, I25.758, I25.759, I25.760, I25.761, I25.768, I25.769, I25.790, I25.791, I25.798, I25.799, I25.82, I25.83, I25.89, I25.9, Z95.1, Z95.5, Z98.61.

AND

Patient encounter during the reporting period (CPT): 99201, 99202, 99203, 99204, 99205, 99212, 99213, 99214, 99215, 99304, 99305, 99306, 99307, 99308, 99309, 99310, 99324, 99325, 99326, 99327, 99328, 99334, 99335, 99336, 99337, 99341, 99342, 99343, 99344, 99345, 99347, 99348, 99349, 99350.

WITHOUT

Telehealth Modifier: GQ, GT

NUMERATOR:
Patients who were prescribed aspirin or clopidogrel.

Definition:

Prescribed - May include prescription given to the patient for aspirin or clopidogrel at one or more visits in the measurement period OR patient already taking aspirin or clopidogrel as documented in current medication list.

(Continued)

FIGURE 2.1. Continued

Numerator Options:

Performance Met: Aspirin or Clopidogrel Prescribed **(4086F)**

OR

Denominator Exception: Documentation of medical reason(s) for not prescribing aspirin or clopidogrel (eg, allergy, intolerance, receiving other thienopyridine therapy, receiving warfarin therapy, bleeding coagulation disorders, other medical reasons) **(4086F with 1P)**

OR

Denominator Exception: Documentation of patient reason(s) for not prescribing aspirin or clopidogrel (eg, patient declined, other patient reasons) **(4086F with 2P)**

OR

Denominator Exception: Documentation of system reason(s) for not prescribing aspirin or clopidogrel (eg, lack of drug availability, other reasons attributable to the health care system) **(4086F with 3P)**

OR

Performance Not Met: Aspirin or clopidogrel was not prescribed, reason not otherwise specified **(4086F with 8P)**

RATIONALE:
Use of antiplatelet therapy has shown to reduce the occurrence of vascular events in patients with coronary artery disease, including myocardial infarction and death.

CLINICAL RECOMMENDATION STATEMENTS:
The following evidence statements are quoted verbatim from the referenced clinical guidelines.
2012 ACCF/AHA/ACP/AATS/PCNA/SCAI/STS Guideline for the Diagnosis and Management of Patients With Stable Ischemic Heart Disease (SIHD)

ANTIPLATELET THERAPY
Treatment with aspirin 75 to 162 mg daily should be continued indefinitely in the absence of contraindications in patients with SIHD. (Class I Recommendation, Level of Evidence: A)
Treatment with clopidogrel is reasonable when aspirin is contraindicated in patients with SIHD. (Class I Recommendation, Level of Evidence: B)
(American College of Cardiology, American Heart Association and American Medical Association, 2014)

Source: CMS 2018a.

III code exists, it must be used in place of an unlisted category I CPT code. An unlisted category I code represents a service or procedure that does not exist in CPT. An example of a category III code is 0101T, *Extracorporeal shock wave involving musculoskeletal system, not otherwise specified, high energy.*

Category III codes may or may not eventually become category I codes and are archived five years after publication or revision in CPT, unless there is demonstrated need that the temporary status is still necessary. If a category III code is archived after five years, and it has not been given a category I status, the appropriate unlisted category I code would then be reported.

Both category II and category III codes are assigned in simple numerical and chronological order and do not reflect the organization of the rest of the CPT book.

Proprietary Laboratory Analyses Codes

In 2016, the CPT Editorial Panel approved the addition of the new Proprietary Laboratory Analyses (PLA) subsection within the Pathology and Laboratory section of the CPT code set. Codes in the PLA subsection will be available to any clinical laboratory or manufacturer that wants to specifically identify their tests. The tests included in the PLA subsection must be commercially available in the US for use on human specimens.

PLA codes are released on a quarterly basis and are published on the CPT public website (see [AMA n.d.a] in the resources section at the end of this chapter). New codes are effective in the quarter following their approval and publication. These codes are alphanumeric codes that end with the letter U. They have been included in the annual update of the CPT codebook since 2018. The PLA codes will be included in the Pathology and Laboratory chapter of the CPT code book. Due to the quarterly update frequency of these codes, users should refer to the online file for the most current listing of the PLA test codes (see [AMA n.d.b] in the resources section at the end of this chapter).

Organization of CPT

As noted above, CPT is organized into specific categories of codes. The codes in the main section (category I codes) are intended to describe procedures and services performed by physicians and other healthcare professionals. The main section of CPT is divided into the following sections:

- Evaluation and management
- Anesthesiology
- Surgery
- Radiology
- Pathology and Laboratory
- Medicine

In addition to these six sections, there is an introduction, an index, and sixteen appendices. The appendices are as follows:

- Appendix A, Modifiers
- Appendix B, Summary of Additions, Deletions, and Revisions
- Appendix C, Clinical Examples
- Appendix D, Summary of CPT Add-on Codes
- Appendix E, Summary of CPT Codes Exempt from Modifier 51

- Appendix F, Summary of CPT Codes Exempt from Modifier 63
- Appendix G, Summary of CPT Codes that Include Moderate (Conscious) Sedation
- Appendix H, Alphabetic Clinical Topics Listing
- Appendix I, Genetic Testing Code Modifiers
- Appendix J, Electrodiagnostic Medicine Listing of Sensory, Motor, and Mixed Nerves
- Appendix K, Product Pending FDA Approval
- Appendix L, Vascular Families
- Appendix M, Renumbered CPT Codes-Citations Crosswalk
- Appendix N, Summary of Resequenced CPT Codes
- Appendix O, Multianalyte Assays with Algorithmic Analyses
- Appendix P, CPT Codes that May Be Used for Synchronous Telemedicine Services

Each of the main CPT sections is further subdivided into subsections.

Evaluation and Management

Evaluation and management (E/M) codes are designed to report physician work as performed in different clinical settings. With a few exceptions, E/M codes are based on the practitioner's documentation of history, physical examination, and medical decision-making. The subsections within the E/M section are as follows:

- Office or other outpatient services
  - New patient
  - Established patient
- Hospital observation services
  - Observation care discharge services
  - Initial observation care
    - New or established patient
  - Subsequent observation care
- Hospital inpatient services
  - Initial hospital care
    - New or established patient
  - Subsequent hospital care
    - Observation or inpatient care services
    - Hospital discharge services

- Consultations

  - Office or other outpatient consultations

    - New or established patient

  - Inpatient consultations

    - New or established patient

- Emergency department services

  - New or established patient
  - Other emergency services

- Critical care services
- Nursing facility services

  - Initial nursing facility care

    - New or established patient

  - Subsequent nursing facility care
  - Nursing facility discharge services
  - Other nursing facility services

- Domiciliary, rest home (for example, boarding home), or custodial care services

  - New patient
  - Established patient

- Domiciliary, rest home (for example, assisted living facility), or home care plan oversight services
- Home services

  - New patient
  - Established patient

- Prolonged services

  - Prolonged physician service with direct patient contact
  - Prolonged physician service without direct patient contact
  - Prolonged clinical staff services with physician or other qualified health care professional supervision
  - Standby services

- Case management services

  - Anticoagulant management
  - Medical team conferences

- Medical team conference, direct (face-to-face) contact with patient and/or family
- Medical team conference, without direct (face-to-face) contact with patient and/or family

- Care plan oversight services
- Preventive medicine services

  - New patient
  - Established patient
  - Counseling risk factor reduction and behavior change intervention

    - New or established patient
    - Other preventive medicine services

- Non-face-to-face services

  - Telephone services
  - Online medical evaluation
  - Interpersonal telephone, internet, and electronic health record consultations
  - Digitally stored data services and remote physiologic monitoring
  - Remote physiologic monitoring treatment management services

- Special evaluation and management services

  - Basic life and/or disability evaluation services
  - Work related or medical disability evaluation services

- Newborn care services

  - Delivery/birthing room attendance and resuscitation services

- Inpatient neonatal intensive care services and pediatric and neonatal critical care services

  - Pediatric critical care patient transport
  - Inpatient neonatal and pediatric critical care
  - Initial and continuing intensive care services

- Cognitive assessment and care plan services
- Care management services

  - Chronic care management services
  - Complex chronic care coordination services

- Psychiatric collaborative care management services
- Transitional care management services
- Advance care planning

- General behavioral health integration care management
- Other evaluation and management services

Anesthesia

The anesthesia section is used to report the administration of anesthesia for designated surgical services, including general, regional, supplementing local, or other supportive services. The anesthesia code reported includes the pre- and postprocedure anesthesia visit, the anesthesia care during the procedure, the administration of fluids and/or blood, and the usual monitoring services, such as EKG, temperature, blood pressure, oximetry, capnography, and mass spectrometry. The leading 0 in each code number is reported. The subsections of the anesthesia section are as follows:

- Head
- Neck
- Thorax (chest wall and shoulder girdle)
- Intrathoracic
- Spine and spinal cord
- Upper abdomen
- Lower abdomen
- Perineum
- Pelvis (except hip)
- Upper leg (except knee)
- Knee and popliteal area
- Lower leg (below knee, includes ankle and foot)
- Shoulder and axilla
- Upper arm and elbow
- Forearm, wrist, and hand
- Radiological procedures
- Burn excisions or debridement
- Obstetric
- Other procedures

Surgery

The surgery section is by far the largest in CPT. It is divided into subsections based on body system. Within each subsection, the next level of subdivision is body part, then type of procedure, and finally body parts within procedures. Examples of subsections include the following:

- General
- Integumentary system
- Musculoskeletal system
- Respiratory system
- Cardiovascular system
- Hemic and lymphatic systems
- Mediastinum and diaphragm
- Digestive system
- Urinary system
- Male genital system
- Reproductive system procedures
- Intersex surgery
- Female genital system
- Maternity care and delivery
- Endocrine system
- Nervous system
- Eye and ocular adnexa
- Auditory system
- Operating microscope

Radiology

Within the radiology section, subsections are based on type of diagnostic or therapeutic procedure and then by body part. The subsections are as follows:

- Diagnostic radiology (includes diagnostic imaging, computed tomography, magnetic resonance imaging, magnetic resonance angiography)
- Diagnostic ultrasound
- Radiologic guidance
- Breast, mammography
- Bone/joint studies
- Radiation oncology
- Nuclear medicine

Pathology and Laboratory

Within the pathology and laboratory section, subsections are based on type of diagnostic procedure performed. Subsections include the following:

- Organ or disease-oriented panels
- Drug assay
- Therapeutic drug assays
- Evocative/suppression testing
- Consultations (clinical pathology)
- Urinalysis
- Molecular pathology
- Genomic sequencing procedures and other molecular multianalyte assays
- Multianalyte assays with algorithmic assays
- Chemistry
- Hematology and coagulation
- Immunology
- Transfusion medicine
- Microbiology
- Anatomic pathology
- Cytopathology
- Cytogenetic studies
- Surgical pathology
- In vivo (for example, transcutaneous) laboratory procedures
- Other procedures
- Reproductive medicine procedures
- Proprietary Laboratory Analyses

Medicine

The medicine section of CPT contains a variety of codes that describe procedures that are not appropriate for reporting elsewhere within CPT. The subsections of the medicine section are as follows:

- Immune globulins, serum or recombinant products
- Immunization administration for vaccines/toxoids
- Vaccines/toxoids
- Psychiatry
- Biofeedback

- Dialysis
- Gastroenterology
- Ophthalmology
- Special otorhinolaryngologic services
- Cardiovascular
- Noninvasive vascular diagnostic studies
- Pulmonary
- Allergy and clinical immunology
- Endocrinology
- Neurology and neuromuscular procedures
- Medical genetics and genetic counseling services
- Adaptive behavior services
- Central nervous system assessments/tests
- Health and behavior assessment/intervention
- Hydration, therapeutic, prophylactic, diagnostic injections and infusions, and chemotherapy and other highly complex drug or highly complex biologic agent administration
- Photodynamic therapy
- Special dermatological procedures
- Physical medicine and rehabilitation
- Medical nutrition therapy
- Acupuncture
- Osteopathic manipulative treatment
- Chiropractic manipulative treatment
- Education and training for patient self-management
- Non-face-to-face nonphysician services
- Special services, procedures, and reports
- Qualifying circumstances for anesthesia
- Moderate (conscious) sedation
- Other services and procedures
- Home health procedures/services
- Medication therapy management services

The subsections are further divided into subcategories, then headings, and finally, procedures/services. For example, procedure 24600, *Treatment of closed elbow dislocation; without anesthesia*, is located within the surgery section, musculoskeletal subsection, humerus (upper arm) and elbow subcategory, fracture and/or dislocation heading. Within procedure groupings, the progression is usually from either proximal to distal or least to most complex.

Inclusion of a procedure code within a particular subsection of CPT does not restrict its use to professionals within that specialty; any professional may report any CPT code. For example, both emergency department physicians and orthopedic surgeons treat fractures and both may report the fracture treatment codes within the musculoskeletal subsection of CPT.

CPT has an Alphabetic Index and a Tabular List. The index contains an alphabetic listing of entries that may include:

- Procedure, service, or examination (for example, appendectomy, physical therapy, electrocardiography)
- Organ or anatomic site (for example, humerus, liver)
- Diagnosis or condition (for example, aortic stenosis, fracture)
- Synonym (for example, Seminin, followed by a note to see Antigen, prostate specific)
- Eponym (for example, Silver procedure, Shelf procedure)
- Abbreviation (for example, EEG, ERCP)

Following each entry is a single CPT code, several CPT codes separated by commas, a series of CPT codes, or a combination of CPT codes. The Alphabetic Index serves as a guide to the Tabular List; it is not recommended to assign a code from the index alone. Each of the suggested codes must be reviewed in its entirety, and the code that most accurately describes the procedure performed should be assigned.

To illustrate, following are the listings in the index for pancreas:

Anastomosis	
With intestines	48520–48540, 48548
Biopsy	48100
Needle Biopsy	48102
Cyst	
Anastomosis	48520–48540
Repair	48500
Debridement	
Peripancreatic tissue	48105
Dilation	
Ampulla of Vater	47542, 43277
Endoscopy	
See Endoscopy, Pancreatic Duct	
Excision	
Ampulla of Vater	48148
Duct	48148
Partial	48140–48146, 48150, 48154, 48160

Peripancreatic Tissue	48105
Total	48155–48160
Lesion	
Ablation	43278
Excision	48120
Needle biopsy	48102
Placement	
Drainage	48000, 48001
Polyp	
Ablation	43278
Pseudocyst	
Drainage	
Open	48510
Percutaneous	48511
Removal	
Calculi (Stone)	43264, 48020
Removal Transplanted Allograft	48556
Repair	
Cyst	48500
Resection	48105
Suture	48545
Transplantation	48160, 48550, 48554–48556
Allograft Preparation	48550–48552
Tumor	
Ablation	43278
Unlisted Services and	
Procedures	48999
X-ray	74300, 74301
Injection Procedure	48400

Principles and Guidelines

The AMA develops guidelines for CPT use. The guidelines may appear in the form of coding notes in several places, including:

- At the beginning of a section. Notes at the beginning of a section apply to all codes within the section and may include information such as:

  - Integral components of a service

- Definitions of terms and codes
- Directions to assign additional codes
  - At the beginning of a subsection
  - Before or following a specific code

In addition, the AMA publishes *CPT Assistant*, a monthly magazine that provides official coding advice, and the annual *CPT Changes: An Insider's View*, a review, with extensive clinical rationales, of the new and revised codes for each year. Only the AMA can develop official guidelines for CPT coding, although CMS and other payers also issue guidelines that relate to the use of CPT for coverage and reimbursement purposes.

The American Hospital Association (AHA) through its Central Office on HCPCS also offers guidance to hospitals on the appropriate use of HCPCS. The AHA has an agreement with CMS for the establishment of an AHA clearinghouse for issues related to the use of certain HCPCS codes. As per the agreement, a responsibility of the AHA Central Office includes providing advice on Level I HCPCS (CPT-4 codes) for hospital providers (AHA 2019).

Guidelines for Reporting E/M Codes

E/M codes are used primarily to describe cognitive physician services. As noted, they are assigned based on documentation of history, physical examination, and medical decision-making, with a few exceptions.

History

CPT defines the history as follows:

- Chief complaint, usually in the patient's own words, is a concise statement of the symptom, problem, condition, diagnosis, or other factor that is the reason for the encounter.
- History of present illness, which in turn is defined in terms of:
  - Location (for example, pain in the right lower quadrant of the abdomen)
  - Quality (for example, pain, stabbing, burning)
  - Severity (for example, pain rated 7 on a scale of 10, or severe pain)
  - Duration (for example, pain lasting for up to an hour)
  - Timing (for example, occurs after meals)
  - Context (for example, pain occurring when lying down)
  - Modifying factors (for example, pain improved with aspirin, rest, and so on)
  - Associated signs and symptoms (for example, pain accompanied by nausea and vomiting)

- Review of systems is an inventory of body systems obtained through a series of questions designed to elicit signs and/or symptoms. The systems as defined by the AMA are:

  - Constitutional (for example, fever, weight loss)
  - Eyes (for example, blurred vision, double vision)
  - Ears, nose, mouth, and throat (for example, diminished hearing, throat pain)
  - Cardiovascular (for example, chest pain, palpitations)
  - Neck (for example, stiffness, swelling)
  - Respiratory (for example, shortness of breath, difficulty breathing)
  - Gastrointestinal (for example, abdominal pain, diarrhea)
  - Genitourinary (for example, difficulty voiding, pain on urination)
  - Musculoskeletal (for example, joint pain, stiffness upon awakening)
  - Integumentary (for example, skin rash, breast pain)
  - Neurological (for example, loss of sensation, dizziness)
  - Psychiatric (for example, feelings of helplessness and hopelessness)
  - Endocrine (for example, heat or cold intolerance)
  - Hematologic/lymphatic (for example, easy bruising, swollen glands)
  - Allergic/immunologic (for example, history of allergies)

- Past history is a review of the patient's past illnesses, treatments, and injuries, including:

  - Prior major illnesses or injuries
  - Prior operations
  - Prior hospitalizations
  - Current medications
  - Allergies (for example, drugs, foods)
  - Age-appropriate immunization status
  - Age-appropriate feeding/dietary status

- Social history is a review of past and current activities and interactions, including:

  - Marital status and/or living arrangements
  - Current employment and past occupational history
  - Use of drugs, alcohol, and tobacco
  - Educational level
  - Sexual history and habits
  - Other relevant social factors

- Family history is a review of medical events in the patient's family, including:

  - Parents' and siblings' morbidity and mortality, especially as related to the presenting concerns or risk of morbidity

- Family history of congenital defects
- Family history of hereditary conditions

Physical Examination

For purposes of CPT, the AMA recognizes the following body areas:

- Head, including face ("head normocephalic, face symmetrical")
- Neck ("range of motion of the neck normal," "no thyroid masses palpable")
- Chest, including breasts and axilla ("chest symmetrical, lungs clear")
- Abdomen ("abdomen flat, no masses palpable")
- Genitalia, groin, and buttocks ("genitalia without masses, groin without palpable nodes")
- Back ("back straight with normal range of motion")
- Each extremity ("right upper extremity in a cast, remainder of extremities without loss of range of motion")

The physical examination also may be defined in terms of organ systems. The following organ systems are recognized:

- Eyes ("pupils equal, react to light and accommodation")
- Ears, nose, mouth, and throat ("ear canals clean, nose without congestion")
- Cardiovascular ("heart sounds normal without murmurs, rubs, or gallops")
- Respiratory ("breath sounds clear to auscultation and percussion")
- Gastrointestinal ("abdomen is flat and soft, without tenderness or masses")
- Genitourinary ("no tenderness of the genitalia")
- Musculoskeletal ("range of motion of all joints within normal limits")
- Skin ("no rashes or areas of discoloration")
- Neurologic ("normal sensation to pinprick and light touch in all dermatomes tested")
- Psychiatric ("alert and oriented to time, place, person, and station")
- Hematologic/lymphatic/immunologic ("no bruising, glandular enlargement")

Medical Decision-Making

Medical decision-making is the most cognitive of the three criteria for assigning E/M codes and the most difficult to quantify. CPT recognizes the following levels of medical decision-making:

- Straightforward

- Minimal number of diagnoses or management options
- Minimal or no data to be reviewed
- Minimal risk of complications, morbidity, mortality

- Low complexity

  - Limited number of diagnoses or management options
  - Limited amount or complexity of data to be reviewed
  - Low risk of complications, morbidity, mortality

- Moderate complexity

  - Multiple diagnoses or management options
  - Moderate amount or complexity of data to be reviewed
  - Moderate risk of complications, morbidity, mortality

- High complexity

  - Extensive diagnoses or management options
  - Extensive amount or complexity of data to be reviewed
  - High risk of complications, morbidity, mortality

The Principle of Counseling

Counseling is defined as being a discussion of one or more of the following topics:

- Diagnostic results, impressions, and/or recommended diagnostic studies
- Prognosis
- Risks and benefits of management
- Instruction for management
- Importance of compliance
- Risk factor reduction
- Patient and family education

If counseling or coordination of care makes up more than 50 percent of a patient encounter, time is a key factor in determining the level of service, rather than the nature of the presenting problem. When counseling is a major part of a patient visit, documentation is very important. The visit note should include the topic of the counseling, the total visit time, the number of minutes spent counseling, and the plan for follow-up.

Guidelines for Coding Critical Care Codes

Although critical care codes are a type of E/M code, they are not defined by documentation of history, physical examination, and medical decision-making. Rather, critical care codes are defined by time, the nature of the problem, and the nature of the treatment.

Critical care services should be reported in conjunction with a critical illness or injury, which is defined as an illness or injury that acutely impairs one or more vital organ systems such that there is a high probability of imminent or life-threatening deterioration in the patient's condition (AMA 2013). CPT goes on to state that critical care service involves decision-making of high complexity to assess, manipulate, and support vital organ system failure and/or to prevent further life-threatening deterioration of the patient's condition. According to CPT, examples of vital organ system failure include, but are not limited to, central nervous system failure, circulatory failure, shock, and renal, hepatic, metabolic, and/or respiratory failure.

Guidelines for Reporting Surgery Codes

The surgery section has a number of unique guidelines. An example is the principle of surgical package.

The Principle of the Surgical Package

Within the surgery section of CPT, the principle of the **surgical package** (also referred to as the global surgical package) applies. This concept is based on a single, readily identifiable procedure that may contain a number of services. Per CPT guidelines, the following services are always included in each operation:

- Local infiltration, metacarpal/metatarsal/digital block, or topical anesthesia
- Subsequent to the decision for surgery, one related E/M encounter on the date immediately prior to, or on the date of, the procedure (including history and physical)
- Immediate postoperative care, including dictating operative notes, talking with family and other physicians or other quality healthcare professionals
- Writing orders
- Evaluating the patient in the postanesthesia recovery area
- Typical postoperative follow-up care (AMA 2018)

Another, slightly different definition for surgical package, as defined by the Medicare program, is as follows:

- Preoperative Visits: Preoperative visits after the decision is made to operate beginning with the day before the day of surgery for major procedures and the day of surgery for minor procedures
- Intraoperative Services: Intraoperative services that are normally a usual and necessary part of a surgical procedure
- Complications Following Surgery: All additional medical or surgical services required of the surgeon during the postoperative period of the surgery because of complications that do not require additional trips to the operating room
- Postoperative Visits: Follow-up visits during the postoperative period of the surgery that are related to recovery from the surgery
- Postsurgical Pain Management: By the surgeon
- Supplies: Except for those identified as exclusions; and Miscellaneous Services - Items such as dressing changes; local incisional care; removal of operative pack; removal of cutaneous sutures and staples, lines, wires, tubes, drains, casts, and splints; insertion, irrigation, and removal of urinary catheters, routine peripheral intravenous lines, and nasogastric and rectal tubes; and changes and removal of tracheostomy tubes
- The surgeon's initial evaluation or consultation will be paid separately (CMS 2018b)

Guidelines for Reporting Separate Procedures

In CPT, a **separate procedure** is commonly part of another, more complex procedure. The guidelines for reporting separate procedures generally apply when one procedure designated as a separate procedure is performed with another procedure rather than with an E/M service. If the separate procedure is an integral part of the other procedure, it is not reported separately. However, when a separate procedure is performed independently or is otherwise unrelated to another procedure performed during the same session, it may be reported separately with an appropriate modifier appended.

Guidelines for Reporting Unlisted Procedure Codes

Unlisted procedure codes appear throughout the CPT system. These codes, many of which end in xxx99, are used to report procedures for which a category I code, a category III code, or a HCPCS code does not exist. When any of the above do exist, they must be used instead of the unlisted procedure code.

When an unlisted procedure code is reported for reimbursement purposes, payers will likely require additional documentation. For a surgical procedure, an operative report is always required, and additional information also may be requested.

Guidelines for Using Modifiers

CPT codes can be customized by the use of one or more **modifiers**, which are listed in appendix A of the CPT code book each year. Modifiers are two-character extensions appended to a CPT code to indicate that a particular event or circumstance modified the service or procedure without changing its basic definition. Modifiers may be used in the following circumstances (this list is not all inclusive):

- A service or procedure has both a professional and a technical component.
- A service or procedure was performed at more than one anatomic site or by more than one physician.
- A service or procedure has been reduced or expanded in scope.
- A service or procedure was performed bilaterally.
- An unusual event occurred during the service or procedure.
- Only part of a service was done.
- An adjunctive service was done.
- A service or procedure was provided more than once.

Like the rest of CPT, modifiers may change in meaning or be deleted through the update process. Most CPT modifiers may be used with physician services, but only select ones can be reported with hospital outpatient services. Within physician services, some modifiers can be used only with E/M codes, others only with surgical codes, and others with all codes. Appendix A in the CPT code book indicates which of these modifiers may be used in each circumstance.

In addition to the CPT modifiers, there are HCPCS Level II modifiers (see chapter 3). These modifiers may also be used with CPT codes. However, relatively few HCPCS Level II modifiers have been approved for hospital outpatient department use.

Guidelines for Using the Semicolon

The **semicolon** has a special meaning in CPT. In order to make the format less cluttered, common information is not repeated. Within a code set, an initial code may contain a procedure description, a semicolon, and additional information. The information to the left of the semicolon applies to that code and all the codes indented under it; the information to the right of the semicolon changes.

For example:

36800	Insertion of cannula for hemodialysis, other purpose (separate procedure); vein to vein
36810	arteriovenous, external (Scribner type)
36815	arteriovenous, external revision, or closure

The complete description for code 36810 is *Insertion of cannula for hemodialysis, other purpose (separate procedure); arteriovenous, external (Scribner type)*, and the complete description for code 36815 is *Insertion of cannula for hemodialysis, other purpose (separate procedure); arteriovenous, external revision, or closure.*

Process for Revision and Updates

Category I codes are updated annually, with January 1 as the effective date for the use of the updated CPT codes. The exception is vaccines, which are released January 1 and July 1. The **CPT Editorial Panel** develops new codes or revisions of existing codes with the assistance of the CPT Advisory Committee. The Editorial Panel is composed of 17 members and they are authorized to revise, update, delete, or modify CPT codes, descriptors, and the rules and guidelines. Of the 17 members, 11 are physicians from various medical specialty societies, with one position reserved for a member with expertise in performance measurement. Further, one physician is nominated from each of the following organizations: Blue Cross and Blue Shield Association, America's Health Insurance Plans, the American Hospital Association, and Centers for Medicare and Medicaid Services (CMS). The other two positions are reserved for two members of the CPT Health Care Professionals Advisory Committee. Advisors also support the work of the CPT Editorial Panel.

Category II codes are updated three times a year. Further CPT category II code changes with "implementation date" are available on the AMA website. The implementation date is three months subsequent to the date of release following code set updates. The Performance Measures Advisory Group (PMAG) reviews their content. The PMAG is an advisory body to the CPT Editorial Panel and is composed of representatives from the AMA, Agency for Healthcare Research and Quality (AHRQ), CMS, The Joint Commission, the National Committee for Quality Assurance (NCQA), and the Physician Consortium for Performance Improvement, with solicited input from various specialty societies and other agencies.

Because they are intended to report emerging technologies and must respond quickly to changes in treatment methods, category III codes are updated semiannually on January 1 and July 1, with effective dates for use six months later. Updates are found on the AMA/CPT website. The most current version of category III codes can be downloaded from the AMA website.

Anyone may submit a request to change CPT codes, including the addition of new codes (in any category), the deletion of old codes, and changes to code descriptors. The process for updating CPT is discussed in detail, and the change form may be downloaded from the AMA website.

Relationship to Other Terminologies, Classification Systems, and Code Sets

Besides CPT, other systems and code sets are in use simultaneously within the US healthcare system. Therefore, there are times where it may be useful to compare them to CPT. For example, ICD-10-PCS is a procedural coding system used by facilities to identify inpatient procedures. ICD-10-PCS is driven by diagnoses and the objectives of the service, whereas CPT is primarily focused on appropriately describing physician work involved in delivering or performing a medical procedure or service. CPT is the standard mandated in the US (see adoption and use cases to follow).

SNOMED CT is another terminology system that interacts with CPT and is the standard for electronic exchange of clinical health information across electronic health record (EHR) platforms. The system is comprised of clinical terminology and definitions and describes clinical documentation that facilitates communication between various EHRs (NIH 2018). More information on SNOMED CT is found in chapter 6.

As previously discussed, CPT is an integral part of the HCPCS. The first part, Level I, is the CPT code set. The second part, Level II, includes those supplies and services that are not covered by a CPT code. HCPCS Level II is covered in chapter 3.

Tools to Access and Use

CPT represents a standardized set of codes, descriptions, and guidelines that describe procedures and services performed by physicians and other healthcare professionals or entities. In addition to the curation and maintenance of the CPT code set, the AMA has created tools to leverage CPT in various environments.

One such tool is CPT Link, which formats CPT content into computer readable and executable sets of data files that enable seamless integration of CPT codes with other data and software and contains computer readable representations of CPT guidelines and parentheticals to promote accurate coding. The product also tracks code changes yearly and quarterly and provides CPT history since 1990. In addition, CPT Link contains bidirectional rules-based SNOMED to CPT maps for reimbursement and meaningful use reporting.

Another tool is the CPT QuickRef app, which is a free-to-download mobile app that provides access to CPT codes and includes an E/M code selection utility based on the CMS 1995 and 1997 guidelines. One can choose to purchase access to additional content, including the 2018 and 2019 code sets, full-color illustrations, and access to the *CPT Assistant* archive.

CPT Assistant is the AMA's official monthly newsletter that educates the industry on proper CPT coding for past, present, and future code set releases. It is used to appeal insurance denials, validate coding to auditors, train staff, and answer day-to-day coding questions. Each monthly issue offers information such as the latest codes and trends in medicine; clinical scenarios that demystify confusing codes; answers to frequently asked questions; anatomical and procedural illustrations; and charts and graphs that add context to codes and guidelines (AMA 1992–2018).

The CPT Network is another tool that provides subscription-based access to CPT coding resources including a database (Knowledge Base) of commonly asked questions and clinical examples. If the answer to a specific question cannot be found in the database, authorized users may submit an electronic inquiry directly to CPT.

All of the resources above are available to coders, healthcare professionals, and entities that use CPT to report medical procedures and services. Oftentimes, CPT is licensed through and bundled into EHR systems that are used to house and maintain patient health records, for reporting claims to third-party payers, and for tracking patient health outcomes or other reporting. There are also various encoder software tools available that enable users to enter in key words describing a medical procedure or service. The utility helps to narrow the search for the appropriate CPT code to report. CMS also provides an online tool that can display calculated relative value units (RVUs) that CMS has determined for physician reimbursement when performing various CPT procedures. Currently there are over 10,000 CPT codes with attached RVUs available (CMS n.d.).

Adoption and Use Cases

Under HIPAA, the US Department of Health and Human Services (HHS) has adopted specific code sets for diagnoses and procedures to be used in all electronic transactions. The Final Rule issued August 17, 2000, names CPT (including codes and modifiers) and HCPCS as the procedure code set for physician services, physical and occupational therapy services, radiological procedures, clinical laboratory tests, other medical diagnostic procedures, hearing and vision services, and transportation services. Public as well as private insurers were required to be in compliance with the August 2000 regulation by October 1, 2002.

Quality-measure developers have adopted CPT as a way to express healthcare performance data used in the measure. CPT is one of the code sets identified in defining certain data elements, such as an encounter or procedure. For example, the AMA is the developer of a number of clinical quality measures (CQMs). Contained within the various measures are data elements that are defined by CPT and thus when reported are used to construct the measure.

Use Case One: Billing Office Surgery

Services provided by physicians and other healthcare professionals are reported using CPT and HCPCS Level II codes in hospital-based outpatient departments, physicians' offices, and other ambulatory settings.

FIGURE 2.2. Reporting codes for physician's claim

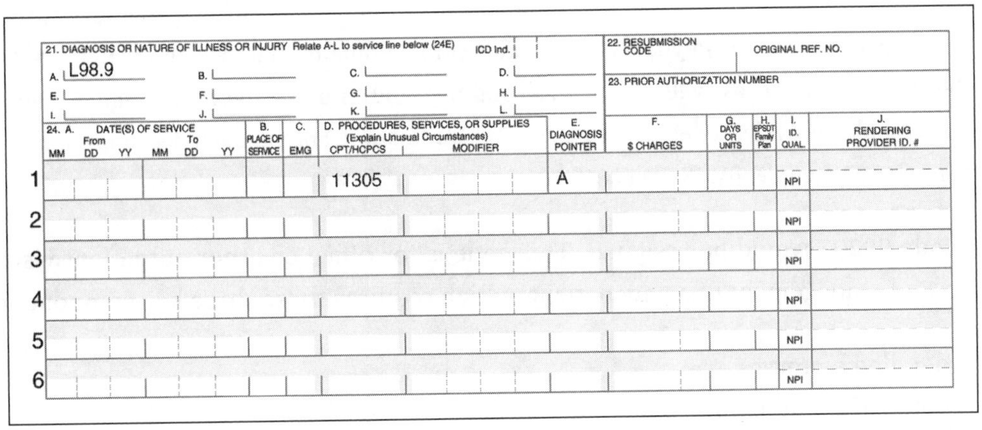
21. DIAGNOSIS OR NATURE OF ILLNESS OR INJURY Relate A-L to service line below (24E) ICD Ind.
A. L98.9 B. C. D.
E. F. G. H.
I. J. K. L.
22. RESUBMISSION CODE ORIGINAL REF. NO.
23. PRIOR AUTHORIZATION NUMBER

24. A. DATE(S) OF SERVICE From MM DD YY To MM DD YY	B. PLACE OF SERVICE	C. EMG	D. PROCEDURES, SERVICES, OR SUPPLIES (Explain Unusual Circumstances) CPT/HCPCS MODIFIER	E. DIAGNOSIS POINTER	F. $ CHARGES	G. DAYS OR UNITS	H. EPSDT Family Plan	I. ID. QUAL.	J. RENDERING PROVIDER ID. #
1			11305	A				NPI	
2								NPI	
3								NPI	
4								NPI	
5								NPI	
6								NPI	

Source: Smith 2019.

As an example for reporting codes, refer to figure 2.2, which is an excerpt from the paper billing form for use by physician offices. In this illustration, assume a patient was seen for a growth on the skin of the foot. The physician documented that the following procedure was performed: shaving of a 0.5 centimeter epidermal lesion of the foot. For billing purposes, Field 21.1 would contain the ICD-10-CM diagnosis code L98.9 (lesion of skin), which explains the reason for the encounter. The services provided would be listed in Field 24D, with CPT code 11305 (shaving). Payers could deny or question the bill if the services do not coincide with the diagnosis.

Use Case Two: Processing the Claim Per Guidelines

Payers process claims according to their medical review policies. These policies often, but not always, follow guidelines published by the AMA and CMS. In the case of E/M services, the payer follows the 1997 Documentation Guidelines for E/M Services.

The E/M codes are designed to classify the cognitive services provided by physicians during hospital and office visits, skilled nursing facility (SNF) visits, and consultations. The various levels of the E/M codes describe the wide variety of skills and the amount of effort, time, responsibility, and medical knowledge that physicians dedicate to the prevention, diagnosis, and treatment of illnesses and injuries as well as the promotion of optimal health. Healthcare facilities such as hospitals also report E/M codes to designate encounters or visits for outpatient services.

In claims processing for physicians, E/M codes are reported to document the professional services provided to patients. The level of medical decision-making is a key factor in the selection of appropriate E/M codes, but the level of decision-making is sometimes difficult to quantify in documentation. Generally, it is preferable that physicians select E/M codes. Coding professionals can then validate and verify the physicians' code selections according to the documentation guidelines developed jointly by the AMA and CMS (Smith 2019, 213–214).

Example:

> A new patient sees Dr. Reynolds in his office complaining of diarrhea and watery stool the previous night, as well as nausea, vomiting, and crampy, lower abdominal pain. Dr. Reynolds provides a detailed history and examination, and medical decision-making of moderate complexity. (Smith 2019, 231)

CPT code 99203 would be assigned. This code is for office or other outpatient visit for the evaluation and management of a new patient, which requires these three key components:

- A detailed history;
- A detailed examination; and
- Medical decision-making of low complexity.

This case could not be upcoded to code 99204 because all three components must be met or exceeded. In this case, the medical decision-making was moderate, but the history and examination were only at a detailed level. The next code, 99204 has higher criteria for history and examination.

To assign CPT code 99204 the following criteria is required:

- A comprehensive history;
- A comprehensive examination; and
- Medical decision-making of moderate complexity.

If the physician practice had submitted a claim with CPT code 99204 with the ICD codes for the patient's diagnosis, suspension or denial of the claim would be a possible outcome. Additional documentation would be requested and subsequently reviewed, and the 1997 guidelines applied. With no justification, the E/M code would have been downcoded to 99203 and paid at that level of service.

CHECK YOUR UNDERSTANDING

1. True or false? The AMA developed CPT primarily to describe medical services and procedures performed by physicians and other healthcare providers.

   a. True
   b. False

2. Which provider below does *not* submit CPT codes for reimbursement for the services indicated?

   a. Physicians for office services
   b. Hospitals for inpatient services
   c. Hospitals for outpatient services
   d. Ambulatory surgery centers for outpatient services

3. CPT category III codes are used to describe:

   a. Emerging technology procedures
   b. Procedures that are widely performed
   c. Procedures that Medicare recognizes as covered entities
   d. All of the above

4. Which of the following statements about category II codes is true?

   a. Category II codes are alphanumeric ending with the letter U.
   b. Category II codes are only used in conjunction with category III codes.
   c. Category II codes describe emerging technologies.
   d. Category II codes support performance measurement.

5. CPT codes are part of a larger system known as:

   a. Healthcare Common Procedure Coding System (HCPCS)
   b. ICD-10-CM
   c. Uniform Hospital Discharge Data Set (UHDDS)
   d. Unified Medical Language System (UMLS)

6. Who may submit a request to make changes to the CPT code set?

   a. Physicians and medical professionals
   b. Device manufacturers and pharmaceutical companies
   c. Public and private individuals
   d. All of the above

REVIEW

1. True or false? Diagnostic radiology codes (70010–76499) are generally assigned on the basis of documentation of history, physical examination, and medical decision-making.

   a. True
   b. False

2. A list of clinical examples is included in which appendix of CPT?

    a. A

    b. B

    c. C

    d. D

3. Which of the following is not a subsection of the radiology section of CPT?

    a. Nuclear medicine

    b. Magnetic resonance imaging

    c. Diagnostic ultrasound

    d. Radiation oncology

4. The Alphabetic Index of CPT includes which of the following types of listings?

    a. Procedures

    b. Diagnoses

    c. Abbreviations

    d. All of the above

5. Which of the following is not a requirement for inclusion of a Category I code in CPT?

    a. Many healthcare professionals across the country must perform the procedure.

    b. The procedure must be FDA cleared, or approved.

    c. Medicare must cover the procedure.

    d. The procedure must be of proven clinical efficacy.

6. True or false? CPT is not used for measurement of quality of care.

    a. True

    b. False

7. Which set of E/M codes below is not assigned based on documentation of history, physical examination, and medical decision-making?

    a. Inpatient consultations

    b. Office visits

    c. Critical care services

    d. Hospital observation services

8. Which circumstance below cannot be reflected with a CPT modifier?

    a. A service or procedure that has both a professional and a technical component

    b. A service or procedure that has been reduced or expanded in scope

c. A service or procedure that does not yet have a specific CPT code

d. A patient that has a bilateral procedure performed

9. CPT is composed of

   a. Category I, category II, and category III codes

   b. Category I and category II codes

   c. HCPCS Level I, HCPCS Level II, and HCPCS Level III codes

   d. Category I and HCPCS Level II codes

10. True or false? CPT codes can be assigned solely from the Index.

    a. True

    b. False

11. What resource helps educate the industry on proper CPT coding for past, present, and future code set releases?

    a. CMS

    b. CPT Assistant

    c. CPT Link

    d. CPT QuickRef app

12. What terminology is the standard used for exchanging clinical information across various EHR platforms?

    a. SNOMED CT

    b. CPT

    c. ICD-10-PCS

    d. ICD-10-CM

References

American Hospital Association (AHA). 2019. About the AHA central office. http://www.ahacentraloffice.org/aboutus/history-role.shtml.

American Medical Association (AMA). 2018. *Current Procedural Terminology (CPT)*, 4th ed. Chicago, IL: AMA.

American Medical Association (AMA). 2013. *CPT Changes 2013: An Insider's View*. Chicago, IL: AMA.

American Medical Association (AMA). 1992–2018. *CPT Assistant*. Chicago, IL: AMA.

Centers for Medicare and Medicaid Services (CMS). 2018a. 2018 Resources: Quality measure specifications. https://qpp.cms.gov/mips/explore-measures/quality-measures?py=2018&search=0067.

Centers for Medicare and Medicaid Services (CMS). 2018b. Internet-Only Manuals (IOMs) Medicare Claims Processing Manual, Chapter 12-Physicians/Nonphysician Practitioners. http://www.cms.gov/Regulations-and-Guidance/Guidance/Manuals/downloads/clm104c12.pdf.

Centers for Medicaid and Medicare Services (CMS). n.d. Overview. https://www.cms.gov/apps/physician-fee-schedule/overview.aspx

National Institute of Health (NIH). 2018. SNOMED CT. https://www.nlm.nih.gov/healthit/snomedct/index.html.

Smith, G. 2019. *Basic Current Procedural Terminology and HCPCS Coding*. Chicago, IL: AHIMA.

Resources

American Medical Association (AMA). n.d.a. AMA website for resources on CPT, category II, and category III CPT codes. Accessed Dec. 20, 2018. https://www.ama-assn.org/practice-management/cpt-current-procedural-terminology.

American Medical Association (AMA). n.d.b. AMA website for the most up to date list of PLA codes. Accessed Dec. 20, 2018. https://www.ama-assn.org/practice-management/cpt-pla-codes.

3

Healthcare Common Procedure Coding System (HCPCS)

June Bronnert, MHI, RHIA, CCS, CCS-P

LEARNING OBJECTIVES

- Discuss the history of the development of the Healthcare Common Procedure Coding System (HCPCS)
- Explain the use and structure of HCPCS
- Differentiate the levels of HCPCS
- Examine the relationship HCPCS has with other classifications, terminologies, and code sets
- Compare tools available to access and use
- Demonstrate how HCPCS is used in an electronic environment

KEY TERMS

- American Hospital Association's Central Office on HCPCS
- American Medical Association (AMA)
- Clinical quality measure (CQM)
- CMS HCPCS Workgroup
- Code on Dental Procedures and Nomenclature (Code)
- Descriptor
- HCPCS Level I
- HCPCS Level II

- Healthcare Common Procedure Coding System (HCPCS)
- Health Insurance Portability and Accountability Act (HIPAA)
- Miscellaneous codes
- Permanent national codes
- Pricing, Data Analysis and Coding (PDAC) contractor
- Temporary national codes

Introduction to HCPCS

The **Healthcare Common Procedure Coding System (HCPCS)** is a standardized system for healthcare providers and medical suppliers to report professional services, procedures, and supplies. The Centers for Medicare and Medicaid Services (CMS) established HCPCS under the **Health Insurance Portability and Accountability Act (HIPAA)** as a required standardized coding system. Public and private insurance programs need the HCPCS Level II system to ensure the providers and suppliers uniformly report services on claims and for meaningful data collection.

HCPCS includes into two principal subsystems: Level I and Level II. **HCPCS Level I** comprises the Current Procedural Terminology (CPT) coding system, a system maintained and published by the **American Medical Association (AMA)**. See chapter 2 for information on CPT. **HCPCS Level II**, often referred to as national codes, are the focus of this chapter. The original composition of HCPCS included a third level known as Level III. Deprecation of Level III HCPCS codes occurred by December 31, 2003, due to evolving industry requirements.

Developer

Standardizing medical procedures, supplies, products, and services necessary for Medicare and Medicaid claims was a key goal in development of HCPCS Level II. Uniform reporting and statistical data collection occurred due to the establishment of HCPCS Level II. The original title of HCPCS reflected the name of the agency that administered the Medicare and Medicaid programs at the time the coding system was established, the HCFA (Health Care Financing Administration) Common Procedure Coding System. When the agency changed its name in 2001 from HCFA to CMS, the coding system was renamed Healthcare Common Procedure Coding System.

CMS has maintained the intention of HCPCS since 1983 regardless of the additions, deletions, and changes to the system. The intention of the system is to meet the operational needs of the Medicare and Medicaid reimbursement programs, not only for reimbursement, but also for benchmarking, trending, planning, and measurement of quality of care.

Purpose

HCPCS (usually pronounced "hick picks") is a collection of codes and **descriptors** used to represent healthcare procedures, supplies, products, and services that are outside the scope of the CPT system (see chapter 2). For example, the code L0130 describes a flexible cervical thermoplastic collar molded to patient. HCPCS Level II's primary purpose supports efficient claims processing and CMS's operational needs.

In 1985, the federal government required physicians to use HCPCS codes to report services provided to Medicare patients, and, in October 1986, CMS required physicians to use HCPCS codes to report services provided to Medicaid patients. Section 9343(g) of the Omnibus Reconciliation Act of 1986 required hospitals (effective July 1, 1987) to report ambulatory surgery services, radiology, and other diagnostic services using HCPCS codes (HCFA 2000).

Content

Level II alphanumeric codes describe professional services, procedures, and supplies. They consist of a single alphabetic letter followed by four numeric digits. In addition to alphanumeric codes, HCPCS Level II includes modifiers to enable qualification of the reported item or service. A HCPCS index, table of drugs, and a file of not otherwise classified (NOC) codes complete the HCPCS Level II coding set. The index and table of drugs list alphabetically the service, supply name, or drug, followed by the code, whereas the NOC file is in code order followed by the descriptor.

The system provides a comprehensive and standardized set of codes that classifies similar healthcare products, supplies, or services into established categories. Although Level II codes are used for billing purposes, decisions regarding the addition, deletion, or modification of HCPCS are made independent of the process for making determinations regarding coverage and payment.

Separate categories of like items or services encompass millions of products from different manufacturers. When submitting a claim, providers and suppliers are required to use one of these codes to identify the items they are billing. The descriptors assigned to codes represent the official definition of the items and services; they do not refer to specific products. The reason the descriptors do not refer to specific products is to avoid the appearance of endorsement of particular products through HCPCS.

Types of HCPCS Level II Codes

There are several types of HCPCS Level II codes. Different organizations are responsible for establishing and maintaining the different types of codes. The **Code on Dental Procedures and Nomenclature (Code)** (see chapter 5) is one type of HCPCS Level II codes. Three other types are permanent, temporary, and miscellaneous codes.

PERMANENT NATIONAL CODES

Permanent national codes are the responsibility of CMS, which makes decisions about additions, revisions, and deletions to the standardized codes used by private and public insurers. **CMS HCPCS Workgroup** manages permanent national codes. The Workgroup is comprised of private and public insurers. Representatives include:

- Medicare
- Medicaid
- Department of Veterans Affairs
- **Pricing, Data Analysis and Coding (PDAC) contractor**

PDAC represents, with input from the durable medical equipment (DME) Medicare Administrative Contractors (MACs), Medicare's durable medical equipment, prosthetic, orthotics, and supplies (DMEPOS) operational needs for processing claims. Members are responsible for reviewing requests for additions, deletions, and revisions to the codes and formulating preliminary coding recommendations for presentation to the public for comment. The Workgroup provides a stable environment for maintaining the standardized coding system. DME MACs and the PDAC assign HCPCS codes to DMEPOS products (PDAC 2016).

TEMPORARY NATIONAL CODES

Temporary national codes provide insurers a mechanism for establishing codes in a short time frame to meet their operational needs before the next annual update. Temporary national codes are independent of the permanent national codes and do not have an expiration date. Temporary codes are subject to replacement by permanent codes. If this occurs, the deleted temporary code is cross-referenced to the new permanent code. Changes to temporary codes occur quarterly. The implementation effective date for temporary code change is included in the update. The date is dependent upon the time needed to prepare CMS's and the contractor's computer systems and issue implementation instructions to suppliers along with user education.

The types of temporary codes are as follows:

- C codes: Established for Medicare's hospital outpatient prospective payment system (OPPS) operational purposes. The codes represent facility services.
- G codes: Used to identify professional healthcare procedures and services for which no CPT code currently exists.
- H codes: Required for Medicaid agencies when state law mandates separate codes for reporting mental health services such as alcohol and drug treatment services.

- K codes: Established for use by the DME MACs when existing permanent national codes do not include the codes needed to implement a DME MAC medical review policy.
- Q codes: Established for claims-processing purposes for various drugs and other types of medical services not identified by national level II codes.
- S codes: Established by private insurers to report drugs, services, and supplies for which there are no national codes. The codes support operational needs of the private sector to implement policies, programs, or claims processing.
- T codes: Created for state Medicaid agencies program administration requirements. The codes describe items for which there are no permanent national codes. Medicare does not use T codes for operational program requirements. Private insurers may elect to use T codes to meet their needs.

MISCELLANEOUS CODES

Miscellaneous codes allow for timely claims submission when a national code that describes the item or service is unavailable. The permission of the Food and Drug Administration (FDA) to market the service or item is separate from establishing a distinct HCPCS Level II code. Miscellaneous codes allow providers timely claims submission for the service or item during the time a new code is under the HCPCS review process. Utilization of miscellaneous codes also helps to avoid the inefficiency of assigning distinct codes for items or services that are rarely furnished or for which few claims are expected.

Services and Products in HCPCS Level II

Alphanumeric Level II codes are grouped into categories. The following sections describe the codes that represent these categories of services and products along with the code modifiers.

A CODES: TRANSPORTATION SERVICES, INCLUDING AMBULANCE, MEDICAL AND SURGICAL SUPPLIES, RADIOPHARMACEUTICALS, AND MISCELLANEOUS

A code services include ground and air ambulance, nonemergency transportation (taxi, bus, automobile, wheelchair van), and ancillary transportation-related fees. Examples include A0225, Ambulance service, neonatal transport, base rate, emergency transport, one way, and A0390, advanced life support (ALS) mileage (per mile).

A codes also describe a range of medical, surgical, and other supplies and accessories related to DME. Medicare's prosthetic devices provisions generally cover DME-related supplies, accessories, maintenance, and repair required for proper DME equipment functioning. The codes describing these services are typically A codes. Examples include A4206, Syringe with needle, sterile 1 cc, each; A4330, Perineal fecal collection pouch with adhesive, each; and a series of codes (A5500–A5513) for diabetic footwear. Special dressings (A6000–A6550) also are included in this area as are supplies of some radiopharmaceutical imaging agents (A9500–A9700). Other imaging agents are included in the C codes (temporary outpatient PPS) section of HCPCS.

B CODES: ENTERAL AND PARENTERAL THERAPY

B codes are for supplies, formulae, nutritional solutions, and infusion pumps. B code examples are as follows:

- B4034, Enteral feeding supply kit; syringe fed, per day; includes but not limited to feeding/flushing syringe, administration set tubing, dressings, tape
- B4150, Enteral formula, nutritionally complete with intact nutrients, includes proteins, fats, carbohydrates, vitamins and minerals, may include fiber, administered through an enteral feeding tube, 100 calories = 1 unit
- B4168, Parenteral nutrition solution; amino acid, 3.5%, (500 ml = 1 unit) home mix
- B9002, Enteral nutrition infusion pump, any type

C CODES: OUTPATIENT PPS (TEMPORARY)

C codes describe drugs, biologicals, and devices used by facilities. C codes are required for facilities reimbursed by OPPS, but other providers or payment systems may recognize the codes on claim forms. Services identified by C codes are eligible for transitional pass-through payments for hospitals and for items classified in new-technology ambulatory payment classifications (APCs) under OPPS. The OPPS defines payment status, such as separately payable, bundled, or non-covered, for individual codes. Report all eligible C codes regardless of payment status.

Included in this section are codes for devices such as infusion pump, non-programmable, temporary (implantable) (C2626), procedures such as magnetic resonance angiography (MRA) without contrast followed by with contrast, chest (excluding myocardium) (C8911), brachytherapy source, non-stranded, gold-198, per source (C1716), and some drugs, such as injection of 1 mg guselkumab (C9029).

D CODES: DENTAL PROCEDURES

D (dental) codes are a separate category of national codes. Chapter 5 addresses the dental code set copyrighted by the American Dental Association (ADA).

E CODES: DURABLE MEDICAL EQUIPMENT

E codes are permanent codes describing DME such as canes (E0105, Cane, quad or three-prong, includes canes of all materials, adjustable or fixed, with tips), crutches (E0117, Crutch underarm, articulating, spring assisted, each), walkers (E0130, Walker, rigid [pickup] adjustable or fixed height), and commodes (E0163, Commode chair, mobile or stationary, with fixed arms). Temporary code sections K and L also describe DME supplies. Examples of other types of equipment included in this section are:

- Decubitus care equipment (E0184, Dry pressure mattress)
- Bath and toilet aids (E0241, Bath tub wall rail, each)
- Hospital beds and accessories (E0295, Hospital bed, semi-electric [head and foot adjustment], without side rails, without mattress)
- Oxygen and related respiratory equipment (E0455, Oxygen tent, excluding croup or pediatric tents)
- Monitoring equipment (E0607, Home blood glucose monitor and E0619, Apnea monitor, with recording feature)
- Safety equipment (E0700, Safety equipment, device or accessory, any type)
- Neurostimulators (for which temporary L codes can also be used), along with infusion supplies (E0776, IV pole), traction (E0860, Traction equipment, over door, cervical)
- Wheelchair accessories (E0968, Commode seat, wheelchair), wheelchairs (E1140, Wheelchair; detachable arms, desk or full-length, swing-away, detachable footrests), and other devices such as power wheelchairs and accessories (for which temporary K codes can also be used)
- Artificial kidney machines also are included in this section (E1594, Cycler dialysis machine for peritoneal dialysis)

G CODES: PROCEDURES/PROFESSIONAL SERVICES (TEMPORARY)

G codes identify professional healthcare procedures and services that are not identified by a CPT code or that use an existing code but need additional details for CMS operational purposes. G codes cover diverse services ranging from quality measure documentation to screening services. Additionally, there are codes for telehealth and codes for complex radiation therapy using robotic linear accelerators. G0105, Colorectal cancer screening; colonoscopy on individual at high risk; G0252, Positron emission tomography (PET) imaging, full and partial-ring PET scanners only, for initial diagnosis of breast cancer and/or surgical planning for breast cancer; and G8452, Beta-blocker therapy not prescribed are examples of services represented by G codes.

H CODES: ALCOHOL AND DRUG ABUSE TREATMENT SERVICES

State Medicaid agencies mandated by state law to establish separate codes for identifying mental health services that include drug and alcohol treatment services use H codes. This section includes detoxification services (H0014, Alcohol and/or drug services; ambulatory detoxification), medication administration (H0033, Oral medication administration, direct observation), prenatal care (H1000, Prenatal care, at-risk assessment), and various therapies (H2032, Activity therapy, per 15 minutes; H2019, Therapeutic behavioral services, per 15 minutes; and H2024, Supported employment, per diem).

J CODES: DRUGS ADMINISTERED OTHER THAN BY ORAL METHOD

J codes include drugs that ordinarily cannot be self-administered, such as drugs administered by other than oral means (J0120–J3590), chemotherapy drugs (J8501–J9999), immunosuppressive drugs (J7500–J7599), and inhalation solutions (J7604–J7799).

CMS publishes the Table of Drugs on the CMS HCPCS website. The table is an alphabetical list of drug names that includes the dosage and administration method along with the J code. Azathioprine, parenteral 100 mg IV J7501 is one example of the drugs listed in the table.

K CODES (TEMPORARY CODES)

K codes were established for use by the DME MAC when current permanent national codes for supplies and certain product categories do not exist or do not contain a sufficient level of detail for DME MACs to administer established medical review policies. K codes identify wheelchairs and wheelchair accessories not listed in the E code section (K0019, Arm pad, replacement only, each). Other examples of K codes are lower extremity orthotics that are not included in the L code section (K0672, Addition to lower extremity orthotic, removable soft interface, all components, replacement only, each), and various miscellaneous codes (K0601, Replacement battery for external infusion pump owned by patient, silver oxide, 1.5 volt, each).

L CODES: ORTHOTIC AND PROSTHETIC PROCEDURES AND DEVICES

L codes include orthotic and prosthetic procedures and devices as well as scoliosis equipment, orthopedic shoes, and most prosthetic implants. Codes in the orthotics section are extremely specific.

Example:

> L0490, TLSO (thoracic-lumbar-sacral orthosis), sagittal-coronal control, one-piece rigid plastic shell with overlapping reinforced anterior, with multiple straps and closures, posterior extends from sacrococcygeal junction and terminates at or before the T9 vertebra, anterior extends from the symphysis pubis to xiphoid, anterior opening, restricts gross trunk motion in sagittal and coronal planes, prefabricated, includes fitting and adjustment.

In addition to spinal orthoses, there are codes for extremity orthoses (L1971, ankle-foot orthosis [AFO], plastic or other material with ankle joint, prefabricated, includes fitting and adjustment), for orthopedic shoes (L3219, Orthopedic footwear, men's shoe, oxford, each), and for repair of orthotic devices (L4205, Repair of orthotic device, labor component, per 15 minutes).

The prosthetic procedures are considered "base," or basic, procedures and may be modified by adding terms and procedures or special materials from the "additions" sections to the base procedure. Although termed *procedures*, these codes are not surgical procedures but rather codes for fabrication of prostheses. Included are codes for prostheses for knee disarticulation (L5150, Knee disarticulation [or through knee], molded socket, external knee joints, shin, SACH foot), additions and replacements to prostheses (L5704, Custom-shaped protective cover, below knee), breast prostheses (L8020, Breast prosthesis, mastectomy form), and elastic support garments. Also included in this section are codes for prosthetic implants such as implantable breast prostheses (L8600, Implantable breast prosthesis, silicone or equal), artificial larynx, any type (L8500), and some joint replacements (L8641, Metatarsal joint implant).

M CODES: MEDICAL SERVICES

M codes include cellular therapy, prolotherapy, intragastric hypothermia, intravenous (IV) chelation therapy, and fabric wrapping of an abdominal aneurysm. These services do not qualify for CPT codes because they are either not of proven efficacy or considered obsolete modalities.

P CODES: PATHOLOGY AND LABORATORY SERVICES

The P codes include chemistry, toxicology, and microbiology tests, screening Papanicolaou procedures, and various blood products. Included in this section are codes for laboratory procedures now considered to be obsolete (for example, P2033, Thymol turbidity, blood), blood products (P9038, Red blood cells, irradiated, each unit), and codes for travel allowances to collect specimens (P9604, Travel allowance one way in connection with medically necessary laboratory specimen collection drawn from homebound or nursing homebound patient; prorated trip charge).

Q CODES (TEMPORARY)

Codes in this section identify supplies such as telehealth, chemotherapy, and hospice care without a CPT code designation. Telehealth Q codes describe the originating site facility while other HCPCS codes related to telehealth describe various telehealth services, such as a consultation. Q codes identify drugs, such as oral antiemetic given in conjunction with chemotherapy, devices and supplies, such as emergency hand pump for use with electronic/pneumatic ventricular assist device. Radiopharmaceuticals, casting and splinting supplies, and skin substitutes are other examples of Q codes.

R CODES: DIAGNOSTIC RADIOLOGY SERVICES

R codes identify transportation of portable x-ray and/or EKG equipment.

S CODES: TEMPORARY NATIONAL CODES (NON-MEDICARE)

Private insurers use S codes to report drugs, services, and supplies for which there are no national codes. The private sector needs the codes to implement policies, programs, or claims processing. The Medicaid program also uses these codes. However, they are not payable by Medicare. An example of an S code is S0317 Disease management program; per diem.

NATIONAL T CODES (TEMPORARY)

State Medicaid agencies use T codes for items for which there are no permanent national codes, but for which codes are necessary to administer the Medicaid program. Medicare does not use T codes, but private insurers may do so. T codes identify a variety of services from home health to nonemergency transportation. Supplies such as incontinence products are another example of what can be found in the T codes.

V CODES: VISION AND HEARING SERVICES

V codes include vision-related supplies, including spectacles, lenses, contact lenses, prostheses, intraocular lenses, and miscellaneous lenses. The codes in this section are very specific as to type of lens.

V codes also describe hearing tests and related supplies and equipment, speech-language pathology screenings, and the repair of augmentative communication systems. Dispensing fees for hearing aids are included as well.

HCPCS MODIFIERS

Modifiers provide supplemental specific circumstantial information to an item or a service described by a HCPCS code. They allow for an enhanced code narrative unique to an individual patient.

In some situations, insurers instruct providers and suppliers to add a modifier to provide additional information regarding the service or item identified by the HCPCS code. For example, ambulance services codes require modifiers. The specific modifier is individual and built for a patient depending upon the patient's origin and destination. The letter *H* identifies hospital while *R* indicates residence. The letter's position determines if the hospital is the patient's origin or destination. The modifier RH indicates the patient's origin was their residence and the destination was the hospital.

Level II HCPCS modifiers are either alphanumeric or two letters and range from A1–ZC. Examples of level II modifiers include:

LT	Left side
RT	Right side
E1	Upper left, eyelid
E2	Lower left, eyelid
F1	Left hand, second digit
F2	Left hand, third digit
LC	Left circumflex coronary artery
LD	Left anterior descending coronary artery
LM	Left main coronary artery
RC	Right coronary artery

Both CPT and HCPCS Level II codes are eligible for level II modifiers. However, by definition, modifiers may be limited to certain HCPCS codes. Modifiers are subject to change quarterly. They can be added, deleted, or revised, similar to temporary Level II HCPCS codes. In accordance with HIPAA rules, CMS requires all providers to report HCPCS modifiers valid at the time a service is performed.

Principles and Guidelines in HCPCS Level II

Level II HCPCS coding guidance depends upon the specific section of codes. The DME MAC provides coding guidance for manufacturers and suppliers on the proper use of the HCPCS codes used to describe DMEPOS used for Medicare billing (PDAC 2016). The **American Hospital Association's Central Office on HCPCS** and CMS established a clearinghouse process that provides coding guidance for the following Level II HCPCS codes: A codes for ambulance services and radiopharmaceuticals; C codes; G codes; J codes; and Q codes, except Q0136 through Q0181 for hospitals, physicians, and other health professionals who bill Medicare. CMS addresses the other HCPCS Level II related questions.

Establishment of a HCPCS code does not guarantee reimbursement of the device, supply, or service rendered. Payers make coverage and payment determinations independent of the HCPCS Level II code creation and maintenance process.

Process for Revision and Updates

Maintenance and distribution of HCPCS Level II codes and modifiers is the responsibility of CMS. It is a multi-step process with various timelines according to the type of requested HCPCS Level II code. Annual updates to permanent codes and quarterly updates to temporary codes determine the maintenance timelines. Requests for HCPCS Level II code changes come from a variety of sources (see figure 3.1 for the HCPCS decision tree for external requests to add or revise codes). The CMS HCPCS website contains downloadable instructions for applicants. All applicants must submit requests by stated timelines for each coding cycle. Applications to

FIGURE 3.1. HCPCS decision tree for external requests to add or revise codes

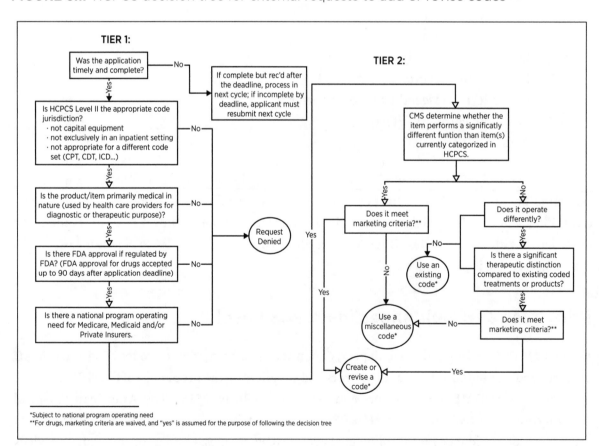

Source: CMS 2018.

create, revise, or discontinue a HCPCS Level II code follow the same CMS recommended format described on the CMS website. Among the items of data required on the application are the following:

- The FDA status of the device or drug, as appropriate
- A description of what the device, drug, or service does
- Whether or not the item is durable
- The usual medical purpose of the item
- Similar items
- Any payment history for the item
- Why there is no appropriate existing code for the item
- Settings in which the item is used

Applicants request at least one of three types of coding modifications to HCPCS Level II codes. The types of requests are:

- Additions: Requests to add new codes occurs when no distinct code describes a product or service. If the CMS HCPCS Workgroup implements a new code, payment determinations are a separate process from establishing a new code. Whether an item identified by a new code is covered is determined by the Medicare law, regulations, and medical review policies and not by assignment of a code.
- Changes to existing code description: Modification requests occur when an interested party believes changing the descriptor for the code provides a better narrative of the device, supply, or service.
- Discontinue an existing code: When an existing code becomes obsolete or is duplicative of another code, a request can be made to discontinue the code.

Timely and properly formatted external recommendations are analyzed by the workgroup during regularly scheduled meetings. The workgroup makes a preliminary coding decision recommendation based upon established criteria. Examples of the criteria are:

- Is the item appropriate for HCPCS Level II jurisdiction?
- Does the Federal Drug Administration (FDA) regulate the product or service?
  - If so, has the FDA approved the product or service?
- Is the product or service significantly different from other products or services currently represented by a HCPCS Level II code?
- Does an existing code describe the item in a coding request? An existing code describes an item in a coding request when it describes products either with functions similar to the item in the coding request or without significant therapeutic distinctions.

- Does an existing code describe products almost the same in function with only minor distinctions?
- Is the item for an inpatient setting or for an item that is not diagnostic or therapeutic in nature?
- Is there sufficient claims activity or volume, as evidenced by three months of marketing activity for non-drug products, for adding or modifying a code? Data should indicate changes will make the system more efficient and warrant the administrative burden.

(CMS 2015)

Discontinuation of a code occurs when the descriptor is obsolete (for example, products no longer are used, or other more specific codes have been added) or duplicative and no longer useful (for example, new codes better describe items identified by existing codes).

If a code already exists, no new or modified code is established. If an existing code describes the item in the coding request, the recommendation is to group the item into the existing code and the code descriptor is modified to reflect the distinctions.

The Medicare Modernization Act included an update to the code revision methodology in 2004 to increase the public input into the maintenance process. The updates included:

Expansion of the public meetings: Public meetings relate to all external requests for HCPCS codes for products, supplies, and services. Notice of Public Meetings for All New Public Requests for Revisions to the HCPCS Coding and Payment Determinations appears in the Federal Register and is posted on CMS website. Obtaining industry and public comments is a primary purpose of the meetings. Public meeting agendas comprise the preliminary CMS HCPCS Workgroup recommendations on the external requests. Advanced published agenda items include descriptions of the coding requests, the requestor, and the name of the product or service. This information provides an opportunity for the public to become aware of coding changes under consideration and provide public input on the proposals. Interested parties may present at the meeting or submit written comments.

Implementation of a reconsideration process: CMS maintains an appeals process for denied new code requests. Denied new code requests have the denial rationale delineated. Applicants have the opportunity for reconsideration of their request during the same coding cycle.

Publication of notice of decisions: The CMS HCPCS website publishes all preliminary recommendations of the CMS HCPCS workgroup prior to public meetings to facilitate effective public discussion and comment.

CMS notifies an applicant of final coding decisions according to established timelines. For permanent HCPCS code requests, CMS is the final decision-making authority. When quarterly updates occur to the temporary codes, the updated files are located on the HCPCS website. Each temporary code section publishes individual quarterly files. For example, G code quarterly update files are independent of C code quarterly update files. All modifications to the HCPCS codes are incorporated into the HCPCS Level II annual update. The file contains code changes to all temporary and national HCPCS codes for the year. The update is published by mid-November on the official HCPCS website.

Relationship with Other Terminologies, Classification Systems, and Code Sets

Given the coverage of HCPCS Level II across professional services, procedures, and supplies, it has a relationship with other systems used to capture similar data. This link to CPT codes, dental codes, and national drug codes is described below.

CPT Codes

CPT is one of the two subsystems of the HCPCS code set. Developed by the AMA in 1966, CPT is a uniform coding system consisting of descriptive terms and identifying codes used primarily to identify medical services and procedures furnished by physicians and other healthcare professionals. Level I codes include five-character codes and two-digit modifiers. Physicians and other healthcare professionals use CPT to identify services and procedures for multiple uses such as reimbursement and quality measure reporting. The AMA makes decisions regarding the addition, deletion, or modification of CPT codes. The Level I HCPCS CPT codes contain their own scope and jurisdiction. Codes needed to report medical supplies, devices, or other services by suppliers other than physicians are typically outside the scope of CPT and are found in HCPCS Level II. See chapter 2 for further details about HCPCS Level I, CPT.

Dental Codes

The Code on Dental Procedures and Nomenclature (Code), which is printed in a manual titled *Current Dental Terminology (CDT)*, establishes uniformity for billing dental procedures and supplies. The ADA, not the CMS HCPCS Workgroup, maintains the system and decides the changes to CDT. While CMS originally published CDT as section D of HCPCS Level II, the ADA distributes this code system. Chapter 5 discusses the details of CDT.

National Drug Codes

The National Drug Codes (NDC) codes establish unique identifiers for human-use drugs. The codes represent manufacturer and specific product information, such as dosage, strength, and packaging. The appropriate HCPCS Level II and NDC codes are required for accurate claims submission. The NDC code provides important drug-specific information while the HCPCS code provides information to determine reimbursement. In order to facilitate accurate reporting of both codes, the PDAC maintains a crosswalk of NDC codes to HCPCS Level II codes for drugs deemed billable to DME MACs (PDAC 2018). The crosswalk supports CMS's claims processing operational needs by providing conversion factors used in determining applicable billings. See Chapter 4 for NDC details.

Tools to Access and Use

While there are many components to Level II HCPC codes, the codes CMS is responsible for maintaining and distributing are located on their website. The annual HCPCS Level II files typically consist of five files with one file focusing on the record layout of the file containing all alphanumeric HCPCS Level II codes for the year. The other files consist of the index, not otherwise classified (NOC) codes, and the table of drugs. Temporary Level II HCPCS code files have their own unique files. The files are organized by type of temporary code, C code or G code, along with the quarter in which the code is effective. For example, G codes effective in April of the current year is a downloadable file separate from C codes effective in April.

Other HCPCS tools to access and use vary depending upon the provider's setting. For example, hospitals typically have HCPCS Level II codes as part of their billing systems charge master file. This file facilitates the selection of supplies and services with the appropriate codes.

CMS and their associated contractors offer various online resources for information related to Level II HCPCS codes. The information may cover payment information based upon CMS coverage determinations for various HCPCS codes. For example, the physician-fee schedule search provides payment policy indicators and relative value units (RVU) for HCPCS codes. The fee schedule for DMEPOS is accessible from CMS contractors' websites.

The CMS Medicare Coverage Database (MCD) includes national and local coverage determinations. The database also contains local articles and proposed national coverage determinations (NCDs). The site provides coverage information along with appropriate Level II HCPCS codes. It is useful for all providers to determine if supplies and services are medically necessary for reimbursement as defined by CMS. There are a number of ways to use the MDC, including quick and advanced searching, access to pre-defined lists of coverage documents, coverage data reports, and the ability to download articles and coverage decisions.

Adoption and Use Cases

In accordance with the Social Security Act, federal laws governing Medicare require CMS to contract with entities to process and pay Medicare claims and associated services.

The Medicare Prescription Drug, Improvement and Modernization Act of 2003 (MMA) mandated significant changes to the Medicare fee-for-service program's administrative structure. Through implementation of Medicare Contracting Reform (or section 911 of the MMA), CMS established multi-state, regional contractors called MACs. MACs are responsible for administering both Medicare Part A and Medicare Part B claims.

The CMS regulation published on August 17, 2000 (45 CFR 162.1002) to implement the HIPAA requirement for standardized coding systems established the HCPCS Level II codes as the standardized coding system for describing and identifying substances, equipment, supplies, or other items used in healthcare services that are not identified by the HCPCS Level I, CPT codes. October 1, 2002, was the deadline for public and private insurers' compliance with the HIPAA regulation.

Clinical quality measure (CQM) developers adopted HCPCS as a way to express healthcare performance. CQMs are tools that help measure and track the quality of healthcare services that eligible professionals, eligible hospitals, and critical access hospitals provide. Selected HCPCS codes represent data elements used in the measure. HCPCS is one of the code sets identified in defining certain data elements such as a procedure or intervention. Contained within the various measures are data elements defined by HCPCS and thus, when reported, identify specific aspects of care the measure identifies. For example, the National Committee for Quality Assurance (NCQA) is the developer of numerous CQMs. Colonoscopy is an NCQA-developed measure containing HCPCS Level II G codes identifying high-risk or non-high-risk individuals receiving colonoscopies.

Use Case One: Billing Physician Services

Physicians use HCPCS codes to describe and bill for a number of different services and procedures. Here is one example: A 14-year-old gymnast felt pain in her leg after vaulting at practice. She was unable to bear any weight on her left leg. Physician exam revealed foot and ankle to be normal. The neurovascular status of the foot was normal. The ankle was nontender and not swollen. An x-ray of the tibia and fibula showed a displaced fracture of the distal fibula. The fracture was reduced, and the patient was placed in a short leg splint molded for her from fiberglass with extensive padding placed over the fracture site. The physician's biller examined the documentation and chose an ICD code for the left distal fracture of the fibula, a HCPCS Level I (CPT) code for the reduction of the fracture, and a HCPCS Level II code for the fiberglass cast supplies (A4590) and submitted them on a claim to the insurance company. Based on the benefits of the parent's insurance plan, the insurance company processed the claim and paid the provider for the supplies and services rendered.

Use Case Two: Creating a Clinical Quality Measure

HCPCS Level II codes are one code system clinical quality measure developers may incorporate in a measure. Electronic clinical quality measures (eCQM) use data from health information technology systems, such as electronic health records (EHRs) to measure healthcare quality. Developers use the web-based Measure Authoring Tool (MAT) to create the desired measure through identification of various data elements. For example, developers identify the annual wellness visit services as one initial population criteria necessary for their measure. The initial population criteria identify all patients evaluated by a specific performance eMeasure who share a common set of specified characteristics within a specific measurement set to which a given measure belongs. Criteria may include specific age groups and diagnostic and procedure codes. The developer selected HCPCS Level II as one of the code systems to investigate. The result was an annual wellness visit value set containing two HCPCS codes: G0438 annual wellness visit includes a personalized prevention plan of service (PPS), initial visit and G0439 annual wellness visit includes a personalized prevention plan of service (PPS), subsequent visit. The developer incorporated this value set representing two HCPCS codes into the eMeasure.

CHECK YOUR UNDERSTANDING

1. True or false? HCPCS was developed to report physician and nonphysician services.

   a. True
   b. False

2. What organization is responsible for development of HCPCS Level II codes?

   a. CMS
   b. AMA
   c. AHA
   d. ADA

3. True or false? HCPCS includes three levels of codes.

   a. True
   b. False

4. The first level of HCPCS consists of:

   a. CPT codes
   b. CDT codes
   c. NDC codes
   d. DSM 5 codes

5. HCPCS Level II codes are also known as:

   a. Local codes
   b. Mandatory codes
   c. National codes
   d. Non-physician codes

REVIEW

1. What organization(s) is (are) responsible for maintenance and distribution of HCPCS Level II codes?

   a. Health Care Financing Administration
   b. American Hospital Association, American Medical Association
   c. American Medical Association, American Nursing Association
   d. Centers for Medicare and Medicaid Services

2. True or false? HIPAA regulations established HCPCS Level II codes as one of the standardized code sets.

   a. True
   b. False

3. How frequently are permanent Level II HCPCS codes updated?

   a. Quarterly
   b. Semiannually
   c. Annually
   d. Monthly

4. Which of the following is not a type of HCPCS Level II temporary code?

   a. G codes
   b. Q codes
   c. T codes
   d. E codes

5. Which of the following organizations makes decisions regarding the modification, deletion, or addition of HCPCS dental codes?

   a. AMA
   b. PDAC
   c. ADA
   d. CMS

6. True or false? Modifiers can be used with both levels of HCPCS codes.

   a. True
   b. False

7. What organization(s) is (are) responsible for providing coding guidance to hospitals on the J codes?

   a. AHIMA and CMS
   b. ADA and AMA
   c. AHA Central Office
   d. CMS

8. True or false? Once the CMS HCPCS Workgroup establishes a HCPCS Level II code as a permanent national code, Medicare recognizes it as a covered and payable service.

   a. True
   b. False

9. Which question is asked in Tier 2 for submissions requesting to add or revise a HCPCS Level II code?

   a. Was the application by the external requester timely?
   b. Is there a national program operating need for Medicare, Medicaid, and/or private insurers?
   c. Is the product/item primarily medical in nature?
   d. Is there a significant therapeutic distinction compared to existing coded treatments or products?

10. A miscellaneous HCPCS Level II code is used:

    a. When no HCPCS Level I code exists
    b. When no HCPCS Level II code exists
    c. After calling the payer for an authorization number
    d. After submission of an application form to CMS for a new code

11. The HCPCS code system is composed of the following:

    a. Level I CPT codes
    b. Level I CPT, Level II HCPCS, and NDC codes
    c. NDC and Level II HCPCS codes
    d. Level I CPT codes and Level II HCPCS codes

12. CMS publishes what online resource for healthcare providers to review individual services or supplies defined as medically necessary for Medicare patients?

    a. Medicare necessity database
    b. Medicare coverage determinations
    c. Medical necessity decision database
    d. Physician fee schedule database

13. When providers submit a Medicare claim for medication, what code(s) are required to be reported?

    a. NDC and HCPCS Level II code
    b. Level I CPT code
    c. HCPCS Level II code
    d. Level I CPT and HCPCS Level II code

14. True or false? HCPCS Level II codes are typically incorporated into a hospital's electronic billing systems.

    a. True
    b. False

15. What section of HCPCS Level II codes identifies drug and alcohol services reported to state Medicaid agencies?

    a. A codes
    b. J codes
    c. H codes
    d. L codes

References

45 CFR 162.1002: Administrative requirements. 2000 (August 17).

Centers for Medicare and Medicaid Services (CMS). 2018. HCPCS decision tree for external requests to add or revise codes. https://www.cms.gov/Medicare/Coding/MedHCPCSGenInfo/downloads/HCPCS_Decision_Tree_and_Definitions.pdf.

Centers for Medicare and Medicaid Services (CMS). 2015. HCPCS Level II Coding Procedures. https://www.cms.gov/Medicare/Coding/MedHCPCSGenInfo/Downloads/HCPCSLevelIICodingProcedures7-2011.pdf.

Health Care Financing Administration (HCFA). 2000. Program Memorandum Intermediaries. Transmittal A-00-09. http://www.cms.hhs.gov/transmittals/downloads/A000960.PDF.

Medicare Pricing, Data Analysis and Coding (PDAC). 2018. NDC/HCPCS crosswalk. https://www.dmepdac.com/crosswalk/index.html.

Medicare Pricing, Data Analysis and Coding (PDAC). 2016. Correct coding - HCPCS coding recommendations from non-Medicare sources. https://www.dmepdac.com/resources/articles/2016/08_03_16b.html.

Resources

American Dental Association. 2018. *CDT 2019: Dental Procedure Codes*. Chicago: ADA. https://www.ada.org/en/publications/cdt.

Centers for Medicare and Medicaid Services and the Office of the National Coordinator. 2018. Guide for Reading Eligible Professional (EP) and Eligible Hospital (EH) eMeasures, Version 4. https://ecqi.healthit.gov/system/files/Guide-for-Reading-Electronic-Clinical-Quality-Measures-v4-0-2018-0504.pdf.

Centers for Medicare and Medicaid Services. 2018. HCPCS - General Information. https://www.cms.gov/Medicare/Coding/MedHCPCSGenInfo/index.html.

Centers for Medicare and Medicaid Services. 2018. HCPCS Coding Questions. https://www.cms.gov/Medicare/Coding/MedHCPCSGenInfo/HCPCS_Coding_Questions.html.

Centers for Medicare and Medicaid Services. 2018. HCPCS Release & Code Set. https://www.cms.gov/Medicare/Coding/HCPCSReleaseCodeSets/index.html.

Centers for Medicare and Medicaid Services. 2018. Welcome to the Medicare Coverage Database. https://www.cms.gov/medicare-coverage-database/.

Centers for Medicare and Medicaid Services. 2013. Transactions and Code Sets Regulations. https://www.cms.gov/Regulations-and-Guidance/Administrative-Simplification/Code-Sets/index.html.

Centers for Medicare and Medicaid Services. n.d. Overview. https://www.cms.gov/apps/physician-fee-schedule/overview.aspx.

CGS. 2018. Look Up a HCPCS Code. https://www.cgsmedicare.com/medicare_dynamic/hcpcs/search.asp

Commonwealth Care Alliance. 2018. National Drug Code (NDC) requirements for physician-administered medications. https://www.commonwealthcarealliance.org/getmedia/6553153a-a906-4072-b5cf-c48f083931a5/Payment-Policy-National-Drug-Code-(NDC)-Requirement_1.

Smith, G. 2019. *Basic Current Procedural Terminology and HCPCS Coding*. Chicago, IL: AHIMA.

4

National Drug Codes (NDCs)

Gary L. Saner

LEARNING OBJECTIVES

- Discuss the history, development, and use of National Drug Codes (NDCs)
- Explain the components of NDCs
- Present the information available in the *NDC Directory*
- Review the process for updating NDCs
- List current principles and guidelines for using NDCs
- Examine the relationship NDC has with other classifications, terminologies, and code sets
- Compare tools available to access and use NDCs
- Demonstrate how NDCs are used in an electronic environment

KEY TERMS

- Drug Listing Act of 1972
- Food and Drug Administration (FDA)
- Federal Food, Drug and Cosmetic Act (FDCA)
- Labeler
- Labeler code
- National Drug Code (NDC)
- *National Drug Code (NDC) Directory*
- Package code
- Product code
- Product trade name
- Structured Product Labeling (SPL)

Introduction to National Drug Codes

The **National Drug Code (NDC)** system is a set of product identifiers maintained and approved by the US **Food and Drug Administration (FDA)** that uniquely identify human drugs and biologics and veterinary drugs. Each drug product listed under Section 510 of the Food, Drug and Cosmetic Act (FDCA) is assigned a unique ten-digit NDC number consisting of three segments: labeler code, product code, and package code. The NDC identifier is used throughout the drug product life cycle from manufacturing, agency listing, importing, supply chain distributing, prescribing, dispensing, administrating, payment, and reimbursing.

This chapter discusses why the NDC system was developed and by what agency. It also describes the components of the codes as they are listed in the *NDC Directory*. Adoption of NDC as a code system and two use cases, including application in the electronic environment, are examined as well. Additionally, NDC's relationships with other classifications, terminologies, and code sets and tools available for access and use are explained.

Developer

Under the direction of the Secretary of the Department of Health, Education, and Welfare, the Commissioner of Food and Drugs established the National Drug Code (NDC) system in 1969 to "...provide an identification system in computer language to permit automated processing of drug data by Government agencies, drug manufacturers and distributors, hospitals, and insurance companies" (FDA 1969, 11157). The initial NDC identifier consisted of a nine-character, three-segment code: Labeler Identity Code (three characters assigned by the FDA), Drug Product Identity Code (four characters assigned by the firm), and Trade Package Identity Code (two characters assigned by the firm). The *NDC Directory* was published by the government "...to provide a complete listing of drugs and their code designations" (FDA 1969, 11157). Some segments of the healthcare industry considered the directories essential for third-party reimbursement programs. However, due to the voluntary nature of the system, it did not meet the needs of the FDA for a complete inventory of all commercially distributed drug products.

The **Federal Food, Drug, and Cosmetic Act (FDCA)** was amended by the **Drug Listing Act of 1972** to make submission of information on all commercially marketed drugs mandatory. The Drug Listing Act required all domestic and foreign firms (manufacturers, repackagers, and labelers) to list with the FDA prescription drug products manufactured, prepared, propagated, compounded, or processed for commercial distribution in the US. The products are identified and reported using the NDC. The Drug Listing Act also dictated expansion of the NDC system to include human over-the-counter (OTC) drugs and veterinary drugs.

As of June 2009, FDA required drug product listings to be submitted electronically in an XML file format using the Health Level 7 (HL7) standard, **Structured Product Labeling (SPL)**. The drug product listing SPL files are transmitted to the FDA via the Electronic Submissions

Gateway (ESG). With a few exceptions, the NDCs and related data elements in the submitted drug product listing SPL files are published by the FDA in the public *NDC Directory*.

Purpose

The FDA NDC drug product identification system facilitates the following activities:

- FDA's management and official identification of drug products commercially marketed in the US
- Identifying drug products during manufacturing, supply chain distribution, and inventory storage, including track and trace efforts
- Prescribing, dispensing, and administering drugs by healthcare professionals
- Documenting patient's drug treatment in their electronic health record (EHR)
- Identifying unique drug products in patient's and public's search for drug product reference information
- Identifying drug products for coverage, billing, payment, and reimbursement by the Centers for Medicare and Medicaid Services (CMS), insurance companies, and other stakeholders
- Enforcing safety of imported drug products by US Customs and Border Protection
- Conducting drug product pharmacovigilance, reporting adverse events, and processing recalls

Content

The NDC identifier is composed of 10 digits divided into three ordered segments: labeler code, product code, and package code. Each numerical segment is separated by a hyphen. Though the overall NDC length is 10 digits, three allowable NDC formats are specified by the FDA that allocate a different number of digits to each segment. The three NDC formats are defined as 4-4-2, 5-4-1, and 5-3-2 (see table 4.1). The FDA allows only one selected product/package format be

TABLE 4.1. NDC format

NDC Format	Labeler Code	Product Code	Package Code	Example NDC
4-4-2	4	4	2	1234-5678-90
5-3-2	5	3	2	12345-678-90
5-4-1	5	4	1	12345-6789-0

Source: FDA 2017.

used for a particular labeler code; for example, if a 5-digit labeler elects to use 5-4-1, the format cannot be switched to 5-3-2.

NDC Labeler Code

The **labeler code**, the first segment of the NDC, is four or five digits and associated to one particular labeler. A **labeler** is any firm that manufactures, repacks, or distributes a drug product. Domestic and foreign firms marketing drug products in the US must obtain a labeler code from the FDA. The FDA assigns a labeler code to each labeler (see table 4.2). For labeler codes 0001 through 9999, the labeler code is four digits; for labeler codes 10000 through 99999, the labeler code is five digits. If a labeler needs additional NDC numbers, the labeler may request additional labeler codes. A labeler may also have multiple labeler codes as the result of mergers and acquisitions.

NDC Product Code

The **product code**, the second segment of the NDC, is three or four digits and identifies a unique product. The product code is assigned by the labeler and identifies a specific strength, dosage form, and formulation of a drug for a particular firm (see table 4.3). Thus, when there are different formulations or different strengths of the same formulation or when drug products share the same formulation but have different product characteristics that differentiate one drug product version from another, a different product code is assigned (FDA 2017).

TABLE 4.2. Examples of NDC labeler codes

Labeler Code	Firm Name
0069	PFIZER LABORATORIES DIV PFIZER INC
0078	NOVARTIS PHARMACEUTICALS CORPORATION
0140	ROCHE LABORATORIES INC.
16837	JOHNSON & JOHNSON CONSUMER INC., MCNEIL CONSUMER HEALTHCARE DIVISION
50580	JOHNSON & JOHNSON CONSUMER INC., MCNEIL CONSUMER HEALTHCARE DIVISION
55513	AMGEN INC.
60793	PFIZER LABORATORIES DIV PFIZER INC
68546	TEVA NEUROSCIENCE INC

Source: FDA 2019.

TABLE 4.3. Examples of NDC labeler and product codes

Labeler Code	Product Code	Firm Name	Brand Name	Strength	Dosage Form	Product Characteristics
50580	730	JOHNSON & JOHNSON, MCNEIL DIVISION	CHILDENS ZYRTEC	5 mg/5 mL	SYRUP	~~~
50580	779	JOHNSON & JOHNSON, MCNEIL DIVISION	ZYRTEC	10 mg/1	CAPSULE	14 mm, Oval, ...
50580	782	JOHNSON & JOHNSON, MCNEIL DIVISION	CHILDENS ZYRTEC ALLERGY	10 mg/1	TABLET, Orally Disintegrating	11 mm, Round, ...
50580	726	JOHNSON & JOHNSON, MCNEIL DIVISION	ZYRTEC ALLERGY	10 mg/1	TABLET, Film Coated	9 mm, Rectangle, ...

Source: FDA 2019; NLM n.d.

NDC Package Code

The **package code**, the third segment of the NDC, is one or two digits and identifies a particular package size and type. The package code is also assigned by the labeler (see table 4.4). The labeler will assign a different package code to differentiate between different quantitative and qualitative attributes of the product packaging (FDA 2017).

NDC Allocation

A new NDC product code must be created if any of the following characteristics change:

- The drug's established name or proprietary name (brand name)
- Any active pharmaceutical ingredient
- The strength of any active pharmaceutical ingredient
- The dosage form
- The drug's status, between prescription and nonprescription, or for animal drugs, between prescription, nonprescription, or veterinary feed directive (VFD) status
- The drug's intended use between human and animal
- The drug's distinguishing characteristics such as size, shape, color, code imprint, flavor, and scoring (if any)

When there is a change only to the package size or type, a new NDC package code must be created and the same product code should be retained unless all available package codes have already been assigned.

TABLE 4.4. Examples of NDC labeler, product, and package codes

Labeler Code	Product Code	Package Code	Firm Name	Brand Name	Strength	Dosage Form	Packsize	Packtype
50580	726	03	JOHNSON & JOHNSON, MCNEIL DIVISION	ZYRTEC ALLERGY	10 mg/1	TABLET, Film Coated	50	BLISTER PACK
50580	726	32	JOHNSON & JOHNSON, MCNEIL DIVISION	ZYRTEC ALLERGY	10 mg/1	TABLET, Film Coated	14	BLISTER PACK
50580	726	38	JOHNSON & JOHNSON, MCNEIL DIVISION	ZYRTEC ALLERGY	10 mg/1	TABLET, Film Coated	45	BOTTLE
50580	726	50	JOHNSON & JOHNSON, MCNEIL DIVISION	ZYRTEC ALLERGY	10 mg/1	TABLET, Film Coated	50	BOTTLE

Source: FDA 2017.

If marketing is resumed for a discontinued drug and no changes have been made to the drug that would require a new NDC, the drug must have the same NDC that was assigned to it before marketing was discontinued.

A particular NDC must not be reused for a drug product that has different characteristics. The NDC must remain associated to a single drug product indefinitely. The NDC uniqueness was instituted with the FDA regulation published in the Federal Register (FDA 2016, 60187). Prior to this regulation, the NDC product code could be reused for a different drug product five years after the expiration date of the discontinued product, or, if there was no expiration date, five years after the last shipment of the discontinued product into commercial distribution. This now obsolete reuse option was exercised by various drug manufacturers in the past and resulted in confusion in historical drug records.

Future Six-Digit NDC Labeler Code

The FDA estimates the labeler code segment in the current 10-digit NDC numbering scheme will be fully allocated between years 2028 and 2032. Knowing that any change to the current NDC formats will cause major effects inside the government and across a great number of industry

TABLE 4.5. Possible future NDC formats

NDC Format	Labeler Code	Product Code	Package Code	Example NDC
6-3-2 (11-digit)	6	3	2	123456-789-01
6-4-1 (11-digit)	6	4	1	123456-7890-1
6-4-2 (12-digit)	6	4	2	123456-7890-12

Source: FDA 2018.

stakeholders, the FDA is starting to investigate possible approaches to continue provisioning NDC labeler codes in the future. Current regulations allow labeler codes to consist of 4, 5, or 6 digits. Though not currently moving forward with any particular strategy, FDA stated that when it runs out of 5-digit labeler codes, it will begin assigning 6-digit labeler codes (FDA 2016, 60170). This regulatory framework allows the FDA to create 11-digit NDC numbers based on a 6-digit labeler code. The possible 11-digit NDC formats are defined as 6-3-2 and 6-4-1 (FDA 2016, 60216). The future, FDA-considered 11-digit NDC format has major issues that need to be resolved as it allows 11-digit NDC numbers to overlap with Health Insurance Portability and Accountability Act (HIPAA) standard 11-digit NDC numbers that are currently used in government and throughout the healthcare industry. Although various approaches are still under evaluation, the FDA is also considering a new, uniform 12-digit NDC with a 6-4-2 format. See table 4.5 for examples of the possible future 11-digit and 12-digit NDC formats.

The conversion of the current 10-digit NDC to a HIPAA standard 11-digit NDC number and its use throughout government and industry is discussed later in this chapter.

NDC Directory

FDA's *National Drug Code (NDC) Directory* is a public repository of NDC numbers and related drug product information populated by domestic and foreign drug labelers that are required to list drugs manufactured, prepared, propagated, compounded, or processed for commercial distribution in the US.

The *NDC Directory* is owned by the FDA and distributed by the Department of Health and Human Services (HHS). The Center for Drug Evaluation and Research within the FDA oversees the *NDC Directory*. It is important to note that the listing of a firm or product in the *NDC Directory* does *not* equate to FDA approval, imply the product is a "drug" as defined by federal law, or mean the product is eligible for reimbursement (FDA 2017).

Having a comprehensive list of drug products supports a variety of compliance activities and health initiatives at the FDA and other federal agencies. The National Drug Code system is utilized extensively for billing and reimbursement purposes, but it also plays a significant role in protecting public health. The FDA relies on registration and listing information for administering key programs. Uses of the *NDC Directory* include verifying drug imports, monitoring adverse drug events, managing drug recalls, monitoring drug shortages and availability, and evaluating the drug impacts of natural disasters or terrorist threats. The *NDC Directory* is also used to determine whether products are being marketed without an approved application, identify the ingredients of marketed drugs, and as a resource for the inspection of drug facilities (OIG 2006).

NDC Directory Content

The *NDC Directory* includes the following drug types:

- Finished Drugs (in final dosage forms):

  - Human Prescription
  - Human OTC
  - Plasma Derivative
  - Cellular Therapy
  - Standardized Allergenic
  - Non-standardized Allergenic
  - Vaccine

- Unfinished Drugs

  - Active Pharmaceutical Ingredients
  - Drugs for Further Processing
  - Bulk for Human and Animal Drug Compounding.

The *NDC Directory* does NOT include the following drug types:

- Approved Drug Product Manufactured Under Contract
- OTC Monograph Drug Product Manufactured Under Contract
- Unapproved Drug Product Manufactured Under Contract
- Animal Drugs
- Blood Products

The current generation of the *NDC Directory* only includes data from electronic submissions of drug product listing SPL files dating back to June 2009. No paper-based drug listing records were migrated into the electronic-based *NDC Directory*. Currently the *NDC Directory* contains over 120,000 drug products and is updated each weekday. Roughly two dozen drug product data elements are included for each listed product. The data elements include the NDC, the labeler company, the proprietary name, dosage form, active ingredient(s), strength and unit, FDA-approved application number, and others.

All data element values published in the *NDC Directory* website are supplied by the labeler's submission of drug product listing SPL files with a few exceptions. Some submitted codes are translated by the FDA to common names, and a few database system fields are created by the FDA. The exemptions are so noted in the list below.

NDC Directory Product Data Elements

The following drug product data elements, with some noted exceptions, are published by the FDA on the *NDC Directory* website. All the drug product data elements listed in table 4.6 are included in a downloadable NDC Product file. Access to the *NDC Directory* website and the downloadable NDC Product file is explained later in this chapter.

TABLE 4.6. Drug product data elements

Data Element	Description
ProductID	A concatenation of Product NDC data element and the document ID value in the submitted drug product listing SPL file. It is created by the FDA system and used as a key field to link records in the NDC Product file and the NDC Package file. It is included only in the NDC Product and NDC Package download files and has no regulatory significance.
Product NDC	Includes the labeler and product code segments of the NDC (repeated in both the NDC Product and NDC Package download files).
Product Type Name	Describes the type of product, such as human prescription drug, and corresponds to the "Document Type" value in the submitted drug product listing SPL file.
Proprietary Name	Also called the **product trade name**, it is the name of the product as chosen by the labeler and submitted in the product listing. Symbols indicating trademarked or registered products were omitted because of computer input capabilities. These deletions are not intended in any way to deprive the labeler of the protection afforded under patent, trademark, registration, or copyright laws or regulations.
Proprietary Name Suffix	Needed to indicate the complete name of the product, often indicates specific characteristics of a product such as extended release (XR). Name suffix is only in the NDC Product download file.
Non-Proprietary Name	Often referred to as the generic name, the nonproprietary name is usually the active ingredient(s) of the product.
Dosage Form Name	Translated by FDA from the Dosage Form Code submitted by the labeler. For example, C42955 translates to lozenge.
Route Name	Translated by FDA from the Route Code submitted by the labeler. For example, C38288 translates to oral.

(continued)

TABLE 4.6. Continued

Data Element	Description
Start/End Marketing Dates	The start date indicates when product marketing started. The end date indicates when the product will no longer be on the market (typically the expiration date of the last lot).
Marketing Category Name	The marketing category is either New Drug Application (NDA), Abbreviated New Drug Application (ANDA), Biological License Application (BLA), OTC Monograph, or another category.
Application Number	Actual NDA, ANDA, or BLA number or Monograph CFR Citation number, or null for unapproved drugs.
Labeler Name	Translated by FDA from labeler code segment in the Product NDC value.
Substance Name (Active Ingredient)	The active ingredient preferred term(s) is translated by FDA from the Unique Ingredient Identifier (UNII) code(s) submitted by the labeler.
Pharm Class	The pharmacological class is the category corresponding to the Substance Name.
DEA Schedule	U.S. Drug Enforcement Administration (DEA) assigned classification number used to grade drugs considered to be controlled substances. The controlled substance schedule values are CI, CII, CIII, CIV, and CV with CI the highest potential of abuse and CV the lowest potential of abuse.
NDC Exclude Flag	The NDC exclude flag, "Y" or "N," is created by the FDA system and indicates if the product has been excluded from the *NDC Directory* due to deficiencies or noncompliance.
Listing Record Certified Through	Created by the FDA system based on recent drug product listing and certification submissions and indicates when the listing record will expire if not updated or certified.

NOTE: Some of the above drug product data elements, that is, Proprietary Name, Proprietary Name Suffix, Route Name, Application Number, Pharm Class, and NDC Exclude Flag, are not included in the data records for *unfinished* drug types.

NDC Directory Package Data Elements

The following drug package data elements, with some noted exceptions, are published by the FDA on the *NDC Directory* website. All the drug package data elements listed below are included in a downloadable NDC Package file. Access to the *NDC Directory* website and the downloadable NDC Package file is explained later in this chapter. In addition to the elements below, ProductID, product NDC, start and end marketing dates, and NDC exclude flag, as described earlier in this chapter, are included.

NDC Package Code

The NDC package code includes the labeler code, product code, and package code segments of the NDC.

Package Description

The package description includes the packaging size and type; it includes multiple levels if they were submitted by the labeler.

Sample Package

The sample package flag, "Y" or "N," indicates if the product package is a sample.

NOTE: Some of the above drug package data elements, that is, Start and End Marketing Dates, NDC Exclude Flag, and Sample Package, are not included in the data records for *unfinished* drug types.

Principles and Guidelines

NDC presentation on a drug label is assigned based on a number of different factors. While the inclusion of the NDC number is merely best practice, other features, such as NDC bar code and product identifier are required.

NDC Number on a Drug Label

"The NDC number is requested but not required to appear on all drug labels and in all drug labeling, including the label of any prescription drug container furnished to a consumer" (21 CFR 201.2). Though not an FDA requirement, industry has generally adopted the "good practice" of placing NDC numbers on drug product labels and labeling.

Example:

"NDC 50580-726-03"

NDC Bar Code on a Drug Label

FDA regulations require the NDC to appear in a linear bar code on the label of a human prescription drug product (21 CFR 201.25(c)). In 2004, the FDA issued a Final Rule requiring that certain human prescription drug and biological products have on their labels a linear bar code that contains, at a minimum, the NDC number (FDA 2004). Those impacted by the rule include manufacturers, repackers, relabelers, and private label distributors of human prescription drug products, biological products, and over-the-counter (OTC) drug products that are dispensed by way of an order and are commonly used in hospitals (FDA 2011).

The NDC is commonly represented using the Universal Product Code (UPC) standard managed by GS1, a standards developing organization. The UPC version that embeds the NDC consists of three components and is 12 digits long without any hyphens (see tables 4.7 and 4.8 and figure 4.1).

- UPC Company Prefix comprised of:

    - UPC Prefix – number "3" (used by default for embedding NDC in UPC)
    - NDC labeler code

- Item Reference comprised of:

    - NDC product code
    - NDC package code

- Check Digit – single digit calculated from previous 11 digits

TABLE 4.7. Example UPC embedding NDC

UPC Prefix	NDC Number (labeler, product, package codes)	Check Digit	UPC
1 Digit	10 Digits	1 Digit	12 Digits Total
3	5058072603	7	350580726037

Source: GS1 2019.

TABLE 4.8. Components of product identifier bar code (GS1 standard)

Component	Application Identifier	Value	Comment
NDC Number (GTIN-14 format)	(01)	00312345678906	Pkg Digit [0] + GS1 Prefix for NDC [03] + NDC [1234567890] + Chk Digit [6]
Serial Number	(21)	SN345678	Up to 20 alphanumeric characters
Lot Number	(10)	LN145	
Expiration Date	(17)	20181127	

Source: GS1 2019.

FIGURE 4.1. NDC embedded in UPC-A linear bar code

3   50580   72603   7

Source: © Gary Saner/Reed Technology and Information Services Inc.

Product Identifier on a Drug Label

Starting November 27, 2018, the Drug Supply Chain Security Act (DSCSA) requires human prescription drugs in finished dosage form to include a Product Identifier on the drug package. The Product Identifier includes:

- Standardized Numerical Identifier (SNI) comprised of:
  - NDC Number – labeler, product, and package codes; 10 digits
  - Serial Number – unique identifier up to 20 alphanumeric characters
- Lot Number
- Expiration Date – FDA recommended formats are YYYY-MM-DD (numerical month) or YYYY-MMM-DD (alpha month) or if there are space limitations, the format can be YYYY-MM (numerical month) or YYYY-MMM (alpha month); use a hyphen or space between segments

The Product Identifier must be presented in both human- and machine-readable formats on each package and homogenous case of product. An example of a human readable product identifier is shown in figure 4.2.

The machine-readable format must be a two-dimensional (2D) data matrix bar code on a package and a linear or 2D data matrix bar code on a homogenous case of product (DSCSA 2013). This serialization Product Identifier is in addition to any other prevailing bar code requirements. Figure 4.3 is an example of a 2D data matrix bar code.

The full Product ID bar code text is a concatenation of the components. An example using the above values is shown in figure 4.4.

FIGURE 4.2. Example product identifier—human readable

NDC: 1234567890
SERIAL: SN345678
LOT: LN145
EXP: 2018-11-27

Source: © Gary Saner/Reed Technology and Information Services Inc.

FIGURE 4.3. Example product identifier—2D data matrix bar code

(01) 00312345678906
(21) SN345678
(10) LN145
(17) 20181127

Source: © Gary Saner/Reed Technology and Information Services Inc.

FIGURE 4.4. Example product identifier—linear bar code

(01)00312345678906(21)SN345678(10)LN145(17)20181127

Source: © Gary Saner/Reed Technology and Information Services Inc.

NDC Number on a Non-drug Label

FDA regulations prohibit placing an NDC number on a non-drug product, that is, a product not subject to 21 CFR Parts 207, 607, or 1271, such as dietary supplements and medical devices. Such placement is considered misbranding and subject to FDA enforcement and penalties (21 CFR 207.37(a)(3)). A few medical devices have been assigned NDC numbers in the past, but the FDA is now exclusively using the Unique Device Identifier (UDI) standard for devices and has conversion dates in place to discontinue the use of NDCs.

HIPAA NDC and NDC11 Format

Triggered by HIPAA legislation, HHS published a regulation in August 2000 that established NDC numbers as the standard medical data code set for reporting drugs and biologics and adopted a uniform 11-digit format of the FDA 10-digit NDC number. The uniform 11-digit format was in turn adopted by the CMS, other government agencies, and the healthcare industry in general including prescribers, dispensers, providers, and payers. Referred to as the HIPAA NDC or NDC11, the 11-digit NDC format is the default format used by pharmacies, hospitals, clinics, CMS, insurance companies, electronic health records (EHR), and other healthcare stakeholders with some exceptions.

The NDC11 is created from a 10-digit NDC number by adding a leading zero to one of the three NDC segments to generate a 5-4-2 format NDC and removing the hyphens (see table 4.9).

Once the hyphens are removed from the NDC11, the NDC11 value cannot always be converted back to the 10-digit NDC.

- If the NDC11 starts with "0" then the starting "0" is the leading "0" added in the conversion because the FDA does not assign any 5-digit labeler codes starting with "0." In this case, the original NDC format was 4-4-2 and the original NDC number can be recreated.
  Example: 02345078901 (NDC11) is 2345-0789-01 (NDC)
- If the NDC11 has only one "0" in position 6 or position 10, then the single "0" is the leading "0" added in the conversion. In this case, the original NDC format can be determined and the original NDC number can be recreated.
  Example: 12345078911 (NDC11) is 12345-789-11 (NDC)
  Example: 12345678901 (NDC11) is 12345-6789-1 (NDC)
- If the NDC11 has a "0" in BOTH position 6 AND position 10, the original NDC format could either be 5-3-2 or 5-4-1. The original NDC cannot be recreated without knowing the history or checking other drug data, for example, the firm's NDC configuration.
  Example: 12345078901 (NDC11) could be 12345-789-01 or 12345-0789-1 (NDC)

TABLE 4.9. Examples of NDC11 conversion from FDA 10-digit NDC

NDC Format	NDC11 Change (add "0")	NDC11 Format	NDC Example	NDC11 Example
4-4-2	**0**xxxx-xxxx-xx	5-4-2	0069-2960-30	00069296030
5-3-2	xxxxx-**0**xxx-xx	5-4-2	50580-726-03	50580072603
5-4-1	xxxxx-xxxx-**0**x	5-4-2	10888-7135-2	10888713502

Source: © Gary Saner/Reed Technology and Information Services Inc.

Process for Revision and Updates

For all FDA submissions discussed in this section, labelers use the electronic HL7 SPL XML file standard transmitted to the FDA via the ESG. FDA's electronic drug registration and listing website and FDA's SPL resources website provide labelers with guidance and instructions on registering and submitting.

Initial NDC Listings

If a firm (labeler) does not have an FDA assigned NDC labeler code or if the assignment was previously done in paper form, then the firm must first submit an NDC Labeler Code Request SPL file to the FDA to receive a labeler code from the FDA's electronic system. The labeler must then allocate product codes and package codes to drug products to create full NDC numbers. If desired, a labeler may submit an NDC number (labeler code and product code segments) via an NDC Reservation SPL file to reserve the number for two years. The initial drug product listing must be submitted in a listing SPL file within three calendar days after the corresponding initial establishment (facility) registration is submitted.

The Food and Drug Administration Safety and Innovation Act (FDASIA), signed into law on July 9, 2012, requires drug firms to submit ongoing annual establishment registrations in the period from October 1 to December 31 of each calendar year (FDA 2013). At the time of annual establishment registration, firms must also list any drugs not previously listed.

Updated NDC Listings

Firms marketing products in the US are required to review and update as necessary their FDA drug listing information twice yearly in June and December. The FDA recommends firms submit drug listing updates at the time of the actual change to keep the information current. The FDA updates the *NDC Directory* daily (weekdays) based on the electronic drug product listing SPL files submitted by the firm to the FDA.

In the event no listing SPL file was submitted, and no listing changes occurred during a calendar year, the labeler must submit a No Change Certification SPL file during October through December period to confirm the active drug listing is accurate and current. Those drug products that should be certified but are not certified by the labeler are flagged as "Uncertified" in the *NDC Directory* and the corresponding drug product details are removed from the published content as of January the following year. A drug product must then be relisted to have the "Uncertified" flag removed and the product data elements displayed.

Relationship with Other Terminologies, Classification Systems, and Code Sets

NDCs have relationships with a variety of related healthcare industry standards including CPT and HCPCS, RxNorm, LOINC, and SNOMED CT.

CPT and HCPCS Level II

The Healthcare Common Procedure Coding System (HCPCS) is used by CMS and private health insurance programs to identify healthcare items and services. HCPCS Level I refers to the Current Procedural Terminology (CPT) numeric code system, copyrighted by the American Medical Association (AMA), which includes medical, surgical, and diagnostic services (see chapter 2). HCPCS Level II codes correspond to services, drugs, procedures, and equipment not covered by Level I CPT codes (see chapter 3).

CMS maintains the HCPCS Level II codes and has assigned some drug NDC numbers to HCPCS Level II codes. As of 2007, the NDC, in combination with the HCPCS code, is required for processing manufacturer drug rebates for physician-administered drugs (CMS 2007). Manufacturers submit average sales price (ASP) data at the 11-digit National Drug Code (NDC) level. Providers mostly use HCPCS codes to bill Medicare for drugs and biologicals. CMS publishes an ASP crosswalk from NDC to HCPCS in the form of an Excel file and updates it quarterly.

RxNorm

The National Library of Medicine (NLM) creates and manages RxNorm, a controlled terminology of US drug products (see chapter 8). The systematic, normalized drug names and unique identifiers established by RxNorm facilitate the precise exchange of drug data across healthcare systems. RxNorm includes branded, generic, prescription, and OTC drug information extracted from drug product listing SPL files loaded into the NLM DailyMed website. RxNorm uses over a dozen terminology sources to build terminology groups, each of which is assigned an RxNorm Concept Unique Identifier (RXCUI). The concepts have multiple attributes, one of which is the NDC number in 11-digit HIPAA format.

LOINC

The Regenstrief Institute manages the Logical Observation Identifiers Names and Codes (LOINC) standard (see chapter 10). LOINC codes are used to identify drug product listing SPL document types and internal section headings in the SPL document. These LOINC codes are embedded in the XML coding and are processed by computer systems; the LOINC codes are not visible to the typical user.

SNOMED CT

SNOMED International owns and manages SNOMED CT (see chapter 6). The use of SNOMED CT codes to describe the patient's medical condition was part of an industry pilot for drug indexing using SPL in 2007 and 2008. The industry pilot was closed in June 2008 with the FDA's decision to index drug SPLs themselves in a phased approach starting with pharmacologic class. The FDA currently indexes pharmacologic class and some other drug attributes, but there is no visible FDA activity to index the medical condition in SPL using SNOMED CT codes.

Tools to Access and Use

The FDA offers the *NDC Directory* information to the public via a web portal, downloadable file packages for finished and unfinished drugs, and a mobile app. In addition to the *NDC Directory*, the NDC is referenced and associated to numerous other drug-related repositories and standards.

NDC Directory Access Tools

NDC numbers and related drug product information in the *NDC Directory* are provided freely to the public and can be accessed in three different venues: their website, downloadable files, and a mobile application.

FIGURE 4.5. NDC directory search

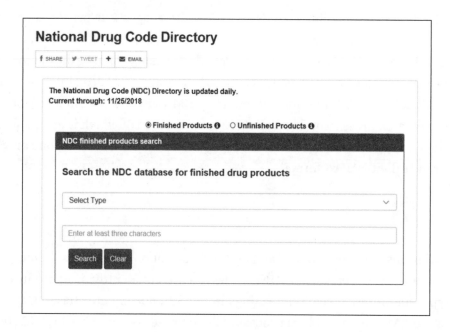

Source: FDA 2019.

- *NDC Directory* Online Website: Information is accessed via an FDA-hosted online portal. The home page provides search functionality based upon: Finished/ Unfinished Products, Proprietary Name, Nonproprietary Name (active ingredient), Application Number, NDC Code, or Labeler (see figure 4.5). Search results are displayed in a tabular format (see figure 4.6).
- *NDC Directory* Data Download: The finished drugs in the *NDC Directory* are available in a downloadable ZIP data file from the FDA *NDC Directory* website in both a spreadsheet XLS and tab-delimited TXT version. Each download ZIP file includes two data files as a paired set, an NDC Product file and an NDC Package file. Most *NDC Directory* data elements are in the product file with a few data elements relative to the package stored in the package file. One row in the product file may correspond to multiple rows in the package file. The file records are linked by a common ProductID field. For more *NDC Directory* data file information, including

FIGURE 4.6. NDC directory search results

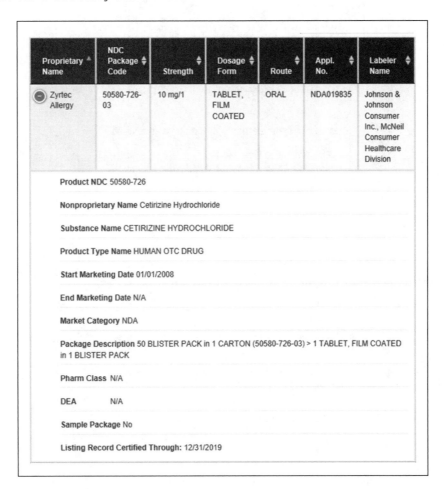

Source: FDA 2019.

file names and descriptions, visit the FDA's National Drug Code Directory website. Figure 4.7 displays the NDC Directory download files for finished drugs.

The unfinished drugs in the NDC Directory are available in a separate, single downloadable ZIP data file from the FDA *NDC Directory* website (see figure 4.8). The downloaded ZIP file contains similar NDC Product and NDC Package files as discussed above in both spreadsheet XLS and tab-delimited TXT versions. The unfinished drug records have an abbreviated list of data elements as compared to the finished drug type records.

- *NDC Express* Mobile App: The *NDC Directory* is offered by the FDA as a free, downloadable mobile application (see figure 4.9).

FIGURE 4.7. NDC Directory download files (finished drugs)

NDC Directory

- NDC Database File - Text Version (Zip Format)
  Last updated:11/23/2018

- NDC Database File - Excel Version (Zip Format)
  Last updated:11/23/2018

- NDC Product File Definitions
  Product File Data Elements, Definitions, and Notes

- NDC Package File Definitions
  Package File Data Elements, Definitions, and Notes

Source: FDA 2017.

FIGURE 4.8. NDC Directory download file (unfinished drugs)

Data Files for Unfinished Drugs

- NDC Unfinished Drugs Database File (Zip Format)
  Last updated:11/23/2018

Source: FDA 2017.

FIGURE 4.9. NDC Express mobile app

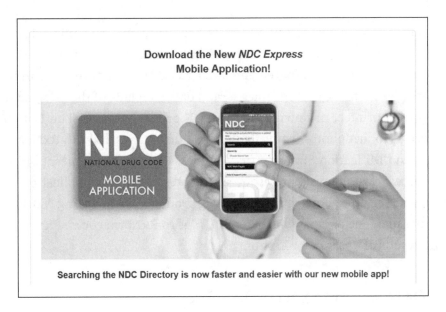

Source: FDA 2017.

NDC Labeler Code List

The FDA provides a downloadable file in XLS format containing FDA-assigned NDC labeler codes and corresponding firm names. The file contains over 10,800 labeler codes. For more information, go to the FDA "Structured Product Labeling Resource" webpage and search for "NDC/NHRIC Labeler Codes."

Drugs@FDA

The FDA provides an online database, Drugs@FDA, searchable by Drug Name, Active Ingredient, or Application Number. Drug product NDCs are typically found in the "How Supplied" section of the label document.

FDA Online Label Repository

The FDA provides an online database of submitted drug product listing SPL files. These files (labels) are used to populate the data elements in the *NDC Directory* and the NSDE file discussed later in this chapter. Basic searches can be performed by NDC Number, Proprietary Name, Active Ingredient, Application Number or Regulatory Citation, Company Name, or Proprietary Name.

NLM DailyMed

The National Library of Medicine (NLM) hosts the DailyMed, an online database of drug product listing SPL files. Users can search over 100,000 drug product listing SPL files by NDC Number, Proprietary Name, Active Ingredient, and Drug Class; an advanced search is also available. All the narrative sections, package images, and data elements of the selected drug product label can be viewed, printed, or downloaded in PDF or XML format. The DailyMed website also provides drug product photos (as available), bulk downloads, links to RxNorm codes, drug Risk Evaluation and Mitigation Strategy (REMS) files, FDA Indexing files, pill identifier tool, and other resources. Two noteworthy resources include 1) multiple application programming interface (API) web services allowing access to drug product data including NDCs and 2) downloadable mapping files, one of which links the SPL files to RxNorm codes. Figure 4.10 shows an example of the results of a search for Lipitor.

NDC SPL Data Elements (NSDE) File

The FDA provides a downloadable XLS format file named NDC SPL Data Elements (NSDE). This file contains some data elements from the submitted drug product listing SPL file and includes the associated NDC11 and Billing Units data elements. The NSDE file is used by CMS in the evaluation to approve or reject prescription drug event (PDE) submissions. The data elements included in the NSDE file are identified below.

FIGURE 4.10. NLM DailyMed

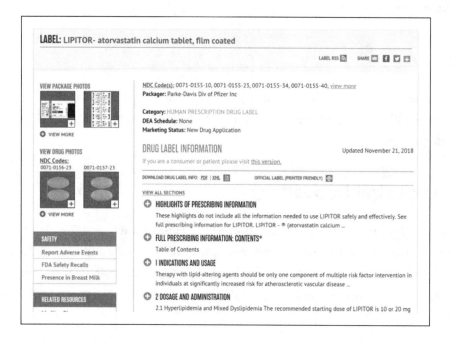

Source: NLM n.d.

- Item Code

  NDC, National Health Related Item Code (NHRIC), or International Society of Blood Transfusion (ISBT) facility and product description code
- Proprietary Name, Dosage Form, Marketing Category, Application Number or CFR citation, Product Type, Marketing Start/End Date
- NDC11

  The NDC11 is a transformed version of the segmented NDC code using the algorithm defined by the National Council for Prescription Drug Programs (NCPDP). Three-segment NHRIC codes have also been transformed following the same algorithm. Two-segment NHRIC and ISBT codes have not been transformed.
- Billing Unit

  The NCPDP developed the Billing Unit Standard to assist in consistent and accurate billing of pharmaceutical products. This data element may contain an NCPDP Billing Unit (gram [GM], milliliter [ML] or each [EA]).

OpenFDA

Since 2014, the FDA has provided a growing list of FDA drug and medical device datasets through APIs. These links provide an on-demand software interface to search and retrieve data from FDA repositories without having to download and update the full database. The FDA has provided API access to the following high-value, structured data repositories:

- Drug Product Labeling (listing SPL files)
- Drug NDC SPL Data Elements (NSDE)
- Drug Adverse Events
- Drug Recall Enforcement Reports
- Medical Device and Food datasets

Animal Drug Product Directory

The FDA offers an independent, downloadable Animal Drug Product Directory organized by NDC number. The repository includes the following data elements from over 9,000 animal drug product listing SPL files submitted since June 2009:

- NDC Number
- Proprietary Name (Trade Name)
- Non-Proprietary Name (Established Name)

- Ingredient List
- Labeler Name
- Product Type
- Marketing Category
- Application Number or Citation
- Link to Animal Drug Product Listing SPL File

Adoption and Use Cases

Drug product regulatory data is distributed from the manufacturer out to a broad landscape of downstream data consumers. Regulatory data flows from the manufacturer, through regulator publication, data aggregators, healthcare providers, and to end users (see figure 4.11). Included in this dataset is the NDC, which accurately identifies the drug product throughout this pathway for both clinical administration and financial activities. With the progression of more content, more structured data, and better technology and systems, the healthcare industry is benefiting from a higher level of quality, increased speed of information, easier and expanded access, and improved data portability, all of which improve the patient's experience and safety.

FIGURE 4.11. Drug product regulatory data flow

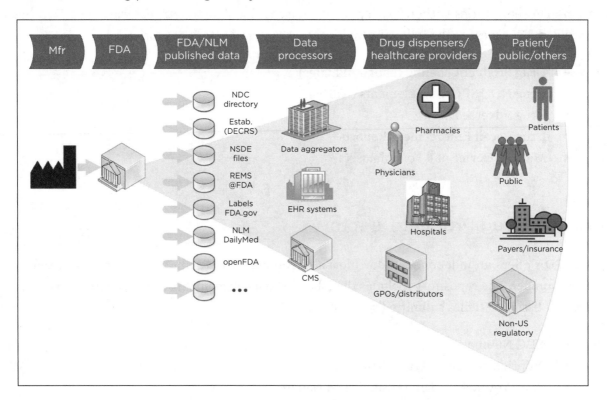

Source: © Gary Saner/Reed Technology and Information Services Inc.

Healthcare Industry Data Flow

Precise product information and advanced technologies are fundamental in automating the processing and exchange of product information. Table 4.10 highlights some of the points where technology facilitates drug product data management.

The NDC identifier on drug products and packages along with increased implementation of Automatic Identification and Data Capture (AIDC) tools enable the technologies highlighted earlier. Sophisticated data aggregation provides a better platform for enhanced support systems and EHR tools. For example, a bar code scan of a drug container at an out-of-state pharmacy while on vacation can quickly and accurately enter data into a support system to:

- Verify the delivered drug product correctly matches the prescribed drug product
- Check for any contraindications with current patient medications
- Alert for any patient allergies
- Check the prescription expiration date
- Check for insurance coverage or CMS reimbursement
- Trigger the billing process and update the inventory
- Record the transaction in the patient's EHR, and so on

The following adoption and use cases illustrate various places where industry has implemented NDC and related drug product data.

TABLE 4.10. Drug product data management

Stakeholders	Responsibilities	Enabling Technology
Manufacturers	Material management and control	Bar codes, readers, robotic handling, vision systems
Distributors	Supply chain logistics	Bar codes, readers, trackers, GPS, environmental sensors
Prescribers	Evaluation, diagnosis	Clinical decision support tools assist indication, contraindication, etc. EHR with current meds with alert, patient allergy alert, patient treatment records
Dispensers	Fulfilment of prescriptions and orders	Inventory systems to pull, verify, record, bill
Providers	Administration	Clinical management systems to ensure accurate, timely, and safe treatment; bill
Payers	Coverage, payments, rebates, reimbursements	Data capture and processing systems for accurate id, quantity, pricing, etc.
Safety	Pharmacovigilance	Data mining, artificial intelligence, analysis

Source: © Gary Saner/Reed Technology and Information Services Inc.

CMS Claims Form CMS-1500

Noridian publishes an official NDC/HCPCS crosswalk. This crosswalk lists the HCPCS Level II codes that have an NDC assigned to them, along with billing unit information. It is updated monthly. As expected, HCPCS codes may be listed more than once, since usually there is not a one-to-one link between an NDC code and a HCPCS Level II code. NDC codes are more specific in that they identify the labeler, product, and package. HCPCS Level II J codes generally identify the drug and dosage. For example, HCPCS code J0290 is listed 53 times in the November 2018 release of the crosswalk. Figure 4.12 is an example from the crosswalk.

CMS New Drug Claims

Section 621(a) of the Medicare Prescription Drug, Improvement, and Modernization Act (MMA) of 2003 included a provision for payment of new drugs or biologicals that are approved by the FDA on or after January 1, 2004, for which a product-specific HCPCS code has not been assigned. The provision further stipulates that the drug or biological be furnished as part of covered outpatient department service under the hospital outpatient prospective payment system. HCPCS code C9399, unclassified drugs or biological, is reported along with the NDC, quantity of the drug that was administered, and the date the drug was provided to the beneficiary (CMS 2009).

CMS Part D Data

NDC numbers are included in the part D data, which is collected by CMS from transactions between pharmacies and Medicare part D sponsors (HHS 2008).

FIGURE 4.12. Example NDC—HCPCS crosswalk

NDC	NDC Mod	HCPCS	HCPCS Mod	Relationship Start Date	Relationship End Date	HCPCS Description	NDC Label	No. of Items in NDC Pkg	NDC Package Measure	NDC Package Type	Route of Administration	Billing Units	HCPCS Amount #1	HCPCS Measure #1	CF	Start Date #1	End Date #1
00002-7140-01		J0130		1/1/2002	12/31/2016	INJECTION ABCIXIM	REOPRO (VIAL) 2 MG/ML	5	ML	VL	IV	ML	10	MG	0.2	1/1/2002	12/31/2016
00002-7335-11		J2941		3/1/2006	99/99/9999	INJECTION, SOMATR	HUMATROPE (WITH STER	1	EA	VL	SC	EA	1	MG	5	3/1/2006	99/99/9999
00002-7335-16		J2941		1/1/2002	2/14/2012	INJECTION, SOMATR	HUMATROPE (W/DILUENT	1	EA	VL	SC	EA	1	MG	5	1/1/2002	2/14/2012
00002-7501-01		J9201		1/1/2002	99/99/9999	INJECTION, GEMCIT	GEMZAR (VIAL) 200 MG	1	EA	VL	IV	EA	##	MG	1	1/1/2002	99/99/9999
00002-7502-01		J9201		1/1/2002	99/99/9999	INJECTION, GEMCIT	GEMZAR (VIAL) 1 GM	1	EA	VL	IV	EA	##	MG	5	1/1/2002	99/99/9999
00002-7510-01		J1817		1/1/2003	99/99/9999	INSULIN FOR ADMIN	HUMALOG (VIAL) 100 U/M	10	ML	VL	SC	ML	50	U	2	1/1/2003	99/99/9999
00002-7511-01		J1815		1/1/2003	99/99/9999	INJECTION, INSULIN	HUMALOG MIX 75/25 (VIA	10	ML	VL	SC	ML	5	U	20	1/1/2003	99/99/9999
00002-7512-01		J1815		11/1/2006	99/99/9999	INJECTION, INSULIN	HUMALOG MIX 50/50 50 U	10	ML	VL	SC	ML	5	U	2	11/1/2006	99/99/9999
00002-7516-59		J1815		1/1/2003	99/99/9999	INJECTION, INSULIN	HUMALOG (CARTRIDGE)	3	ML	CT	SC	ML	5	U	20	1/1/2003	99/99/9999

Source: Noridian 2018.

State Medicaid Rebates

The Deficit Reduction Act (DRA) of 2005 requires all state Medicaid agencies to collect rebates from drug manufacturers for covered physician-administered (or physician-provided) drugs. Physician-administered drugs include any outpatient drug that is administered (or provided) to a patient with a reimbursement claim from a provider instead of a pharmacy. According to the DRA, covered drugs are not restricted to injectable drugs, but include any physician-administered drug regardless of the method of administration. The DRA also requires covered drugs be reported with the NDC on the CMS-1500 and UB-04 claim forms as well as on the 837 electronic transactions. Effective January 1, 2007, the types of practice sites required to report NDCs on claims include, but are not limited to, physician offices, clinics, and outpatient hospital departments (CMS 2012). Medicare primary claims will also require NDCs with HCPCS codes.

Drug Transaction Reporting

The NDC system is the HIPAA standard medical data code set for reporting drugs and biologics for retail pharmacy transactions. The HHS Secretary had also adopted this code set as the standard for reporting drugs and biologics for institutional and professional claims. However, the February 2003 Final Rule on Health Insurance Reform: Modifications to Electronic Data Transaction Standards and Code Sets repealed this requirement. The final rule does not identify a standard medical data code set for reporting drugs and biologics in nonretail pharmacy transactions. However, absence of a code set does not preclude the use of NDCs. A health plan could require a provider to use either of the applicable code sets, NDC or HCPCS, permitted by the implementation guides (CMS 2019). In other words, covered entities could continue to report drugs and biologics as they prefer and agree on with their trading partners, using either the NDC or HCPCS code set.

ASC X12 Claims Transaction 5010

The Accredited Standards Committee X12 (ASC X12) defined transactions include the Health Care Claim: Professional (837P), 005010X222A1 and Health Care Claim: Institutional (837I), 005010X223A2, hereinafter referred to as "5010."

With the implementation of ASC X12 Version 5010, the reporting of the NDC changed. The 11-digit NDC (5-4-2 format) must be used and therefore leading zeros should be incorporated as necessary to the labeler, product, or package segment of the NDC. The Workgroup for Electronic Data Interchange (WEDI) has provided guidelines for reporting the NDC quantity. Per their guidance, the quantity reported is based on the NDC description, which provides the unit of measure, and the dosage administration (WEDI 2014). For example, a patient is given an injection in the physician's office of 250 mg Ampicillin sodium, which is reconstituted from a 500 mg vial of powder, which translates into the following:

> HCPCS code J0290, Injection, Ampicillin sodium, 500 mg
> NDC: 00781-9407-78 (strength number/unit for this NDC is 500 mg/1)
> HCPCS unit: 1
> NDC quantity: 0.5
> Unit of measure: UN
> (WEDI 2014)

CDC Immunization Repository

The Centers for Disease Control and Prevention (CDC) track immunizations at the National Center of Immunization and Respiratory Diseases (NCIRD). Immunization data is managed in Immunization Information Systems (IIS) that store individual history and geographical population data. To support the immunization registry and related activities, NCIRD consolidates vaccine information in a database and makes it available via a public portal and as downloadable XLS, PDF, or TXT files. CDC publishes the NDC Crosswalk Table that charts vaccine data elements, Unit of Sale NDC11 (the saleable unit, for example a carton of 5 syringes), and Unit of Use (the container that holds the vaccine, for example a syringe) NDC11 (see figure 4.13).

FIGURE 4.13. CDC Immunization NDC Crosswalk

Sale NDC11	Sale Proprietary Name	Sale Labeler	Start Date ▴	End Date	Sale GTIN	Sale Last Update	Use NDC11	No Use NDC	Use GTIN	Use Last Update	CVX Code	CVX Description	MVX Code
00005-0100-02	Trumenba	Wyeth Pharmaceutical Division of Wyeth Holdings LLC, a subsidiary of Pfizer Inc.	11/5/2014		00300050100027	7/19/2018	00005-0100-01	False	00300050100010	7/3/2018	162	meningococcal B, recombinant	PFR
00005-0100-05	Trumenba	Wyeth Pharmaceutical Division of Wyeth Holdings LLC, a subsidiary of Pfizer Inc.	11/5/2014		00300050100058	7/30/2018	00005-0100-01	False	00300050100010	7/3/2018	162	meningococcal B, recombinant	PFR
00005-0100-10	Trumenba	Wyeth Pharmaceutical Division of Wyeth Holdings LLC, a subsidiary of Pfizer Inc.	11/5/2014		00300050100102	7/13/2018	00005-0100-01	False	00300050100010	7/3/2018	162	meningococcal B, recombinant	PFR
00005-1970-50	Prevnar	Wyeth Pharmaceutical Division of Wyeth Holdings Corporation, a subsidiary of Pfizer Inc.	3/1/2000	12/31/2011		5/30/2018	00005-1970-49	False		5/30/2018	100	pneumococcal conjugate PCV 7	WAL

Use Case One: Meeting Federal Drug Reporting Requirements

To comply with the Drug Listing Act of 1972, Rx, a company that manufactures, markets, and distributes drugs in the US, must register and list all drug products with the FDA. As part of the process, Rx uses their assigned NDC Labeler Code to create the NDC for their drug products. Rx Company electronically submits information on final marketed drugs to the FDA in the Structured Product Labeling (SPL) standard via the Electronic Submission Gateway. The FDA then inputs the NDC and information submitted as part of the listing process into the Drug Registration and Listing System database. To create the National Drug Code Directory, the FDA uses information from the database, including the NDCs. The FDA uses the *NDC Directory* to verify drug imports, monitor adverse drug events, manage drug recalls, and evaluate the drug impacts of natural disasters or terrorist threats. The *NDC Directory* is also used to identify the ingredients of marketed drugs and as a resource for the inspection of drug facilities.

Use Case Two: Billing a Physician-Administered Medication

The DRA requires Medicaid providers to report the 11-digit NDC on the electronic transaction when billing drug items administered in outpatient offices, hospitals, and other clinical settings. Here is an example of a circumstance when an NDC would be billed.

Dr. Med saw an 11-year-old male patient with a cough that started 3 days ago, growing progressively worse. The patient reported that he coughs when walking short distances. Peak flows have been around 200 at home but hard to measure due to coughing. His personal best is 300. He has been using Albuterol MDI with little success. Peak flows at the clinic were 200, 210, 200 with coughing. Pulse Ox was 97. Albuterol 0.5 cc aerosol via nebulizer was given with resulting peak flows of 230, 240, and 220 and repeat nebulizer at 0.5 cc in minutes showed improvement to 250. At the conclusion of the visit, Dr. Med diagnosed the patient with acute asthma exacerbation and sent him home to continue with Albuterol 2 puffs QID. The clinic's biller submits the bill to the state Medicaid agency and includes the ICD code for the acute asthma exacerbation, the CPT codes for the evaluation and management service and nebulizer treatment, and the HCPCS Level II for the Albuterol. The NDC number, 21695-0245-20, corresponding to the Albuterol was also reported on the claim.

CHECK YOUR UNDERSTANDING

1. Product names used in the *NDC Directory* are usually supplied by:

   a. Retail pharmacies

   b. AMA

   c. AHA

   d. Firms (labelers)

2. Labeler codes may be composed of:

   a. 3 digits, 4 digits
   b. 4 digits, 4 digits
   c. 4 digits, 5 digits
   d. 5 digits, 5 digits

3. What organization was responsible for development of the National Drug Codes?

   a. AHA
   b. The Joint Commission
   c. FDA
   d. CMS

4. True or false? The NDC11 format was a result of the Drug Listing Act.

   a. True
   b. False

5. True or false? There is a one-to-one link between an NDC code and a HCPCS Level II code.

   a. True
   b. False

REVIEW

1. The Deficit Reduction Act of 2005 requires physicians submitting claims to State Medicaid agencies to provide which codes for reimbursement of physician-administered drugs?

   a. ICD-10-CM and NDC
   b. ICD-10-CM and NCPDP
   c. HCPCS and NDC
   d. HCPCS, NDC, and RxNorm

2. True or false? A new NDC product code must be created when there is a change only in the package size or type.

   a. True
   b. False

3. The NDC identifier consists of:

   a. Labeler code and product code

   b. Product code and package code

   c. Labeler code, product trade code, and product code

   d. Labeler code, product code, and package code

4. Which NDC format is not found in the *NDC Directory*?

   a. 5-4-1

   b. 5-4-2

   c. 5-3-2

   d. 4-4-2

5. Which NDC component is assigned by the FDA?

   a. Labeler code

   b. Nonproprietary name

   c. Product code

   d. Product trade name

6. What is the correct conversion of NDC code 0069-5420-66 to the 11-digit format?

   a. 0069-5420-066

   b. 0069-05420-66

   c. 69-5420-00066

   d. 00069-5420-66

7. True or false? The FDA uses the *NDC Directory* for verifying drug imports.

   a. True

   b. False

8. True or false? A listing of a product in the FDA's *NDC Directory* means the drug is FDA approved.

   a. True

   b. False

9. How often is the *NDC Directory* updated?

   a. Every day

   b. Every weekday

   c. Every Monday

   d. Every Friday

10. Which NDC components are assigned by the labeler?

    a. Labeler code and product code

    b. Product code and package code

    c. Product code and product trade name

    d. Labeler code and package code

References

21 CFR201.2: Drugs and devices; National Drug Code numbers. 2016 (Aug 31).

21 CFR201.25(c): Drugs and devices; National Drug Code numbers. 2016 (Aug 31).

21 CFR207.37(a)(3): Drugs and devices; National Drug Code numbers. 2016 (Aug 31).

Centers for Medicare and Medicaid Services (CMS). 2019. Frequently Asked Questions. https://questions.cms.gov/faq.php?id=5005&faqId=1813.

Centers for Medicare and Medicaid Services (CMS). 2012 (September 25). Medicare Shared Systems Modifications Necessary to Accept and Crossover to Medicaid National Drug Codes (NDC) and Corresponding Quantities Submitted on CMS-1500 Paper Claims. MLN Matters Article. http://www.cms.hhs.gov/MLNMattersArticles/downloads/MM5835.pdf.

Centers for Medicare and Medicaid Services (CMS). 2009 (February 13). Pub 100-20 One Time Notification, Transmittal 446. http://www.cms.gov/Regulations-and-Guidance/Guidance/ Transmittals/downloads/R446OTN.pdf.

Centers for Medicare and Medicaid Services (CMS). 2007 (December 21). Pub 100-04 Medicare Claims Processing Manual, Transmittal 1401. http://www.cms.gov/Regulations-and-Guidance/Guidance/Transmittals/downloads/R1401CP.pdf.

Department of Health and Human Services (HHS). 2008 (May 28). Final Rule on Medicare Program; Medicare Part D Claims Data. *Federal Register*. http://www.cms.gov/Medicare/ Prescription-Drug-Coverage/PrescriptionDrugCovGenIn/Part-D-Regulations.html.

Drug Supply Chain Security Act (DSCSA). 2013. Public Law 113-54.

GS1. 2019 (January). GS1 general specifications: The foundational GS1 standard that defines how identification keys, data attributes and barcodes must be used in business applications. https://www.gs1.org/docs/barcodes/GS1_General_Specifications.pdf.

National Library of Medicine (NLM). n.d. *DailyMed*. https://dailymed.nlm.nih.gov/dailymed/index.cfm.

Noridian. 2018 (November). NDC/HCPCS Crosswalk. https://www.dmepdac.com/crosswalk/index.html.

Office of Inspector General (OIG). 2006 (August). The Food and Drug Administration's National Drug Code Directory. http://oig.hhs.gov/oei/reports/oei-06-05-00060.pdf.

U.S. Food and Drug Administration (FDA). 2019. National Drug Code Directory Searchable Database. https://www.accessdata.fda.gov/scripts/cder/ndc/index.cfm.

U.S. Food and Drug Administration (FDA). 2018 (November 5). Public Hearing: Future Format of the National Drug Code. https://www.fda.gov/Drugs/NewsEvents/ucm574488.htm.

U.S. Food and Drug Administration (FDA). 2017. *National Drug Code Directory*. http://www.fda.gov/drugs/ informationondrugs/ucm142438.htm.

U.S. Food and Drug Administration (FDA). 2016 (August 31). Requirements for foreign and domestic establishment registration and listing for human drugs, including drugs that are regulated under a biologics license application, and animal drugs. *Federal Register* 81(169):60170–60224.

U.S. Food and Drug Administration (FDA). 2004 (February 26). Final Rule on Bar Code Label Requirement for Human Drug Products and Biological Products. *Federal Register*. https://www.federalregister.gov/articles/2004/02/26/04-4249/ bar-code-label-requirement- for-human-drug-products-and-biological-products#h-4

U.S. Food and Drug Administration (FDA). 1969 (July 2). National Drug Code system. *Federal Register* 34(126):11157.

U.S. Food and Drug Administration Center for Drug Evaluation and Research. 2013 (April). Drug Registration and Listing System. http://www.fda.gov/Drugs/Guidance ComplianceRegulatoryInformation/ DrugRegistrationandListing/default.htm.

U.S. Food and Drug Administration Center for Drug Evaluation and Research. 2011 (August). Guidance for Industry: Bar Code Label Requirements Questions and Answers. http://www.fda.gov/downloads/ BiologicsBloodVaccines/GuidanceCompliance RegulatoryInformation/Guidances/UCM267392.pdf.

Workgroup for Electronic Data Interchange (WEDI). 2014 (October 28). NDC reporting requirements in health care claims. https://www.wedi.org/docs/resources/ndc-reporting-requirements-in-health-care-claims.pdf?sfvrsn=0.

Resources

Department of Health and Human Services. 2003 (February 20). Final Rule on Health Insurance Reform: Modifications to Electronic Data Transaction Standards and Code Sets. *Federal Register*. http://www.aspe. hhs.gov/admnsimp/FINAL/FR03-8381.pdf.

5

Current Dental Terminology (CDT)

Mark W. Jurkovich, DDS, MBA, MHI

LEARNING OBJECTIVES

- Explain the development and purpose of dental procedural terminology
- Determine what information is contained in CDT Code
- Describe the components of a CDT Code
- Discuss the process for updating the CDT Code
- Examine the relationship between CDT and diagnostic coding systems in dentistry
- Compare tools available to access and use
- Demonstrate how CDT is used in an electronic environment

KEY TERMS

- Alphabetical Index
- American Dental Association (ADA)
- CDT Coding Companion
- Code Maintenance Committee (CMC)
- Council on Dental Benefit Programs (CDBP)
- Current Dental Terminology (CDT)
- Electronic dental record system (EDR)
- Numeric Index
- Systematized Nomenclature of Dentistry (SNODENT)

Introduction to Current Dental Terminology

The dental procedure code set called the Code on Dental Procedures and Nomenclature is generally referred to as the CDT Code, and is published as **Current Dental Terminology (CDT)**. This code set is recognized as the standard dental procedural code reference for dentists practicing in academic, clinical, and administrative settings. This chapter reviews the Code on Dental Procedures and Nomenclature with discussions of its development, history, purpose, principles, relationships, availability, and maintenance. CDT is updated and published annually.

Developer

The CDT Code was developed and is published by the **American Dental Association (ADA)**. The ADA was founded in 1859 and provides advocacy, facilitates research, and promotes professional development to the dentistry profession throughout the US.

The CDT Code was first published in the *Journal of the American Dental Association* (JADA) in 1969. JADA published six iterations until the seventh version, which became effective on January 1, 1991. This version was published in a separate educational manual titled *Current Dental Terminology*, 1st edition (CDT-1).

Development of CDT-1 began in 1986 when the **Council on Dental Benefit Programs (CDBP)** decided to develop an educational manual that would include a standard set of codes describing dental procedures. The CDBP is "the ADA agency dedicated to promoting quality dental care through the development, promotion and monitoring of the dental benefit programs for the public, and by development and maintenance of dental coding systems and quality assessment and improvement tools and methodologies" (ADA n.d.). It was thought that an educational manual would enable dentists to document and report the care rendered to their patients and also provide dental practices with valuable instructive resources on how to report and process insurance claims. The manual was developed with support from dentists, dental office staff, and the healthcare insurance industry.

The latest edition of the CDT Code is in effect for the entire calendar year, January 1 to December 31. It is revised, as needed, during each calendar year and issued for use beginning January 1 of the following year. Editions of CDT now correspond to the current year. For instance, CDT 2019 is valid during the year 2019.

In 1999, the ADA and the Centers for Medicare and Medicaid Services (CMS) entered into a license agreement for the electronic and print use of CDT. Although CDT is included in the CMS Healthcare Common Procedural Coding System (HCPCS) Level II code set, only the ADA makes decisions on CDT code modification. In 2000, under authority granted by the Health Insurance Portability and Accountability Act of 1996 (HIPAA), the CDT code was deemed the federally mandated terminology for reporting dental services rendered on electronic claims to third-party payers. The ADA owns all property rights, title, and interest in CDT. The ADA's Council on Dental Benefit Programs oversees the maintenance and development of CDT.

Purpose

"The purpose of the CDT Code is to achieve uniformity, consistency and specificity in accurately documenting dental treatment" when reporting dental procedures in claims to third-party payers (ADA 2019a). The CDT Code is used most often for efficient processing of dental benefit claims and to populate an electronic health record (EHR). As indicated by CDT's stated purpose, documentation is also an important function of CDT. It is used in recording treatment rendered in both electronic and paper health records.

Content

The preface to the CDT manual provides instructions on how to use the manual. The three components of a dental procedure code are defined and include: Procedure Code, Nomenclature, and Descriptor. The manual is divided into sections, which are discussed in the following subsections.

Section 1: Code on Dental Procedures and Nomenclature (CDT Code)

Section 1 includes 12 dental service categories. Each category contains the applicable five-character alphanumeric codes. Under each category heading the individual codes are described in detail utilizing the three components described in the Preface of the CDT manual. The service categories and code series are as follows:

Service Category		Code Series
I.	Diagnostic	D0100–D0999
II.	Preventive	D1000–D1999
III.	Restorative	D2000–D2999
IV.	Endodontics	D3000–D3999
V.	Periodontics	D4000–D4999
VI.	Prosthodontics, removable	D5000–D5899
VII.	Maxillofacial Prosthetics	D5900–D5999
VIII.	Implant Services	D6000–D6199
IX.	Prosthodontics, fixed	D6200–D6999
X.	Oral & Maxillofacial Surgery	D7000–D7999
XI.	Orthodontics	D8000–D8999
XII.	Adjunctive General Services	D9000–D9999

This section also includes a "Classification of Materials." Numerous materials are used in the fabrication of dental restorations. Major categories of these materials are discussed in Section 1 to help the user determine the precise code and term to utilize.

Section 2: CDT Code Changes Mark-Up

Section 2 provides a detailed overview of the revisions to procedure code nomenclatures and descriptors changed from the previous version of the Code. This includes new, revised, and deleted codes, as well as any editorial changes. Editorial changes are made when clarification is needed without any change in the CDT Code entry's purpose or scope (ADA 2019b, 97).

Section 3: Alphabetical Index to the CDT Code

Section 3 is the **Alphabetical Index**, which provides a listing of codes by subcategory, nomenclature, or relationship along with the page(s) where the CDT code(s) are found. It can be used to identify all of the codes that might be used for a specific procedure or procedures. Cross-references are provided to another term as well as notations when a separate code is not assigned.

Section 4: Numeric Index to the CDT Code

Re-introduced in 2014, the **Numeric Index** is a complete listing of every CDT code, making it possible to look up the code numerically and be provided with the page where the code can be found. The index also includes a notation to indicate if the code is new, revised, or deleted or an editorial change has been made.

Principles and Guidelines

Principles and guidelines are found within CDT and the **CDT Coding Companion**. Published by the ADA, the CDT Coding Companion provides advice on using the CDT Code by providing definitions, coding scenarios, and questions and answers for each of the 12 dental service categories. See the Tools for Access and Use sections of this chapter for more information.

Discussed below are the guidelines that apply to sections 1 and 3 of the CDT manual.

Section 1: Code on Dental Procedures and Nomenclature

Dental service and procedure codes are organized first by the 12 procedure categories, then by procedural subcategories, followed by code number with its associated nomenclature. Narrative descriptors are optional and may be added to subcategories or to a dental procedure code.

TABLE 5.1. Components of dental procedure code D0210

Procedure Code	Nomenclature	Descriptor
D0210	intraoral - complete series of radiographic images	A radiographic survey of the whole mouth, usually consisting of 14–22 periapical and posterior bitewing images intended to display the crowns and roots of all teeth, periapical areas, and alveolar bone.

Source: ADA 2019b.

An individual CDT Code entry includes at least the first two of the following three components:

1. *A dental procedure code* is a five-character alphanumeric code that begins with the letter D and is followed by four numerals. Each code identifies a specific dental procedure.
2. A *nomenclature* is a concise written definition of a dental procedure code.
3. A *descriptor* is an optional written narrative that provides additional information on the intended use of a dental procedure code.

Table 5.1 provides an example of the three components for procedure code D0210.

Changes in the current version of the CDT Code are identified by two symbols. A bullet symbol (•) identifies a new procedure code, and a triangle symbol (▲) identifies a revision to a code nomenclature, code descriptor, or both. The change symbols are included before the appropriate code number, nomenclature, and descriptor. Deleted codes, nomenclature, and/or descriptors are listed in Section 2 of the manual. For certain procedure codes, when the nomenclature of a code includes a "by report" notation, the CDT manual instructs a dental procedure narrative description be reported with the claim submission.

Examples of such codes include unspecified dental procedures and those with nomenclature specifically indicating the need to report additional information. Unspecified codes are available for all the categories. The dental treatment narrative description then can be used for claim-processing purposes by third-party payers.

The ADA instructs a licensee that a code nomenclature may be abbreviated only when printed on billing forms that have space limitations and advises that code descriptors cannot be modified by a licensee.

Table 5.2, a listing from the CDT 2019 Manual, provides a review of CDT Code categories and subcategories.

Section 3: Alphabetical Index to the CDT Code

The Alphabetical Index lists dental terms in alphabetical order. The dental code and the appropriate page number(s) follow each dental term in the index. The page number(s) following the

TABLE 5.2. Code categories and subcategories

Category of Service	Code Series	Subcategories

I. Diagnostic	D0100–D0999	Clinical oral evaluations
		Pre-diagnostic services
		Diagnostic imaging
		    Image capture with interpretation
		    Image capture only
		    Interpretation and report only
		    Post processing of image or image sets
		Tests and examinations
		Oral pathology laboratory

II. Preventive	D1000–D1999	Dental prophylaxis Topical fluoride treatment (office procedure) Other preventive services Space maintenance (passive appliances) Space maintainers
III. Restorative	D2000–D2999	Amalgam restorations (including polishing) Resin-based composite restorations—Direct Gold foil restorations Inlay/onlay restorations Porcelain/ceramic inlays/onlays include all indirect ceramic and porcelain type inlays/onlays Resin-based composite inlays/onlays must utilize indirect technique Crowns—single restorations only Other restorative services
IV. Endodontics	D3000–D3999	Pulp capping Pulpotomy Endodontic therapy on primary teeth Endodontic therapy (including treatment plan, clinical procedures, and follow-up care) Endodontic retreatment Apexification/recalcification Pulpal regeneration Apicoectomy/periradicular services Other endodontic procedures
V. Periodontics	D4000–D4999	Surgical services (including usual postoperative care) Non-surgical periodontal services Other periodontal services
VI. Prosthodontics (removable)	D5000–D5899	Complete dentures (including routine post-delivery care) Partial dentures (including routine post-delivery care) Adjustments to dentures Repairs to complete dentures Repairs to partial dentures Denture rebase procedures Denture reline procedures Interim prosthesis Other removable prosthetic services

TABLE 5.2. Continued

Category of Service	Code Series	Subcategories
VII. Maxillofacial prosthetics	D5900–D5999	Carriers

VIII. Implant services	D6000–D6199	Pre-surgical services
		Surgical services
		Implant supported prosthetics
		    Supporting structures
		    Implant/abutment supported removable dentures
		    Implant/abutment supported fixed dentures (Hybrid prosthesis)
		    Single crowns, abutment supported
		    Single crowns, implant supported
		    Fixed partial denture retainer, abutment supported
		    Fixed partial denture retainer, implant supported
		Other implant services

IX. Prosthodontics, fixed	D6200–D6999	Fixed partial denture pontics Fixed partial denture retainers—inlays/onlays Fixed partial denture retainers—crowns Other fixed partial denture services
X. Oral and maxillofacial surgery	D7000–D7999	Extractions (includes local anesthesia, suturing, if needed, and routine postoperative care) Other surgical procedures Alveoloplasty—preparation of ridge Vestibuloplasty Excision of soft tissue lesions Excision of intra-osseous lesions Excision of bone tissue Surgical incision Treatment of closed fractures Treatment of open fractures Reduction of dislocation and management of other temporomandibular joint dysfunctions Repair of traumatic wounds Complicated suturing (reconstruction requiring delicate handling of tissues and wide undermining for meticulous closure) Other repair procedures
XI. Orthodontics	D8000–D8999	Limited orthodontic treatment Interceptive orthodontic treatment Comprehensive orthodontic treatment Minor treatment to control harmful habits Other orthodontic services
XII. Adjunctive general services	D9000–D9999	Unclassified treatment Anesthesia Professional consultation Professional visits Drugs Miscellaneous services Non-clinical procedures

Source: ADA 2019b.

listing designates where to locate pertinent code information in one or more sections of the manual. In some instances, a dental term is further specified by the inclusion of additional information for appropriate code assignment. Some of the dental terms refer users to see another dental term in the index. Finally, the index notes "No separate code" for certain dental terms, which instructs the user not to assign a CDT code.

Process for Revision and Updates

Revisions to the Code are effective and published annually. This is a change from the biennial publication of past years. In 2001, the Code Revision Committee (CRC) was established to maintain the CDT Code. The Committee has now been replaced by the **Code Maintenance Committee (CMC)**, which includes representatives from third-party payers such as the America's Health Insurance Plans and the National Association of Dental Plans (NADP), the American Dental Association, dental specialty organizations, the Academy of General Dentistry, and the American Dental Education Association. The delegates from these entities cast votes to accept or decline CDT code changes, additions, or deletions. However, the ADA Bylaws indicate responsibility for CDT Code maintenance falls to the CDBP (ADA 2019a).

The ADA manages and provides staff to coordinate the technical review and revision process. Members of the dental profession, third-party payers, or other users of the CDT manual may submit a code change request at any time. The date received will determine which edition of the manual could contain the revision, if approved. Requests received after the published closing date will be considered for the next edition. The ADA provides detailed instructions, guidelines, evaluation criteria, and a CDT Code Action Request form used to apply for a new procedure code or revise a current procedure code nomenclature or descriptor. In addition, each submitter must agree to and submit a Copyright Assignment Agreement for the proposed revision, change, or deletion to be considered. Each change request requires the submitter to complete the CDT Code Action Request form and then return it, via e-mail, to the ADA CDBP for consideration. Submission and Evaluation Guidelines are published on the ADA website.

The goal for incorporating new codes is to reflect clinical dentistry advancement and to include revisions that can be recognized and adopted by all users of the CDT Code. Each updated edition includes a summary section of CDT code additions, deletions, and revisions.

If necessary, the ADA will produce an errata listing after printing the CDT manual. This will be available on the ADA website.

Relationship with Other Terminologies, Classification Systems, and Code Sets

CDT defines procedures that are provided by dental clinicians. With rare exceptions, currently limited to Medicaid plans in a few states, CDT codes are the only codes needed to adjudicate a claim. For the remainder of claims, dental benefit companies require submission of tooth numbers and surfaces, where appropriate, but only CDT is necessary as a code set.

As noted above, some Medicaid claims, varying by state, also require a "diagnosis" code that is part of the ICD-10-CM classification system. Below is an example:

> Diagnosis: ICD-10-CM code K02.62, Dental caries on smooth surface extending into dentin

Dental caries is generally treated with a tooth restoration. In this case it could be one of many CDT codes, from D2140 to D2394 or many other CDT codes in the D2000 series. Other CDT codes such as those in the D7000 or D8000 series would not be associated with this particular ICD-10-CM code. In this way, there is a loose relationship between ICD-10-CM diagnostic codes and CDT.

Another internationally used and recognized terminology is SNOMED CT. SNOMED CT contains a variety of concepts including findings, disorders, observations, and procedures. SNOMED CT does contain dental procedure concepts. There are many differences between the procedures in SNOMED CT and those contained in CDT and there is no correlation between the identifiers in the two sets. There is no recognized map between these two code sets. Thus, SNOMED CT concepts and identifiers cannot be used for claims submission to dental insurance plans or payers in the US. An informal subset of SNOMED CT terms that contains mostly findings and observations (and only a very few procedures) is known as the **Systematized Nomenclature of Dentistry (SNODENT)**. SNODENT is an American National Standards Institute (ANSI) standard terminology.

In the past decade, dental schools have begun to use and teach the use of diagnostic codes more frequently. This includes SNODENT and a subset known as SNO-DDS, a harmonization of SNODENT and its previous version, Dental Diagnostic System (DDS) codes. Like the example above, these again are loosely associated with CDT but tend to have fewer associated codes when compared to ICD-10-CM codes due to the greater granularity of SNODENT and SNO-DDS.

CDT also has a relationship with HCPCS. CMS established HCPCS for healthcare providers and medical suppliers to report professional services, procedures, and supplies. CDT is one type of HCPCS Level II codes (see chapter 3 for more on HCPCS). While CMS originally published CDT as section D of HCPCS Level II, this is no longer the case.

Tools to Access and Use

Today, CDT is available in three versions. There is the printed version, most often referred to as the CDT manual. There is also an electronic version, an exact duplicate of the printed version except available electronically and printable in a PDF format. Finally, CDT is available as a searchable application for use on phones or tablets.

The current CDT 2019 manual no longer contains the type of background information that older versions of the manual did. Instead, there is now a CDT 2019 Coding Companion. It provides information on CDT organization, how to request changes, the various components of CDT, and examples of the relationships between CDT and ICD-10-CM codes through a cross-walk. It also includes information to assist in properly submitting either dental or medical claims for dental services. The Coding Companion is available in print or electronic editions. Figure 5.1 is an example of one of the coding scenarios included to assist with proper coding.

FIGURE 5.1. Coding scenario #4

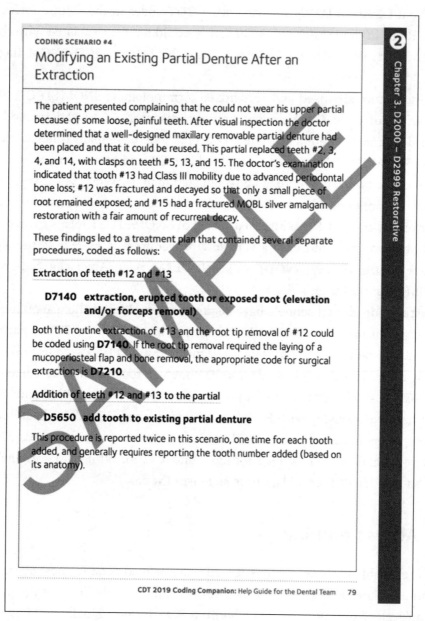

Source: 2019c.

Though not universal, the overwhelming majority of dental clinics use an **electronic dental record system (EDR)** designed specifically for dental use. While a smaller percentage of dental clinicians use their systems to record clinical care, virtually all use it for accounting purposes and documentation of services provided. The EDRs used in dentistry generally include a database specifically for CDT that is updated by the EDR vendor to keep up with the latest CDT release.

These EDRs will access their built-in CDT database to allow ease of documentation as well as either sending claims electronically or printing them on paper for those that are insured. CDT and its associated nomenclature are often also used to provide patients with information on their billing statements as well as for projected treatment (treatment plans).

When submitting a claim electronically, dental offices can usually choose between using a "claims clearinghouse" or submitting it directly to the dental benefit plan through a web portal. A clearinghouse is a company that acts as an intermediary between healthcare providers and payers for electronic claim submission. The overwhelming majority of these claims are submitted through a clearinghouse because this is normally a built-in feature of an EDR. Submitting directly to each dental benefits company generally requires many more key strokes and additional time.

EDR vendors and firms that provide services for e-claims (claims "clearinghouses") are required to have a commercial license if they use CDT. The license includes CDT files provided electronically that can be readily adapted to the data structures used in their systems.

Adoption and Use Cases

In accordance with the Social Security Act, federal laws governing Medicare require CMS to contract with entities to process and pay Medicare claims and associated services.

The CMS regulation published on August 17, 2000 (45 CFR 162.1002) to implement the HIPAA requirement for standardized coding systems established the HCPCS Level II codes as the standardized coding system for describing and identifying substances, equipment, supplies, or other items used in healthcare services that are not identified by the HCPCS Level I, CPT codes. Public and private insurers were required to be in compliance with the August 2000 regulation by October 1, 2002.

Under the authority granted by HIPAA, the CDT code was deemed the federally mandated terminology for reporting dental services rendered on electronic claims to third-party payers.

Use Case One: Billing Dental Services

To be compliant with HIPAA, dentists use CDT codes to describe and electronically submit a claim for a number of different services and procedures.

For example, Patient A, who has a dental benefit (insurance) plan, visited the dentist, and had all four wisdom teeth (third molars) extracted under local anesthesia. The dental practice bills services on the dental claim using CDT codes representing the specific type of procedure for the tooth removed, the tooth number, the fee billed by service, and the date of service for each procedure. No Descriptor is included on the claim form, whether electronic or paper. The tooth number included on the dental claim per service allows the carrier to determine: 1) if a particular service is covered for a particular tooth (some are not); and 2) whether the service was performed on the particular tooth in the past. For Patient A, the procedure codes with their associated tooth numbers that would be billed are shown below.

Procedure Code	Tooth #
D7220	01
D7210	16
D7230	17
D7240	32

Use Case Two: Processing Dental Benefit Claim

Third-party payers process claims according to their policies and the benefits of the patient's insurance plan. For example, in Use Case One, the dental payer would receive the claim for oral surgery services. After verifying the patient's eligibility and group or plan, the payer would pay benefits determined by:

- whether the reported CDT code is a covered benefit;
- what the coverage level for each CDT code should be;
- if a deductible is applicable to the particular service rendered;
- if the patient has exceeded any yearly or plan benefit, if applicable;
- whether the rendering provider participated in the payer's network and if so what fee schedule to utilize; and
- whether to pay the provider (assignment of benefits) or member, based on an indicator on the dental claim, or plan contract.

Upon review of the claim's information, the dental payer determined the CDT codes were a covered benefit and processed the claim according to the patient's benefit plan.

CHECK YOUR UNDERSTANDING

1. What organization holds all property rights, title, and interest in CDT?

   a. Centers for Medicare and Medicaid Services (CMS)
   b. American Dental Association (ADA)
   c. America's Health Insurance Plans
   d. Blue Cross/Blue Shield Association

2. Which of following information is included in the CDT Code manual?

   a. Dental Procedure Code Components
   b. Listing of Categories of Services
   c. Section on Changes to the CDT Code
   d. All of the above

3. Which of the following CDT service categories includes professional visits?

   a. Diagnostic D0100–D0999
   b. Preventive D1000–D1999
   c. Adjunctive General Services D9000–D9999
   d. Miscellaneous Services D9910–D9999

4. True or false? Unspecified codes are not available in the Code manual.

   a. True
   b. False

5. Which component of a CDT code is not always required?

   a. Dental procedure code
   b. Nomenclature
   c. Descriptor
   d. None of the above

REVIEW

1. Who is responsible for overseeing the maintenance and development of the CDT Code?

   a. Centers for Medicare and Medicaid Services (CMS)
   b. Code Revision Committee (CRC)
   c. Blue Cross Blue Shield Association
   d. Council on Dental Benefit Programs of the American Dental Association

2. Which of the following is a required component that provides a written definition of a dental procedure code?

   a. Terminology
   b. Descriptor
   c. Nomenclature
   d. Subcategory

3. True or false? A bullet symbol identifies a new procedure code in the current version of the CDT Code.

   a. True
   b. False

4. Revisions to the CDT Code are published and effective:

   a. Annually
   b. Biennially
   c. Quarterly
   d. Every three years

5. True or false? Only dentists may complete the code change request forms.

   a. True
   b. False

6. The CDT codes are a mandated standard for reporting dental procedures and services under the

   a. Health Information Technology for Economic and Clinical Health Act
   b. Health Insurance Portability and Accountability Act
   c. Council on Dental Benefits Programs
   d. Affordable Care Act

7. Who contributed to the initial development of the CDT Code?

   a. Dentists
   b. Dental schools
   c. The federal government
   d. All of the above

8. True or false? A dental procedure code consists of a five-character alphanumeric code.

   a. True
   b. False

9. Dental codes are first organized by:

   a. Sections
   b. Subcategories
   c. Service categories
   d. Code number and nomenclature

10. True or false? Each updated edition of the CDT Code includes a summary section of CDT code additions, deletions, and revisions.

    a. True
    b. False

References

45 CFR 162.1002: Administrative requirements. 2000 (Aug. 17).

American Dental Association (ADA). 2019a. Code on Dental Procedures and Nomenclature (CDT Code). https://www.ada.org/en/publications/cdt.

American Dental Association (ADA). 2019b. *CDT 2019 Dental Procedure Codes*. Chicago, IL: ADA.

American Dental Association (ADA). 2019c. *CDT 2019 Companion: Help Guide for the Dental Team*. Chicago, IL: ADA.

American Dental Association (ADA). n.d. Understanding organized dentistry. https://www.modental.org/docs/librariesprovider30/members/Students/stud_adaunderstandorgdent.pdf?sfvrsn=4.

Part II

Other Terminologies and Classification Systems

SNOMED Clinical Terms (SNOMED CT)

Mary H. Stanfill, MBI, RHIA, CCS, CCS-P, FAHIMA

LEARNING OBJECTIVES

- Explore the purpose of SNOMED CT
- Summarize the content and organizational structure of SNOMED CT
- Interpret principles and guidelines applied to SNOMED CT content
- Identify the process for ongoing development of SNOMED CT
- Describe the SNOMED International governance structure and the role of National Release Centers
- Examine the relationship of SNOMED CT with other terminologies
- Compare current tools to access and use SNOMED CT
- Explain current uses and adoption of SNOMED CT
- Demonstrate how SNOMED CT is used in an electronic environment

KEY TERMS

- Attributes
- Concepts
- Concept identifier
- Concept orientation
- Concept permanence
- Configurable
- Cross map
- Derivative work

- Description
- Editorial Guide
- Extension
- Fully specified name (FSN)
- General Assembly
- Granularity
- Hierarchy
- | is a | relationship
- Management Board
- Namespace identifier
- National Release Center (NRC)
- Open tooling framework (OTF)
- Post-coordination
- Pre-coordination
- Preferred term (PT)
- Reference set (RefSet)
- Reference terminology
- Relationships
- Root concept
- SNOMED Clinical Terms (SNOMED CT)
- SNOMED CT Identifier (SCTID)
- SNOMED International
- Technical Implementation Guide (TIG)
- Understandable, Reproducible, Useful (URU) principle

Introduction to SNOMED CT

SNOMED Clinical Terms (SNOMED CT) is a reference terminology with comprehensive coverage of diseases, clinical findings, etiologies, and procedures and outcomes used by physicians, dentists, nurses, allied health professionals, veterinarians, and others. According to **SNOMED International**, SNOMED CT is "the most comprehensive, multilingual clinical terminology in the world" (SNOMED International 2018a). SNOMED International is the organization that owns and maintains SNOMED CT. SNOMED CT is a resource with comprehensive, scientifically validated clinical content that enables consistent, processable representation of clinical content in electronic health records (EHRs).

SNOMED CT contributes to the improvement of patient care by underpinning the development of systems that accurately record health care encounters. It provides a standardized way to represent clinical phrases captured by clinicians and enables automatic interpretation to facilitate better communication, interoperability in electronic health record exchange, and clinical decision support functionality. SNOMED CT is designed to capture clinical information for use in an EHR system (SNOMED International 2019). It adds processable meaning to an electronic health record, thus enabling effective, meaningful representation of clinical information. As a result, it plays a pivotal role in worldwide endeavors to deliver cost-effective, high-quality healthcare.

SNOMED CT is one of a suite of designated standards for use in US federal government systems for the electronic exchange of clinical health information, and the Office of the National Coordinator for Health Information Technology (ONC) names SNOMED CT as one of the standards for the entry of structured data in certified EHR systems (ONC 2015). SNOMED CT is also being implemented internationally as a standard within other SNOMED International Member countries. According to SNOMED International, SNOMED CT has been developed collaboratively to ensure it meets the diverse needs and expectations of clinicians worldwide and is now accepted as a common global language for health terms (SNOMED International 2018b).

This chapter explores the purpose of SNOMED CT and describes the content, structure, principles, guidelines, and development, as well as tools and applications for deployment. The chapter also explores SNOMED CT adoption and use to provide an understanding of how SNOMED CT is used.

Developer

SNOMED began as SNOP (Systematized Nomenclature of Pathology), and later extended into other medical fields. First released in January 2002, SNOMED CT combined the strength of SNOMED Reference Terminology (SNOMED RT) in the basic sciences, laboratory, and specialty medicine, including pathology, with the richness of Clinical Terms Version 3, the National Health Service's terminology work in primary care. In 2007, the responsibility for the ownership, maintenance, and distribution of SNOMED CT was transferred from the College of American Pathologists to the International Health Terminology Standards Development Organisation (IHTSDO), a nonprofit organization based in Denmark. In 2017, IHTSDO adopted the trade name of SNOMED International (SNOMED International 2018c).

Purpose

The general purpose of SNOMED CT is to provide a consistent way of indexing, storing, retrieving, and aggregating clinical data from structured electronic health records. SNOMED CT is not a classification. Classifications, by nature, are designed to classify like things together. In contrast, SNOMED CT is designed to uniquely identify clinical information consistently and in great detail, or **granularity**. With SNOMED CT, the objective is to describe the clinical circumstances of a healthcare encounter in a machine-readable format (that is, in unique numeric concept identifiers).

FIGURE 6.1. SNOMED CT's ability to identify clinical content

The following is an example of the SNOMED CT concept identifiers for the content noted.
Office visit for a 64-year-old established female patient being seen for review and follow-up of non-insulin dependent diabetes, obesity, hypertension, and chronic right-sided congestive heart failure. Complains of shortness of breath and admits to dietary noncompliance. Patient's heart failure is assessed (blood pressure measured, level of activity assessed, clinical signs and symptoms of volume overload assessed, respiratory status assessed, and weight recorded). She is counseled concerning diet and current medications adjusted.

In this scenario, SNOMED CT identifies the following concepts:

- 81531005|Type II Diabetes mellitus type 2 in obese (disorder)|
- 59621000|Essential hypertension (disorder)|
- 66989003|Chronic right-sided congestive heart failure (disorder)|
- 267036007|Dyspnea (finding)|
- 185349003|Encounter for check up (procedure)|
- 129832003|Noncompliance with dietary regimen (finding)|
- 46973005|Blood pressure taking (procedure)|
- 398636004|Physical activity assessment (procedure)|
- 422834003|Respiratory assessment (procedure)|
- 424753004|Dietary management education, guidance, and counseling (procedure)|
- 182838006|Change of medication (procedure)|

With a classification system such as ICD-10-CM, a coding professional assigns a code. This is not done with SNOMED CT. SNOMED CT is embedded in the EHR system and works behind the scenes to identify the clinical concepts in the health record in machine-readable format. See figure 6.1 for an illustration of SNOMED CT and its ability to identify clinical content.

It is expected that numerous systems, working together in concert, would be required to support an efficient and effective clinical information system and to handle the administrative needs of a healthcare organization. Although ideally suited for clinical purposes, SNOMED CT is not suitable for certain administrative needs. For example, SNOMED CT would be difficult to use in a reimbursement system because of its tremendous amount of content granularity. A classification system such as ICD with its ability to aggregate data is more suitable for claims processing. SNOMED CT is designed for use in the underlying clinical information system to identify and tag data at the point of input so that it can be used for various purposes.

Purposes of SNOMED CT, for example, are to:

- Capture clinical data at the appropriate level of detail
- Minimize the need for repetitive data entry at varying levels of granularity
- Reduce the risk of different interpretations via unambiguous descriptions
- Facilitate communication among care providers
- Retrieve, transmit, and analyze data consistently
- Facilitate continuity of care
- Reduce repetition across the continuum of care

- Enable efficient searching
- Facilitate point-of-care decision support
- Allow application of logical processing

The Computer-based Patient Record Institute (CPRI) studied the ability of nomenclatures to capture information for computerized patient records. While CPRI no longer exists as a separate entity, the Healthcare Information and Management Systems Society (HIMSS) assumed its mission. During its existence, CPRI determined that SNOMED is the most comprehensive reference terminology for coding the contents of the patient record and facilitating the development of computerized patient records (Chute et al. 1996; Campbell et al. 1997). The more recent version, SNOMED CT, is even better suited to fulfill this purpose.

The purpose of SNOMED CT is to enable the consistent recording and documentation of clinical concepts, with clear relationships between concepts, in an EHR. SNOMED CT helps ensure comparability of data records by multiple practitioners across diverse platforms and systems using computer programs. The use of an EHR improves communication and increases the availability of relevant information. If clinical information is stored in ways that allow

TABLE 6.1. Benefits of SNOMED CT enabled health records

	Benefits
SNOMED CT enabled health record benefits to individuals	Allows precise recording of clinical information. By using many descriptions for a single clinical concept, SNOMED CT allows tailoring for individual care settings while maintaining consistency. Represents health information to support clinical care by encoding statements about the health and healthcare of an individual patient, without forcing arbitrary categories. Supports the sharing of appropriate information with other care providers in a way that allows common understanding and interpretation. Allows accurate and comprehensive searches that identify patients who require follow-up or changes in treatment based on revised guidelines.
SNOMED CT enabled health record benefits to populations	Provides a mechanism to aggregate and analyze clinical information for specific populations. Facilitates early identification of emerging health issues, monitoring of population health and responses to changing clinical practices. Enables the delivery of relevant data to support clinical research and contribute evidence for future improvements in treatment.
SNOMED CT enabled health records support evidence-based care	Enables evidence-based healthcare decisions with links to enhanced clinical guidelines and protocols at the point of care for individual cases. Reduces the cost of inappropriate and duplicative testing and treatment. Limits the frequency and impact of adverse healthcare events. Raises the cost-effectiveness and quality of care for individuals and populations.

Source: SNOMED International 2017a, 6.

meaning-based retrieval, the benefits are greatly increased. Refer to table 6.1 for benefits of SNOMED CT enabled health records.

Content

SNOMED CT has a broad scope of coverage. It includes concepts representing the wide range of types of information that need to be recorded in clinical records. SNOMED CT includes a vast array of clinical concepts beyond diagnoses and procedures. SNOMED CT includes clinical concepts that cover disorders, findings, procedures, body structures, pharmacy products, and other concepts that encompass all of healthcare.

With this level of detail available, it is not surprising that the size of SNOMED CT far surpasses that of any single classification. The July 2018 release of SNOMED CT contained 340,659 active concepts, approximately a million English descriptions, and several million relationships (SNOMED International 2018d). In comparison, ICD-10-CM contains approximately 72,000 diagnosis codes, and ICD-10-PCS contains approximately 79,000 procedure codes.

The SNOMED CT content is represented using three types of components:

- Concepts
- Descriptions
- Relationships

Derivative works that help in the uptake and use of SNOMED CT include:

- Reference sets (RefSets)
- Language or dialect preferences to use particular descriptions
- Cross maps to other code systems and classifications
- Other relevant metadata to support use of SNOMED CT components

Documentation, such as the Editorial Guide, also accompanies a SNOMED CT release.

Concepts

Concepts are the basic units of SNOMED CT and are defined as unique units of knowledge created by a unique combination of characteristics. In essence, a concept is a specific idea or thought. It may have more than one term associated with it, but it cannot have more than one meaning. In SNOMED CT, a unique number known as the **concept identifier** is assigned to each concept. For example, the word *cast* can have a number of different meanings. Among other things, it can refer to a physical object (rigid material molded to the body) or an abnormal urinary product (precipitated product from the kidney tubules found in urine). Each of these concepts represents a unique expression of thought and is assigned its own unique concept identifier.

Concepts are structured according to logic-based representations of meanings. In computer science terms, codes are organized in a directed acyclic graph. Each code (or concept in the case of SNOMED CT) is represented by a node in the graph and each relationship is represented by an arrow. For example, in the graph presented in figure 6.2, bacterial pneumonia is a unique concept with a unique concept identifier, infective pneumonia is a separate unique concept with its own unique concept identifier, and there is a directed relationship between them.

Concept identifiers are unique, machine-readable strings of digits. The minimum length is 6 digits; the maximum is 18 digits, with concept identifiers most commonly 8 or 9 digits. The identifiers themselves hold no inherent meaning associated with the digits, that is, there is nothing in the integer to indicate what it means. Since concept identifiers do not have embedded meaning or digit restrictions, even when the knowledge about a concept changes, the concept identifier remains the same. Other SNOMED CT components also have unique identifiers; however, the concept identifier has a specific role as the code used to represent the meaning in clinical records, documents, messages, and data.

FIGURE 6.2. SNOMED CT relationships graph

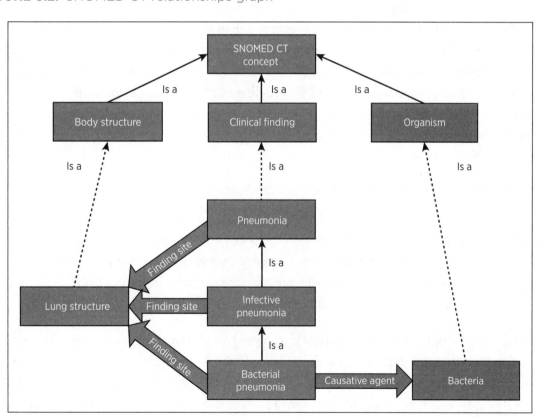

Source: SNOMED International 2018e.

Descriptions

SNOMED CT **descriptions** link appropriate human-readable terms to concepts. Descriptions are the terms or text for the concept. A concept can have several associated descriptions, each representing alternative text that describes the same clinical idea.

Examples of varying descriptions linked to the same concept of pain in throat (concept identifier 162397003):

Fully specified name: Pain in throat (finding) (description identifier 543537013)

Preferred term for the English language, US dialect: Pain in throat (description identifier 253240010)

Synonym: Sore throat (description identifier 2164213014)

Synonym: Throat pain (description identifier 253237010)

Synonym: Pain in the pharynx (description identifier 253239013)

Synonym: Throat discomfort (description identifier 253238017)

Synonym: Pharyngeal pain (description identifier 2164214015)

Synonym: Throat soreness (description identifier 2164212016)

Each distinct description is assigned a unique description identifier. A description is always attached to a specific concept. In the example above, there is one concept identifier (162397003) but, as shown, a distinct description identifier for each of these varying text descriptions.

Since a description is attached to a concept, a unique description identifier is used for terms that hold different meanings. For example, the term *immunosuppression* may mean different things. It could be a procedure or it could be a finding that the person is immunosuppressed. As illustrated in the example below, there are two different meanings and two different description identifiers for this term so even though the term is the same, there are two different description identifiers in SNOMED CT.

Example

concept identifier 86553008 Immunosuppression (type = procedure)

description identifier = 507152014 Immunosuppression (procedure)

concept identifier 38013005 Immunosuppression (type = clinical finding)

description identifier = 63394015 Immunosuppression (finding)

SNOMED CT has a built-in framework to manage different languages and dialects. Each translation of SNOMED CT includes an additional set of descriptions, which link terms in another language to the same SNOMED CT concepts. SNOMED CT concepts and relationships are language-independent, while language-dependent descriptions make SNOMED CT a multilingual terminology. SNOMED CT is available today in US English, UK English, Spanish, Danish, and Swedish. SNOMED CT includes a SNOMED CT Starter Set translation package that has a minimum core set of terms translated in languages other than English to assist in the implementation of SNOMED CT. The March 2018 release, for example, contains the following language sets: French, German, and Chinese (SNOMED International 2018f). Full translations of SNOMED CT into Canadian French, Lithuanian, and several other languages are currently underway (SNOMED International 2017a, 16).

Relationships

Relationships are a type of connection between two concepts, that is, a source concept and a destination concept. SNOMED CT relationships link each concept to other concepts that have a related meaning. These relationships provide formal definitions and other characteristics of the concept. Values of a range of relevant attributes make up the defining characteristics of a concept and include 116680003 |is a (attribute)| relationships and defining attribute relationships (SNOMED International 2018g) both of which are described below. These relationships characterize concepts and give them their meaning. Every SNOMED CT concept except the root concept has at least one relationship to another concept. Relationships are used to logically define the meaning of a concept in a way that can be processed by a computer.

Subtype relationships are the most widely used type of relationship. They are known as the | **is a** | **relationship** (also called supertype-subtype or parent-child relationship). Almost all active SNOMED CT concepts are the source of at least one | is a | relationship. The | is a | relationship states that the source concept is a subtype of the destination concept. SNOMED CT relationships are directional and the | is a | relationship read in the reverse direction states that the destination concept is a supertype of the source concept. In this manner, | is a | relationships link certain concepts to other concepts where one is a part of the meaning of the other. The | is a | relationship must always be known to be true. Concepts are always related by | is a | relationship to the concept directly above them in the **hierarchy**. The following 115580003 | is a | (attribute) relationships are represented by the arrows in figure 6.2:

- Bacterial pneumonia | is a | Infective pneumonia
- Infective pneumonia | is a | Pneumonia
- Pneumonia | is a | Clinical Finding
- Clinical Finding | is a | SNOMED CT Concept
- Bacteria | is a | Organism
- Lung Structure | is a | Body Structure
- Body Structure | is a | SNOMED CT Concept

Attributes represent characteristics or aspects of a concept's meaning to make its meaning more detailed. An attribute relationship contributes to the definition of the source concept by associating it with the value of a defining characteristic. The characteristic (attribute) is specified by the relationship type and the value is provided by the destination of the relationship.

For example, the defining attribute relationships for the concept bacterial pneumonia shown in figure 6.2 are finding site (the name of the type of relationship), lung structure (the value or destination of the relationship), causative agent (the name of the type of relationship), and bacteria (the value or destination of the relationship). Unlike | is a | relationships, which are used to define concepts, the applicability of each type of attribute is limited to a defined domain and range. For example, the allowed attributes for 91723000 |Anatomical structure (body structure)| are (SNOMED International 2018g):

123005000 |Part of (attribute)|
272741003 |Laterality (attribute)|
733928003 |All or part of (attribute)|
733930001 |Regional part of (attribute)|
733931002 |Constitutional part of (attribute)|
733932009 |Systemic part of (attribute)|
733933004 |Lateral half of (attribute)|

Example:

The following defining relationships are specified for the concept identifier 21719001 "Allergic rhinitis due to pollen."

is a	Seasonal allergic rhinitis
is a	Allergic disorder by allergen type
Finding site	Structure of mucous membrane of nose
Associated morphology	Inflammation
Causative agent	Pollen
Clinical course	Seasonal course
Pathological process	Allergic process
Due to	Type 1 hypersensitivity response
Due to	Allergic reaction caused by pollen
Due to	Atopic reaction

Figure 6.2 illustrates not only | is a | relationships but also the causative agent and finding site attribute relationships. The graph indicates that for every instance of bacterial pneumonia, there is a causative agent relationship to particular bacteria and likewise for bacterial pneumonia, there is a finding site of lung structure. SNOMED CT description logic definitions put these together to define bacterial pneumonia as an infective pneumonia with causative agent bacteria and the lung structure as the finding site. Thus the combination of applicable SNOMED CT defining relationships provides a computer-readable definition of a concept.

Reference Sets

Reference sets (RefSets) are a standard way to maintain and distribute additional non-defining information about defined groups of SNOMED CT components. The components included in the group share a common characteristic such as language, specialty, user, or context and are grouped together for a particular purpose. RefSets are important as they can be used in SNOMED CT enabled applications to constrain, configure, and enhance functionality to match requirements for different use cases. RefSets can be a simple list of concepts or a group of concepts that go together. They can also be tagged to denote the type of group or use (such as general, granular, or the specific purpose). Note that RefSets are not necessarily mutually exclusive. The contents of ReSets may overlap.

There are different types of RefSets. For example, Language RefSets identify characteristics of terms according to the language in which they are being used. A Simple RefSet is a subset that is defined extensionally, by enumeration. It contains included and excluded SNOMED CT content that can be used in a particular country, organization, specialty, or context (SNOMED International 2017b). A query RefSet is a subset that is defined intentionally using rules, defined in a query, to determine inclusion. The query, run on the content of SNOMED CT, results in a subset of components, which can be represented as a Simple RefSet. Ordered lists and navigational hierarchies are represented as either Ordered Component RefSets or Ordered Association RefSets. These reference sets order data in sensible ways by priority, or by some readily understood convention that can simplify hierarchies for browsing and allow the user to more readily navigate SNOMED CT. Figure 6.3 provides an example of an ordered component reference set.

FIGURE 6.3. Ordered component reference set example

Ordered reference set example

Fingers sorted A-Z

127053016 |Thumb|
136021011 |Fourth finger|
138873019 |Second finger|
108884010 |Third finger|
21356012 |Fifth finger|

Fingers sorted logically using an ordered component reference set

referencedComponentId	order
127053016 |Thumb|	1
138873019 |Second finger|	2
108884010 |Third finger|	3
136021011 |Fourth finger|	4
21356012 |Fifth finger|	5

Source: SNOMED International 2018h.

Cross Maps

Cross maps are part of the derivative works that help in the uptake and use of SNOMED CT. Cross mappings enable SNOMED CT to effectively reference other terminologies and classifications. Each cross map matches SNOMED CT concepts with values in another coding scheme that is called the "target scheme." Thus a cross map links a single SNOMED CT concept to one or more values in a target coding scheme (such as ICD-10-CM). SNOMED CT supports simple, complex, and extended mappings. Simple maps, where there is a one-to-one relationship between a SNOMED CT concept and code in a target scheme, are represented using a Simple Reference Map Set. Complex and Extended Map Reference Sets enable the representation of maps from a single SNOMED CT concept to either a combination of codes or a choice of codes in the target scheme.

As explained earlier in this chapter, the comprehensive, granular nature of SNOMED CT makes it ideal for data input into an EHR. It is capable of capturing the necessary level of clinical detail required for patient care and clinical decision support. However, this granular detail makes it difficult to use for many administrative purposes, such as claims processing. Use of a mapping of SNOMED CT to administrative code sets solves this difficulty.

SNOMED CT provides a technical structure that supports rule-based processing. It is designed to support semi-automated cross mapping to other terminologies or coding schemes. A cross map links the content from one classification or terminology scheme to another. Maps allow data collected for one purpose to be used for another purpose. For example, SNOMED CT mapped to ICD-10-CM facilitates the translation of more granular clinical data into less granular classifications that can be used for administrative and statistical purposes. The map provides an approximation of the closest ICD code or codes that best represent the SNOMED CT concept. This simplifies coding and data-entry processes, which is expected to lower costs and minimize errors.

Examples of maps include:

- SNOMED CT to ICD-10
- SNOMED CT to ICD-10-CM
- SNOMED CT to ICD-0-3
- GP/FP SNOMED CT to ICPC-3

The IHTSDO developed a rule-based approach to mapping from SNOMED CT to ICD-10. This approach was adopted by the National Library of Medicine (NLM) for development of its map to ICD-10-CM. Due to differences in granularity, emphasis, and organizing principles between SNOMED CT and ICD-10-CM, it is not always possible to have a one-to-one map between a SNOMED CT concept and an ICD-10-CM code. To address this challenge, the NLM adopted the following IHTSDO rules-based approach. When there is a need to choose between alternative ICD-10-CM codes, each possible target code is represented as a map rule (the essence of "rule-based mapping"). Related map rules are grouped into a map group. Map rules within a map group are evaluated in a prescribed order, based on contextual information and co-morbidities. Each map group will resolve to at most one ICD-10-CM code. In the event that a SNOMED CT concept requires more than one ICD-10-CM code to fully represent its meaning, the map will consist of multiple map groups. The scope of this mapping effort included all active pre-coordinated SNOMED CT concepts within three hierarchies (Clinical findings, Events, and Situations with Explicit Context). A priority list of clinically important concepts was identified based on existing subsets, including the CORE Problem List subset (which is described later in this chapter). As of 2018, the priority SNOMED CT concepts in the US Extension are mapped to ICD-10-CM (NLM 2018a). Over 123,000 SNOMED CT source concepts are mapped to ICD-10-CM targets (NLM 2018b).

Additional maps are in development. For example, SNOMED International has established a SNOMED CT to ICD-10-PCS mapping project group that includes participation from US, Spain, and Belgium. The group has studied various ways of automatically mapping the two terminologies. Reportedly, 86% of the top 100 most commonly used ICD-10-PCS codes can be fully represented with post-coordinated SNOMED CT concepts (Fung et al. 2017).

Documentation

There is a wealth of documentation available to facilitate use of SNOMED CT. Documents include formal specifications of SNOMED CT as well as guidance on use and implementation. Documentation is available in a web-browsable format, in pdf, or both.

One such document is the SNOMED CT **Technical Implementation Guide (TIG)**. The TIG provides a general overview of technical topics related to SNOMED CT implementation and is an entry point to individual guides on more specific topics. This document serves as a roadmap to documentation of direct interest to those developing software applications and systems that use SNOMED CT. Clinical knowledge is not required, although some background is helpful to understand the application context and needs. The TIG contains guidelines and advice on SNOMED CT implementation, including implementation types, levels, and services. It also provides an overview of SNOMED CT components and derivatives as well as other topics that relate to the use of SNOMED CT to represent instances of clinical information (SNOMED International 2018e).

The SNOMED CT **Editorial Guide** is another often-used document. The Editorial Guide is intended for clinical personnel, business directors, software product managers, and project leaders. Information technology experience can be helpful, though not necessary, to interpret the guidance. The Editorial Guide is intended to explain SNOMED CT's capabilities and uses from a content perspective. The guide provides detailed information about the rules by which SNOMED CT content is authored. It describes editorial policies regarding the purpose, scope, authoring principles, requirements, concept model, hierarchies, terming, and other policies related to the content in SNOMED CT. It is primarily intended to guide those who are responsible for editing the content of the International Release, but secondarily is important for those creating extensions (SNOMED International 2018g). The overarching intention of this guide is to support communication among those who are actively creating definitions, as well as those who are advising, consulting, or providing feedback on SNOMED CT in a variety of capacities.

The SNOMED CT Starter Guide provides a practical and useful starting point from which anyone with a general interest in healthcare information can begin learning about SNOMED CT. The intended audience includes clinical personnel, business directors, software product managers, and project leaders who are involved in the acquisition, implementation, and use of SNOMED CT and SNOMED CT-enabled applications in their organizations. This guide is intended to provide new as well as experienced users with an overview and illustrations of SNOMED CT's capabilities and uses from a content perspective. Examples of topics covered include SNOMED CT Logical Model, SNOMED CT Concept Model, and SNOMED CT Expressions (SNOMED International 2017a). The detailed structures of SNOMED CT are documented more fully in the TIG, and the details of the content model and principles used to edit the terminology are documented more fully in the Editorial Guide.

SNOMED International maintains SNOMED CT documentation and makes it available via the internet in the SNOMED CT document library (SNOMED International 2018i). A wealth of documentation beyond the TIG, Editorial Guide, and Starter Guide described here is available. See table 6.2 for examples of some of the additional SNOMED CT documentation.

TABLE 6.2. Examples of additional SNOMED CT documentation

Document	Description
National Release Center Guide	This guide offers a practical starting point for SNOMED International Members. It provides guidance on National Release Center (NRC) responsibilities and the relationships between NRCs, SNOMED International, implementers, and users within a Member country or territory.
Vender Introduction to SNOMED CT	This introduction to SNOMED CT focuses primarily on the needs of vendors and developers of healthcare systems and applications.
Extensions Practical Guide	This guide presents the purpose, process, and principles of creating, distributing, and managing SNOMED CT extensions.
Reference Sets Practical Guide	This guide presents the purpose, process, and principles of creating, distributing, and managing SNOMED CT reference sets.
ICD-10 Mapping Technical Guide	This guide explains the process used for mapping SNOMED CT to ICD-10 and provides guidance on this process.
Release File Specification	This specification defines the file formats in which SNOMED CT is distributed to SNOMED International Members and Affiliates.
Compositional Grammar	This specification defines a standard syntax for representing individual clinical meanings using SNOMED CT expressions.

Source: SNOMED International 2018i.

Structure

To achieve its intended purpose, SNOMED CT must not only contain an incredible amount of content, but it also must be organized in such a way that the underlying meanings of concepts and expressions are represented consistently. The fact that SNOMED CT is a reference terminology is one of the characteristics that make it more than just a huge list of medical terms. A **reference terminology** is a controlled terminology employing a set of terms and relationships that capture and define the meaning of each concept. Controlled means that the content of the terminology is managed carefully to ensure that it is structurally sound, biomedically accurate, and consistent with current practice.

A controlled terminology is key to a functional electronic health record. "The single greatest obstacle to comparable data remains medical terminology. Failure to adopt and embrace a common terminology will doom outcomes research and data-driven clinical guideline development" (Chute et al. 1994). In Chute's opinion, clinical data gathered without a controlled terminology are not comparable and thus rendered meaningless.

All terminology or classification systems use hierarchies to organize the information. For example, ICD has a monohierarchical structure where an item is classified in only one place. In ICD-10-CM, for example, carpal tunnel syndrome is classified to the nervous system chapter. In contrast, SNOMED CT is polyhierarchical, meaning the placement of the concept in the hierarchies is based on the underlying medical concepts represented. Thus, the concept "carpal tunnel syndrome" is a not only a disorder of the nervous system but also a soft tissue disorder and an extremity disorder.

At the top of a SNOMED CT hierarchy are very broad concepts and those below are more specialized or specific. The top of the SNOMED CT hierarchy is the **root concept**, |SNOMED CT concept|. The root concept is a single special concept that represents the root of the entire content in SNOMED CT. Subtypes of the root concept are "top-level concepts" (SNOMED International 2018e). The top-level concepts are the parent concepts and they have many subtype children and subtype descendants. As one goes down the hierarchy from the root concept and then the top-level concepts, the concepts become increasingly granular. Since SNOMED CT concepts lower in the hierarchy are more specific, this allows detailed clinical data to be recorded and later accessed or aggregated at a more general level. Table 6.3 provides an illustration of this concept model. Table 6.4 provides a brief description and examples of elements contained in top-level hierarchies.

From this exploration of the content of SNOMED CT, it is evident that the basic principles underlying the SNOMED CT structure are:

- SNOMED CT is concept-based.
- Each concept represents a unit of meaning.

- Each concept has one or more human language terms that can be used to describe the concept.
- Every concept has interrelationships with other concepts that provide logical, computer-readable definitions.

Defining relationships link concepts within a hierarchy. Every concept has at least one relationship to another concept. Certain concepts are assigned additional relationships to explicitly describe the concept's essential characteristics. Thus, the basic structural elements of SNOMED CT are concepts, hierarchies, descriptions, and relationships. These elements are necessary to precisely represent and provide clinical information across the scope of healthcare. Understanding the principles underlying the SNOMED CT structure is critical to understanding the terminology and its design for use in EHRs.

Another important aspect of the SNOMED CT structure is that it is **configurable**. The ability to create reference sets allows SNOMED CT to be configured and optimized to meet specific requirements, such as creating terminology subsets and value sets. SNOMED CT is a deep and detailed clinical terminology with a broad scope. However, some groups of users will need additional concepts, descriptions, or subsets to support national, local, or organizational needs.

The **Extension** mechanism allows SNOMED CT to be customized to address the terminology needs of a country or organization that are not met by the International Edition. An extension may contain components (such as concepts, descriptions, or relationships) or reference sets used to represent subsets, maps, or language preferences. Extensions can include content required to support national, local, or organizational needs that may not have international relevance or may not meet the editorial guidelines for inclusion in the International Edition (SNOMED International 2018j). Table 6.5 provides examples of use cases for extension content.

TABLE 6.3. The SNOMED CT Concept Model

Organization	Example
Root concept	SNOMED CT concept
Top-level concept	Clinical finding
Subtype of clinical finding	Disease
Subtype of disease	Disorder of Respiratory system
Subtype of disorder of respiratory system	Disorder of Lung
Subtype of disorder of lung	Pneumonia
Subtype of pneumonia	Infective pneumonia
Subtype of infective pneumonia	Bacterial pneumonia

Source: SNOMED International 2018e.

TABLE 6.4. SNOMED CT top-level hierarchies

Hierarchies	Examples
Clinical finding Contains the subhierarchies of Finding and Disorder Represents the result of a clinical observation, assessment, or judgment Important for documenting clinical disorders and examination findings	Finding: Swelling of arm Disorder: Pneumonia
Procedure Concepts that represent the purposeful activities performed in the provision of healthcare	Biopsy of lung Diagnostic endoscopy Fetal manipulation
Observable entity Concepts represent a question or procedure that can produce an answer or result	Gender Tumor size Ability to balance
Body structure Concepts include both normal and abnormal anatomical structures Abnormal structures are represented in a subhierarchy as *morphologic abnormalities*	Lingual thyroid (*body structure*) Neoplasm (*morphologic abnormality*)
Organism Coverage includes animals, fungi, bacteria, and plants Concepts represent organisms of etiologic significance in human medicine Necessary for public health reporting and used in evidence-based infectious disease protocols	Hepatitis C virus Streptococcus pyogenes Acer rubrum (red maple) Felis silvestris (cat)
Substance Covers a wide range of biological and chemical substances Includes foods, nutrients, allergens, and materials Used to record the active chemical constituents of all drug products	Dust Estrogen Hemoglobin antibody Methane Codeine phosphate
Physical object Concepts include natural and man-made objects Focus on concepts required for medical injuries	Prosthesis Artificial organs Vena cava filter Colostomy bag
Physical force Concepts are directed primarily at representing physical forces that can play a role as mechanisms of injury Includes motion, friction, electricity, sound, radiation, thermal forces, and air pressure	Fire Gravity Pressure change
Event Concepts represent occurrences that result in injury Exclude all procedures and interventions	Flash flood Motor vehicle accident

(*continued*)

TABLE 6.4. Continued

Hierarchies	Examples
Environment/geographical location Includes all types of environments as well as named locations such as countries, states, and regions	Cameroon Islands of North America Burn center Cancer hospital
Record artifact Includes items created by an individual for the purpose of providing others with information about events or states of affairs	Health record Death certificate
Social context Contains social conditions and circumstances significant to healthcare Includes family and economic status, ethnic and religious heritage, and lifestyle and occupations	Economic status (*social concept*) Asian (*ethnic group*) Clerical supervisor (*occupation*) Donor (*person*) Thief (*lifestyle*) Judaism (*religion/philosophy*)
Situation with explicit context To represent medical information completely, it is sometimes necessary to attach additional information to a given concept. If this information changes the concept's meaning, it is known as context. This category contains concepts that carry context embedded within them.	No family history of stroke Nasal discharge present Suspected epilepsy
Staging and scales Contains concepts naming assessment scales and tumor staging systems	Glasgow coma scale (*assessment scale*) Alcohol use inventory (*assessment scale*) Dukes staging system (*tumor staging*)
SNOMED CT Model Component (metadata) Contains the link assertion and attribute subhierarchies	Has explanation (link assertion) IS_A (attribute) Associated morphology (attribute)
Pharmaceutical/biological product Contains drug products	Diazepam 5-mg tablet (product)
Qualifier value Contains concepts used as values for SNOMED CT attributes	Unilateral (qualifier value) Left (qualifier value) Puncture – action (qualifier value)
Special concept Concepts that have been retired, i.e., inactive, and concepts that exist only to support navigation	Erroneous concept (inactive concept) Oral administration of treatment (navigational concept)
Specimen Concepts that are obtained for examination or analysis	Urine specimen obtained by clean catch procedure (specimen) Calculus specimen (specimen)

Source: SNOMED International 2018g.

TABLE 6.5. Extension use case examples

Use Case	Examples
Translating SNOMED CT	Adding terms used in a local language or dialect Adding terms used by a specific user group such as patient-friendly terms
Configuring the terminology for specific use cases	Specifying pick lists to be used for data entry Specifying groups of components for reporting and analytics Linking components to clinical knowledge resources
Managing content gaps	Adding components that are missing in the International Edition Adding concepts that are only relevant to a local context
Mapping between SNOMED CT and other code systems	Representing maps between SNOMED CT concepts and ICD-10-CM codes
Extending the expressivity of SNOMED CT	Extending the concept model by introducing new attributes to meet specific data retrieval use cases

Source: SNOMED International 2018j.

The logical design of a SNOMED CT extension is technically consistent with that of the International Edition. Both represent and version SNOMED CT components and reference sets in release files that conform to release specifications. National and local extensions are managed by SNOMED International Members or Affiliates who have been issued a namespace identifier by SNOMED International (SNOMED International 2018j).

Components in extensions are identified using an item identifier of one to eight digits and a seven-digit namespace identifier. The namespace is a part of the **SNOMED CT Identifier (SCTID)** that is controlled by the organization that provides the extension identifier. In the SCTID for an extension component represented in figure 6.4, the partition identifier indicates that the SCTID is part of an Extension and the seven digits following the Extension item identifier are a **namespace identifier** that is allocated to the organization authorized to issue Extensions. The namespace identifier 1000124 is assigned to the NLM. The extension namespace ensures that SCTIDs do not collide with other SCTIDs and can be traced to an authorized originator. In

FIGURE 6.4. SCTID for the US national extension component

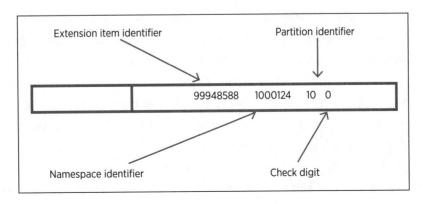

this manner, SNOMED CT extensions are fully integrated with the SNOMED CT International Release, avoiding the need for customized processing of local codes.

SNOMED CT Expressions

Redundancy within a terminology occurs when the same information can be expressed in two different ways. Using synonymous terms (for example, heart attack and myocardial infarction) represented with distinct description identifiers but a single concept identifier is one way in which SNOMED CT handles redundancy. Because SNOMED CT is so large and comprehensive, it is also possible to represent the same clinical issue with two different SNOMED CT concepts. For example, the concept for the disorder "angina" and the concept for the clinical finding of "ischemic chest pain" could be considered clinically equivalent depending upon the context.

SNOMED CT also allows for the **pre-coordination** and **post-coordination** of terms. Pre-coordination is often used to represent a commonly used clinical term as a single concept; post-coordination is when concept identifiers are combined to convey clinical meaning (SNOMED International 2016). For example, "fracture of tibia" can be expressed as either a pre-coordinated single concept identifier or as a combination of concept identifiers: bone structure of tibia and clinical finding fracture. A combination of pre-coordinated and post-coordinated concept identifiers is often used to facilitate the capture and representation of clinical documentation. In this manner, SNOMED CT can represent clinical phrases even when a single SNOMED CT concept does not capture the required level of detail. Pre-coordinated concepts are useful when representing issues commonly documented. Post-coordinated concepts allow for the detailed capture of less commonly reported clinical issues. Post-coordination greatly increases the depth of detail that SNOMED CT can represent without having to include every possible specific site for every possible disorder via a concept. For example, the 2017 release of SNOMED CT does not contain a concept that represents "laparoscopic removal of device from abdomen." However, it is possible to represent this clinical idea using the following post-coordinated expression.

68526006|removal of device from abdomen|:425391005|using access device|= 6174004|laparoscope|

It is important for users of SNOMED CT to be aware that there are multiple ways to express clinical ideas within the terminology and to manage the redundancy when developing EHR systems. The SNOMED CT concept model provides constraints for pre-coordinated and post-coordinated expressions for consistency across distributed SNOMED CT content. The logic on which the SNOMED CT concept model is based allows alternative representation of the same or similar information to be recognized and compared. The SNOMED CT Compositional Grammar specification and guide document (SNOMED International 2016) provides the syntax for representing SNOMED CT expressions that are both human readable and machine parsable. For example, the following two distinct representations can be computed to have the same meaning:

|pneumococcal pneumonia| refined by |finding site| |right upper lobe of lung|
|right upper lobe pneumonia| refined by |causative agent| |streptococcus pneumoniae|

Post-coordinated expressions may be created at run-time by selection of individual facets of a concept; for example, to indicate the nature and location of a fracture for a particular bone and, where relevant, whether the bone affected is on the right or left. Some applications generate post-coordinated expressions using natural language processing. Alternatively, post-coordinated expressions can be selected via a user interface where data entry options are tied to the expression. In these cases, the user may not be aware that the information is being captured in a post-coordinated form.

Principles and Guidelines

By the late 1990s, the limitations of existing schemes, based on terms organized with hierarchical codes, were well recognized. Several authors in the medical informatics community published papers laying out formal requirements for a new generation of healthcare terminologies designed for use in the EHR. Nearly 20 requirements in total are outlined in two key papers (Cimino 1998; Campbell et al. 1999). SNOMED RT and SNOMED CT were designed to be compliant with the principles laid out in these scientific papers, including principles for content, structure, and terminology management processes.

Concept Orientation and Permanence

Two of the key principles are **concept orientation**, which means concepts are based on meanings and not words, and **concept permanence**, which means that the identifiers that represent the concept are not reused and thus meanings do not change.

SNOMED CT allows the recording of data at the appropriate clinical level of detail. The user is not forced to record information at a level of detail that is either too general or too specific. As a guideline, it is preferable to record data at a more specific level if to do so is practical and consistent with clinical practice.

As mentioned earlier, every SNOMED CT concept has a unique numeric concept identifier. The concept identifier can be from 6 to 18 digits long and is computer readable. Concept identifiers are without embedded meaning and without digit restrictions. They are unique identifiers that will not change. This means that if a concept identifier is entered into a patient record, the meaning is futureproofed; if the knowledge about a concept changes, the meaning of the original concept identifier will not change. Instead, a concept identifier will be created for the changed concept.

The SNOMED CT Editorial Guide includes a style guide, which specifies, for example, acceptable abbreviations and punctuation, as well as authoring principles, specific guidelines, and criteria to determine whether new content should be added to SNOMED CT. General naming conventions specify that terms and names must be consistent, unambiguous, follow natural (or human) language when possible, and be clear for translation purposes. There is specific guidance for defining a **fully specified name (FSN)**, which is an unambiguous way to name a concept that also uniquely describes a concept and clarifies its meaning, versus a **preferred term (PT)** (SNOMED International 2018g). Not being a commonly used term or natural phrase, the FSN would not appear in the human-readable clinical record. However, the PT represents a common word or phrase used by clinicians to name a concept in clinical practice or in the literature. Only one of the available synonyms can be designated as preferred. The PT varies according to language and dialect, a description may be preferred in some dialects, acceptable in others, or not used in another (SNOMED International 2018g). Depending on the computer application, the PT may be the synonym selected for display, although each application is assumed to allow for independently determining the most appropriate display term for a given situation.

Example:

> FSN: | Pharyngectomy (procedure) |
>
> PT for the English language, US dialect: | Pharyngectomy |
>
> Synonym: | Excision of pharynx |
>
> Synonym: | Pharynx excision |

Interoperability

SNOMED CT is developed and maintained with the overarching goal of creating and sustaining semantic interoperability of clinical information. To support interoperability, SNOMED International has specified a standard SNOMED CT compositional grammar form that is both human readable and computer processable. Figure 6.5 provides an example to illustrate the SNOMED CT compositional grammar. The concept represented in figure 6.5 is a salpingo-oophorectomy, with laser excision of the right ovary and diathermy excision of the left fallopian tube. This is represented in a post-coordinated expression that is defined with a number of attribute groups. The grouping and the syntax make it possible to tell on which structure

FIGURE 6.5. Example of SNOMED CT compositional grammar

```
71388002 |procedure| :
{ 260686004 |method| = 129304002 |excision - action| ,
  405813007 |procedure site - direct| = 20837000 |structure of right ovary| ,
  424226004 |using device| = 122456005 |laser device| }
{ 260686004 |method| = 261519002 |diathermy excision - action| ,
  405813007 |procedure site - direct| = 113293009 |structure of left fallopian tube| }
```

Source: SNOMED International 2016.

the laser excision was used and on which structure the diathermy excision was used. If compositional grammar rules are followed, it is possible to compute similarities and subtype relationships between different expressions, which is key to effective meaning-based retrieval of post-coordinated expressions.

Three basic operational criteria also support semantic interoperability. The **Understandable, Reproducible, Useful (URU) principle** is followed by SNOMED CT modelers when assessing whether content is creating and sustaining semantic interoperability (SNOMED International 2018g). URU refers to:

- **U**nderstandable: The meaning must be able to be communicated in a manner that can be understood by an average healthcare provider without reference to inaccessible, hidden, or private meanings.
- **R**eproducible: It is not enough for one individual to say that he or she understands a meaning. It must be shown that multiple people understand and use the meaning in the same way.
- **U**seful: The meaning must have some demonstrable use or applicability to health or healthcare.

Referential integrity and conformity with editorial principles are important considerations in determining if a request for SNOMED CT additions or changes should be accepted for inclusion in any SNOMED CT edition. It is important to ensure that every addition of or modification to SNOMED CT concepts conform to the rules specified by the concept model.

Development and Maintenance

SNOMED CT is well maintained and updated in collaboration with subject matter experts to represent current clinical knowledge. The content of SNOMED CT evolves with each release. The types of changes made include new concepts, new descriptions, new relationships between concepts, and new reference sets, as well as updates and retirement of any of these components. Drivers of these changes include changes in understanding of health and disease processes; introduction of new drugs, investigations, therapies, and procedures; and new threats to health as well as proposals and work provided by SNOMED CT users. Content development is directed to address current and emerging priorities. The SNOMED CT development process incorporates the efforts of a team of terminologists, and a documented scientific process that focuses on the aforementioned URU principle is followed. Content is defined and reviewed by multiple editors, with additional experts consulted, as necessary, to review the scientific integrity of the content. The quality improvement process is open to public scrutiny and vendor input to ensure the terminology is truly useful within healthcare applications.

SNOMED International encourages a broad community of interested parties to participate openly in the collaborative developments that enhance the design of SNOMED CT and its content. Development efforts involve diverse clinical groups and medical informatics experts. The SNOMED CT Content Request Service (CRS) allows users to request new content as well as content changes to SNOMED CT (SNOMED International 2018k). This service is directly accessible by National Release Centers (NRC) in Member countries and recognized Terminology Authorities within organizations that are actively collaborating with SNOMED International. Organizations within Member countries can submit their requests for additions and changes to the NRC. In some cases, requests with particular local relevance may be added to a National Extension. The NRC forwards requests that it considers have international relevance to SNOMED International for a decision. If a request is deemed to have a high priority, it should result in action in the next release cycle. However, requests that require significant changes that would impact other content may take longer.

Though SNOMED CT is continuously updated to meet user needs, revisions to the International version of SNOMED CT are released twice a year on the 31st of January and the 31st of July. Each release includes updates to the SNOMED CT core (concepts, descriptions, and relationships) as well as derivative works and related documentation. Updates are driven by user requirements based on priorities set by SNOMED International with input from advisory bodies and guidance from the Content Committee. The Extensions may be released at the same time as the International Edition but in some cases are released on different dates and at different intervals.

Governance Structure

SNOMED International, the trading name of IHTSDO, is an association governed by a **General Assembly**. As of October, 2018, SNOMED International had 35 Members spanning five continents. Members can be either an agency of a national government or another body endorsed by an appropriate national government authority within the country it represents. Members pay a license fee, which varies based on national wealth, to SNOMED International. The governance structure is outlined in figure 6.6. The General Assembly is the highest authority in SNOMED International. It is responsible for "assuring that the purpose, objects and principles of the association are pursued and that the interests of SNOMED International are safeguarded" (SNOMED International 2017a, 60). The general assembly is made up of a representative from each of the Member countries. Each Member country has one nominated representative, who has one vote in the general assembly.

The general assembly turns over the management responsibilities of the organization to the **Management Board**. The Management Board is a much smaller group; it was reduced from 10 to 7 voting Members in 2017. Members have the opportunity to nominate delegates to the Management Board. The Management Board directs the association and has the responsibility for strategic direction and key business decisions. The Management Board also appoints the Chief Executive Officer (CEO), who has the day-to-day responsibility for running the organization.

Each Member country is also entitled to choose a representative to the Member Forum. The Member Forum acts as an advisory body to the Management Board. The Member Forum is a conduit for communication to and from Member countries. For example, the Member Forum facilitates contact between countries with similar needs and priorities for SNOMED CT content. The Member Forum can also raise issues of concern to the Management Board and is asked by the Management Board to provide feedback on specific items. The vendor liaison forum likewise is an advisory body to the Management Board. The vendor forum is made up of experts who utilize SNOMED CT in vendor applications. The purpose of this forum is to advise on ways to facilitate use of SNOMED CT in vendor applications.

As part of its commitment to an open terminology development process, SNOMED International provides a collaborative working space and sponsors additional advisory bodies,

FIGURE 6.6. Governance

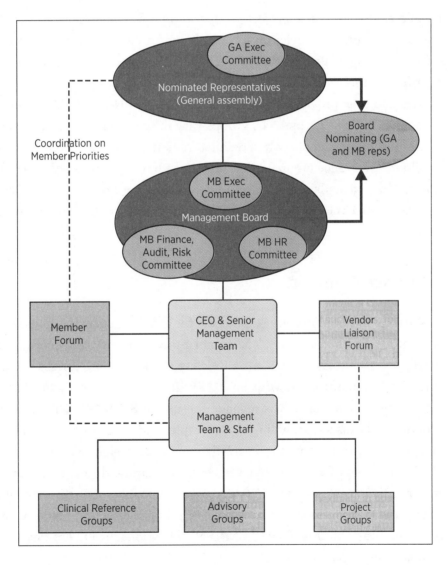

Source: SNOMED International 2017a, 59.

TABLE 6.6. Examples of project and clinical reference groups

Project Groups	Clinical Reference Groups
Cancer Synoptic Reporting Project Group Nutrition Care Process Terminology Clinical Project Group Diabetes Project Group	Anesthesia Dentistry Emergency Medicine General Practice/Family Practice Mapping Medical Devices Nursing Pathology and Laboratory Medicine Pharmacy

Source: SNOMED International 2018l.

including multiple advisory groups, project groups, and clinical reference groups. The role of each advisory group is to provide advice on specific defined areas. Project groups are of a limited duration and focus on a particular task and project plan. These are open to participation and are resourced according to the project needs. Clinical reference groups are focused on delineated clinical specialties and they provide clinical input to support SNOMED CT development. See table 6.6 for examples of these groups. The groups vary in scope, ranging from providing input about the direction of the terminology to a detailed review of specific nomenclature domains. For example, a clinical reference group (such as nursing, pharmacy, or anesthesia) may focus on information needs for a particular clinical area and provide advice on the scope of coverage, the creation of hierarchies, semantic structure, and scientific accuracy of the content for the purpose specified.

National Release Centres

Members of SNOMED International are responsible for distributing, extending and supporting the use of SNOMED CT in their country. The organization or agency that coordinates this role in each country is referred to as the **National Release Center (NRC)**. NRCs provide a single point of contact for communications with SNOMED International and other Member countries. Within their own countries, NRCs manage the use of SNOMED CT and communicate with stakeholders and licensees, including, for example, end users in healthcare institutions. The NRC is responsible for customizing, specializing, and releasing the terminology for each country. Clinical terminology has many things in common worldwide, but also some things that are unique and specific to each country. SNOMED International is structured to allow cooperation and collaboration on an international scale, including interaction between the different national release centers as well as feedback from local and national health entities, and yet allows for specializations to meet specific needs.

The NLM is the US Member of SNOMED International and, as such, is the NRC that distributes SNOMED CT at no cost in accordance with the Member rights and responsibilities outlined by SNOMED International. Licensees of the Unified Medical Language System (UMLS) Metathesaurus have access to SNOMED CT as part of the UMLS Metathesaurus, where it is linked to many other biomedical terminologies and natural language processing tools (NLM 2018b). Additionally, UMLS licensees have free access to SNOMED CT in its native file formats, downloadable directly from the UMLS terminology services (UMLS 2018).

Versioning and History Tracking

Updates deliver important benefits for users, but changes also create challenges. SNOMED CT provides a robust versioning mechanism that allows historically consistent views of all earlier versions from a single full release file. Release file specifications delineate common features of all release files as well as naming conventions for release packages and files (SNOMED International 2018h). A specific file format is defined to document both component release file specifications and reference set release file specifications. This means, in a given release, new concepts, new descriptions, new relationships between concepts, and new reference sets, as well as updates and retirement of any of these components, are specifically identified consistent with the required structure for all release files. The same file formats are used for SNOMED CT extensions. For example, the file format specifications for concepts include an effective time field that specifies the date (time) that the concept was changed or addressed in the released version. It also includes an "active" field that specifies whether the concept was made active or inactive at the date specified in the effective time field. Similar fields are used for relationships and the like, thus providing an elegant mechanism to track explicit changes in each version.

Different release types are provided to facilitate installation and updates of SNOMED CT in computer applications. A full release contains every version of every component that has ever been released prior to or in the current edition. This release provides the complete history of every component of SNOMED CT at any time since its first release. These files are extremely large, with only a small portion representing an actual change in the current edition. In contrast, a delta release includes only those components that have been changed in some manner (such as created or inactivated) since the previous release. This is a much smaller file and is useful to update an application. Lastly, a snapshot release contains the most recent version of every component released up to the time of the snapshot. The snapshot release is useful for a simple installation but does not provide a history of the components. Each release type is useful and every SNOMED CT International edition includes all three release types to allow users to choose the most appropriate release type for their particular use case. Extensions are available as a full release and may be available in other release types.

Relationship with Other Terminologies, Classification Systems, and Code Sets

SNOMED International actively collaborates with other standards development organizations to facilitate the use of SNOMED CT with other terminology and classification systems. These efforts include both mapping and aligning content development with other standards to enhance consistency in meaningful data capture and information exchange. SNOMED International has multiple well-defined relationships with other organizations (SNOMED International 2018m).

One such collaborative relationship exists between SNOMED International and the World Health Organization (WHO). The two organizations worked together to harmonize SNOMED CT and ICD-11. The collaboration was undertaken to create a common ontology so that clinicians globally can use SNOMED CT in the electronic record for clinical information and users can then link to ICD-11 for information related to mortality and morbidity, billing, public health, epidemiology, and so on. Despite the fact that the basic architecture of a classification such as the WHO's ICD is very different from a terminology such as SNOMED CT, the goal was to ensure that they are "synergistic and not antagonistic" to make it easier to use them together (Ustun et al. 2015). The project involved developing a harmonization process and testing it on a named subset from the ICD-11 Foundation. See chapter 7 on ICD-11 for more information. Participants in the project determined that the semantic alignment of SNOMED CT with the ICD-11 classification to support computable semantic interoperation, while possible, requires further work. SNOMED International and WHO continue to collaborate but no further work is being done on the common ontology.

A cooperative agreement also exists between the developers of Logical Observation Identifiers Names and Codes (LOINC), maintained by the Regenstrief Institute Inc., and SNOMED International. They are working together to limit duplication of effort and focus limited resources on enhancements that serve the practical needs of the growing number of users of LOINC and SNOMED CT (SNOMED International 2018m). LOINC has a strong focus on laboratory medicine test order and result reporting, while SNOMED CT has a broad coverage of medical concepts. Linking the two, and minimizing duplication between them, will ensure they work better together so that users can query various lab tests and parts of tests in LOINC in a novel way based on SNOMED CT's robust hierarchies and definitions. In general, LOINC is used to represent the observation being collected (the "question") and SNOMED CT is used for the observation value (the "answer"). The organizations are working together to create and maintain a detailed map of the over 45,000 laboratory LOINC terms to SNOMED CT (SNOMED International 2018m).

Additional examples of the collaborative relationship between SNOMED CT and other terminologies include SNOMED International's partnerships with the International Council of Nurses (ICN) and the American Medical Association (AMA). ICN and SNOMED International developed, and continue to maintain, equivalence tables between the International Classification of Nursing Practice (ICNP) and SNOMED CT for both nursing diagnoses and nursing interventions (SNOMED International 2018m). The AMA and SNOMED International also have a collaborative agreement to coordinate on the design and development of Current Procedural Terminology (CPT) products and SNOMED CT products. They are working together to share tools and expertise related to the development and maintenance of their respective standards with the mutual goal to improve current content to better support existing and emerging uses of health data (SNOMED International 2018m). These harmonization efforts and collaborative activities facilitate adoption and use of SNOMED CT.

Tools to Access and Use

SNOMED International provides a number of tools and services that are made available to the public and have been developed within the **Open Tooling Framework (OTF)** (SNOMED International 2018n). The OTF is an open framework that provides tools for the SNOMED CT community. It includes standardized application programming interfaces (APIs) that provide fundamental software services for business applications.

Open Tooling Framework Modules

The OTF includes core modules, plugin modules, and infrastructure modules, which collectively provide functionality that underpins terminology business functions. The core modules are the foundation of the OTF and include the following:

- Terminology Query Module: used to query official releases of SNOMED CT
- Terminology Editing Module: used to store changes made during the editing process
- Identifier Management Module: used to look up an SCTID, or an array of SCTIDs
- Release Process Module: used to release a version of the terminology, or an extension
- Refset Services Module: used for the storage and back-end processing of reference sets

Plugin modules represent a specific set of business use cases. An example of a plugin module is the Mapping Module, which provides the functionality to allow users to produce complex maps between SNOMED CT and other terminologies. There are at least a half-dozen plugin modules in production, with still more in development.

Infrastructure modules are not necessarily specific to the terminology domain and are used for much more generic purposes. For example, the workflow module is used by an organization to implement a customized workflow that meets its specific needs. The user administration infrastructure module allows role-based access controls to enable a collaborative environment. These tools and applications support the SNOMED CT production life cycle as well as the systems that are used to support SNOMED International, its Members, and the community of practice.

Subsets of SNOMED CT, developed for specific uses, are tools that help in the uptake and use of SNOMED CT. Examples described below include the CORE Problem List subset, the Nursing Problem List subset, and the Route of Administration subset.

CORE Problem List Subset

A subset developed by the clinical observations recording and encoding (CORE) project identifies concepts most useful for documentation and encoding of clinical information at the summary level. The CORE Problem List Subset includes SNOMED CT concepts and codes that can be used for the problem list, discharge diagnoses, or reason for encounter. The original subset, released in 2009, was based on datasets collected from large healthcare institutions that utilize controlled vocabularies for data entry. Concepts in the subset were selected based on their actual frequency of usage in clinical databases. The subset has been maintained and released each year since 2009, with the August 2018 release derived from the SNOMED CT July 2018 version, for example (NLM 2018c).

Nursing Problem List Subset

The nursing problem list subset is intended to facilitate the use of SNOMED CT as the primary coding terminology for nursing problems used in care planning or other summary level nursing documentation. Spearheaded by the IHTSDO Nursing Work Group Problem List Project Team, this subset was first released with the April 2011 version. The August 2017 version includes 673 SNOMED CT concepts (NLM 2017a).

Route of Administration Subset

The Route of Administration subset is a listing of the current set of SNOMED CT terms related to the location of administration for clinical therapeutics. This subset includes SNOMED CT terms used in the Drug Listing section of Structured Product Labeling (SPL). The SPL is a document markup standard approved by Health Level Seven (HL7) and adopted by the FDA as a mechanism for exchanging product and facility information. It also defines a SNOMED CT subset for documentation and encoding of clinical information regarding substance administrations (NLM 2017b).

SNOMED CT Browsers

A range of online and offline SNOMED CT browsers are available to explore and search SNOMED CT content. SNOMED International provides an online browser that is available to anyone for reference purposes (SNOMED International 2018o). This browser is designed to be compatible with Internet Explorer and includes access to the International Edition as well as a variety of local Extensions, such as Australian, Belgian, Canadian, Danish, Netherlands, Swedish, United Kingdom, United States, and Uruguay. Various third parties have also developed websites or applications that allow a person to view the content of SNOMED CT (SNOMED International 2018p). For example, the NLM free online browser provides a mechanism to search for and display SNOMED CT content that is included in the UMLS Metathesaurus (UMLS 2018). The user can expand searches to include synonymous terms from over 100 Metathesaurus vocabulary sources. SNOMED CT browsers are not designed or licensed for use in EHRs or any other production systems, but they are extremely useful to explore SNOMED CT content.

Adoption and Use Cases

Good information is essential for effective health and healthcare. The safe and appropriate exchange of clinical information is necessary to ensure continuity of care for patients across different times, settings, and providers. Today's health information systems include functions to allow for collection of a variety of clinical information, linked to clinical knowledge bases, information retrieval, data aggregation, analyses, exchange, and other functions. SNOMED CT provides a standards-based foundation for these functions. Information systems can use the concepts, hierarchies, and relationships as a common reference point. Furthermore, specific applications can focus on a restricted set of SNOMED CT concepts, such as those related to ophthalmology. These RefSets can be used to present relevant parts of the terminology, depending on the clinical context and local requirements. This means that a drop-down list to select diagnoses in an electronic health record in a mental health facility can be tailored to that setting. Similarly, RefSets can be developed to provide appropriate medication lists for nurses in community care.

Users of SNOMED CT might include:

- Clinicians (end users of EHRs)
- Software designers, system developers who incorporate SNOMED CT into the application
- Vendors and suppliers of software systems
- System implementers (provider organizations)
- Healthcare professionals who want to influence the terminology to represent their field
- Governments and other policymakers who see the need to specify what kind of information they are interested in collecting through a standardized terminology
- Researchers who want to collect data

In short, SNOMED CT adds processable meaning to an EHR, thus enabling effective, meaningful representation of clinical information. As a result, it plays a pivotal role in worldwide endeavors to deliver cost-effective, high-quality healthcare.

SNOMED CT has been implemented in a variety of ways that differ in the extent to which they harness particular features of the terminology. Some of the most common uses of SNOMED CT in healthcare include capturing processable clinical information, real-time decision support, ranging from simple flagging of contraindications to presenting guidelines, batch-mode decision support, including identifying chronic diseases or risk factors that require intervention, and meaning-based retrieval and reuse of clinical information, thereby enabling interoperability.

An example of clinical decision support is the use of alerts to identify specific clinical contraindications in the administration of thrombocytopenia therapy after a stroke. In this example, the hierarchies of SNOMED CT enable complex reasoning to support the defined decision support rule. The SNOMED CT concept |stroke| is synonymous with |cerebrovascular accident| and subsumes all lower-level concepts including |paralytic stroke|, |thrombotic stroke|, and the like. This means that decision support queries are easier to develop and implement because they do not need to identify all the individual terms and codes that may be relevant. SNOMED CT is used for clinical decision support in a number of organizations including Kaiser Permanente and the Duke University Medical Hospital. Kaiser Permanente also uses SNOMED CT to identify potential cohorts for clinical trials (SNOMED International 2017a, 42).

SNOMED International hosts a website to capture and share information on how SNOMED CT is used around the world (SNOMED International 2018q). The website provides a mechanism to register a specific SNOMED CT deployment as well as search functionality to find out where SNOMED is used. For example, in the United States, SNOMED CT is imbedded in problem lists in the EHR, enabling sharing of standardized problems across different healthcare settings. It is also used in EHR templates for hospital-based emergency surgical care, making the templates more efficient based on the fewest, most precise SNOMED CT terms.

SNOMED CT is one of a suite of designated standards for use in US federal government systems for the electronic exchange of clinical health information. It was named a required standard in the interoperability specifications by the Health Information Technology Standards Panel (HITSP). HITSP explicitly named SNOMED CT as an industry-standard vocabulary for the meaningful use Medicare and Medicaid EHR incentive programs. The capabilities matrix, from the HIT Policy Committee and HIT Standards Committee for meaningful use measures and standards, identified SNOMED CT more often than any other vocabulary standard (HITSP 2011). Examples of clinical content where SNOMED CT was the HITSP standard include:

- Clinical problem, diagnosis and condition
- Symptom
- Encounter, intervention, and procedure
- Substance
- Device
- Laboratory and diagnostic study test result

The Meaningful Use Stage 2 final rule defined a Common Meaningful Use Data Set for all summary of care records, including an impressive array of structured and coded data to be formatted uniformly and sent securely during transitions of care, upon discharge, and to be shared with the patients themselves. SNOMED CT was named as the standard for several of the items in the data set.

Currently, SNOMED CT remains one of the standards specified in the Common Clinical Data Set (CCDS). For example, smoking status must be coded using one of the eight specified SNOMED CT codes (ONC 2018a). SNOMED CT is also named as the standard to represent problems and is one of the standards that may be used to represent procedures. Thus, ONC adopted SNOMED CT as a standard for the entry of structured data in certified electronic health record systems. The ONC 2018 Interoperability standards advisory (ISA) process identifies SNOMED CT as the standard for multiple specific interoperability standards and implementation specifications, including, for example, representing patient allergies, intolerances, and allergic reactions, as well as representing patient medical encounter diagnoses (ONC 2018b).

Use Case One: Capturing and Reporting Smoking Status

The *ONC HIT Standard, Implementation Specifications, and Certification Criteria for EHR Technology*, 2015 edition includes certification criteria to both create and receive the Common Clinical Data Set Summary record (ONC 2018c). The CCDS requires that the patient's smoking status be included and coded in one of eight specified SNOMED CT codes (ONC 2018a). The 2014 test procedure for smoking status evaluated the capability of an EHR to enable a user to electronically record, change, and access the smoking status of a patient using SNOMED CT codes. With the 2015 edition, the criterion was essentially unchanged since the CCDS requires exchange of smoking status using the same SNOMED CT codes. The eight SNOMED CT concept codes listed below are the specified standard.

Description	SNOMED CT ID
Current every day smoker	449868002
Current some day smoker	428041000124106
Former smoker	8517006
Never smoker	266919005
Smoker, current status unknown	77176002
Unknown if ever smoked	266927001
Heavy tobacco smoker	428071000124103
Light tobacco smoker	428061000124105

An EHR vendor seeking certification must successfully create and receive the CCDS reflecting smoking status. Therefore, the EHR functionality must be able to:

- Electronically record patient smoking status
- Electronically change patient smoking status
- Electronically access patient smoking status

One of the meaningful use core measures for both eligible professionals and hospital and critical care hospitals under meaningful use stage 2 was that smoking status be recorded as structured data for more than 80 percent of all unique patients 13 years old or older. More recently, under the merit-based incentive payment system (MIPS), healthcare providers who want to qualify for the Medicare EHR incentive program (meaningful use) will use the functionality in a certified EHR system to electronically record, change, and access the smoking status of their patients (ONC 2017).

Use Case Two: Enabling Clinical Decision Support

A public health agency wants to ensure widespread vaccination for influenza and defines criteria for who should, or should not, receive the vaccine. One of the criteria, for example, is that those with heart disease are at higher risk and therefore should receive the vaccine.

A physician group wants to send a vaccination reminder to all of its patients with heart disease. The problem is that the health record will identify these individuals differently, not necessarily stating "heart disease." Some records might say, for example, "coronary arteriosclerosis," in which case the computer would not recognize these patients as having a heart disease. The physician group might attempt to identify patients using reimbursement classification codes, but that would require manually selecting every code in the classification that might be considered a heart disease. This would be a lengthy list of codes and leaves significant room for error.

However, this physician group has SNOMED CT embedded in the electronic health record; therefore, the decision support program can employ a logic-based search to retrieve all patients with a SNOMED CT concept code that has an | is a | relationship to heart disease. The concept in the patient record may be very granular (coronary arteriosclerosis in native artery) or much less specific (coronary sclerosis) but will be retrieved regardless based on the definitional relationship to heart disease. This search will generate a patient list for vaccine reminders. Thus, SNOMED CT provides an automated way to identify all the patients in the practice who have a type of heart disease and need a vaccine this year.

CHECK YOUR UNDERSTANDING

1. Fill in the blank. _____ is when a combination of concept identifiers are joined to convey clinical meaning.

2. True or false? SNOMED CT was specifically designed to capture and organize clinical information for use in the electronic health record environment.

   a. True
   b. False

3. True or false? Pre-coordinated concepts are most useful for capturing less commonly reported clinical issues with greater detail.

   a. True
   b. False

4. Because of its tremendous amount of content, SNOMED CT is a poor choice for what function?

   a. Reimbursement
   b. Medical research
   c. Application in the EHR environment
   d. Documentation of clinical concepts

5. The URU principle requires that all SNOMED CT concepts be:

   a. Uniform, reproducible, useful
   b. Understandable, relevant, uniform
   c. Understandable, reproducible, useful
   d. Understandable, reproducible, uniform

REVIEW

1. What are the main SNOMED CT components?

   a. Attributes, concepts, and codes
   b. Codes, concepts, and hierarchies
   c. Concepts, descriptions, and relationships
   d. Descriptions, relationships, and identifiers

2. Which of the following is *not* a derivative work?

   a. Extensions
   b. RefSets
   c. Cross maps
   d. Hierarchies

3. A motor vehicle accident is an example from which SNOMED CT hierarchy?

   a. Physical force
   b. Event
   c. Context-dependent category
   d. Observable entity

4. True or false? Every SNOMED CT concept has at least one relationship to another concept.

   a. True
   b. False

5. Which of the following is *not* an example from the hierarchy "social context"?

   a. Economic status
   b. Gender
   c. Occupation
   d. Ethnic group

6. True or false? SNOMED CT and the WHO's ICD-11 are fully harmonized.

   a. True
   b. False

7. Which of the following is the unique text assigned to a concept in SNOMED CT that completely describes that concept?

   a. Standard phrase
   b. Fully specified name
   c. Common description
   d. Unique identifier

8. SNOMED CT is a designated standard for all of the following but one. Which of the following does NOT include SNOMED CT as a standard?

   a. HIPAA transaction code sets
   b. HITSP interoperability specifications

    c. ONC EHR certification standards

    d. US federal government for electronic exchange of health information

9. True or false? Every concept except the root concept in SNOMED CT is related by at least one | is a |relationship.

    a. True

    b. False

10. SNOMED CT | is a | relationships serve what purpose?

    a. To further define the concept

    b. To provide a pointer from a concept that is no longer active

    c. To give additional attributes about the concept

    d. All of the above

References

Campbell, J. R., P. Carpenter, C. Sneiderman, S. Cohn, C. G. Chute, and J. Warren. 1997. Phase II evaluation of clinical coding schemes: Completeness, taxonomy, mapping, definitions, and clarity. *Journal of American Medical Informatics Association* 4:238–251.

Campbell, K. E., B. Hochhalter, J. Slaughter, and J. Mattison. 1999 (December). Enterprise issues pertaining to implementing controlled terminologies. IMIA WG 6 Conference, Phoenix, AZ.

Chute, C., et al. 1994 (April 26). Multi-institutional test bed for clinical vocabulary. Grant application to U.S. Department of Health and Human Services.

Chute, C. G., S. P. Cohn, K. E. Campbell, D. E. Oliver, and J. R. Campbell. 1996. The content coverage of clinical classifications. *Journal of the American Medical Informatics Association* 3:224–233.

Cimino, J. J. 1998. Desiderata for controlled medical vocabularies in the 21st century. *Methods of Information in Medicine* 37(4–5):394–403.

Fung, K. W., J. Xu, F. Ameye, A. R. Gutierrez, and A. D'Have. 2017. Achieving logical equivalence between SNOMED CT and ICD-10-PCS surgical procedures. *AMIA Annual Symposium Proceedings* 2017:724-733. eCollection PMID: 29854138. Published online 2018 (Apr 16).

HITSP. 2011. Recommendations from the HIT Policy Committee and HIT Standards Committee for Meaningful Use Measures and Standards. HITSP Capabilities Matrix. http://publicaa.ansi.org/sites/apdl/hitspadmin/Matrices/HITSP_09_N_448_2011.pdf.

National Library of Medicine (NLM). 2018a (March). SNOMED CT to ICD-10-CM Map https://www.nlm.nih.gov/research/umls/mapping_projects/snomedct_to_icd10cm.html

National Library of Medicine (NLM). 2018b (September). SNOMED CT United States edition https://www.nlm.nih.gov/healthit/snomedct/us_edition.html.

National Library of Medicine (NLM). 2018c (June). The CORE Problem List Subset of SNOMED CT. https://www.nlm.nih.gov/research/umls/Snomed/core_subset.html

National Library of Medicine (NLM). 2017a (December). Nursing Problem List Subset of SNOMED CT. https://www.nlm.nih.gov/research/umls/Snomed/nursing_problemlist_subset.html.

National Library of Medicine (NLM). 2017b (January). SNOMED CT Route of Administration Subset. https://www.nlm.nih.gov/research/umls/Snomed/roa_subset.html.

Office of National Coordinator for Health Information Technology (ONC). 2018a. 2015 edition Common Clinical Data Set (CCDS) Reference Document. https://www.healthit.gov/sites/default/files/ccds_reference_document_v1_1.pdf.

Office of National Coordinator for Health Information Technology (ONC). 2018b. 2018 Interoperability Standards Advisory. https://www.healthit.gov/isa/sites/isa/files/2018%20ISA%20Reference%20Edition.pdf.

Office of National Coordinator for Health Information Technology (ONC). 2018c. 2015 Edition Test method. https://www.healthit.gov/topic/certification-ehrs/2015-edition-test-method.

Office of National Coordinator for Health Information Technology (ONC). 2017. Meaningful Use. https://www.healthit.gov/topic/federal-incentive-programs/meaningful-use.

Office of the National Coordinator for Health Information Technology (ONC). 2015. 2015 Edition Health Information Technology (Health IT) Certification Criteria, 2015 Edition Base Electronic Health Record (EHR) Definition, and ONC Health IT Certification Program Modifications. https://www.federalregister.gov/documents/2015/10/16/2015-25597/2015-edition-health-information-technology-health-it-certification-criteria-2015-edition-base

SNOMED International. 2019. 5-Step briefing. https://www.snomed.org/snomed-ct/five-step-briefing.

SNOMED International. 2018a. What is SNOMED CT? https://www.snomed.org/snomed-ct/what-is-snomed-ct

SNOMED International. 2018b. https://www.snomed.org/snomed-ct.

SNOMED International. 2018c. IHTSDO adopts trading name of SNOMED International. https://confluence.ihtsdotools.org/display/ILS/2017/01/04/IHTSDO+Adopts+Trading+Name+of+SNOMED+International

SNOMED International. 2018d. SCT Worldwide. https://www.snomed.org/snomed-ct/snomed-ct-worldwide.

SNOMED International. 2018e. Technical Implementation Guide. https://confluence.ihtsdotools.org/display/DOCTIG/3.1.3.+Relationships

SNOMED International. 2018f. SNOMED CT Starter Set Translation package alpha Release Notes–March 2018. https://confluence.ihtsdotools.org/display/RMT/SNOMED+CT+Starter+Set+Translation+package+Alpha+Release+Notes+-+March+2018#SNOMEDCTStarterSetTranslationpackageAlphaReleaseNotes-March2018-2Background

SNOMED International. 2018g. SNOMED CT Editorial Guide. https://confluence.ihtsdotools.org/display/DOCEG/2.4.1.1+Body+Structure+Attributes+Summary

SNOMED International. 2018h. SNOMED CT Release File Specifications. https://confluence.ihtsdotools.org/display/DOCRELFMT/5.2.9+Simple+Map+Reference+Set

SNOMED International. 2018i. SNOMED CT Document Library. https://confluence.ihtsdotools.org/display/DOC/Guides

SNOMED International. 2018j. SNOMED CT Extensions Practical Guide. https://confluence.ihtsdotools.org/display/DOCEXTPG/1+Executive+Summary

SNOMED International. 2018k. SNOMED CT Content Request Service Guidance Documents. https://confluence.ihtsdotools.org/display/SCTCR/CRS+Guidance+Documents

SNOMED International. 2018l. Clinical Engagement. Directory–Clinical Reference Groups. https://confluence.ihtsdotools.org/display/CP/Directory+-+Clinical+Reference+Groups

SNOMED International. 2018m. Our Partners. https://www.snomed.org/snomed-international/our-partners

SNOMED International. 2018n. SNOMED International Open Tooling Framework. https://ihtsdo.github.io/index.html

SNOMED International. 2018o. SNOMED CT Browser for Internet Explorer Compatibility. http://browser.ihtsdotools.org/index-ie.html

SNOMED International. 2018p. Document Library. SNOMED CT Browsers. https://confluence.ihtsdotools.org/display/DOC/SNOMED+CT+Browsers+-+Downloadable

SNOMED International. 2018q. SNOMED in Action https://www.snomedinaction.org/

SNOMED International. 2017a. SNOMED CT Starter Guide. https://confluence.ihtsdotools.org/display/DOCSTART?preview=/28742871/47677485/doc_StarterGuide_Current-en-US_INT_20170728.pdf

SNOMED International. 2017b. Practical Guide to Reference Sets. https://confluence.ihtsdotools.org/display/DOCRFSPG/5.1.+Simple+Reference+Set

SNOMED International. 2016. SNOMED CT Compositional Grammar Specification and Guide v2.3.1. https://confluence.ihtsdotools.org/display/DOCSCG

Unified Medical Language System (UMLS). 2018. UMLS Terminology Services. https://uts.nlm.nih.gov/home.html.

Ustun, B., J. Case, C. Chute, A. Rector, J Campbell, and H. Solbrig. 2015 (November). "Experience in harmonization of ICD-11 and SNOMED CT: Not just mapping." Presented at AMIA 2015 Annual Symposium, San Francisco, CA.

Resources

Al-Hablani, B. 2017 (Winter). The use of automated SNOMED CT clinical coding in clinical decision support systems for preventative care. *Perspectives in Health Information Management*: 14.

Bronnert, J., J. Daube, G. Joop, K. Peterson, T. Rihanek, R. Scichilone, and V. Tucker. 2014. Optimizing data representation through the use of SNOMED CT. *Journal of AHIMA* 85(3):48–50.

Ceusters, W. and J. P. Bona. 2017. Analyzing SNOMED CT's historical data: Pitfalls and possibilities. *AMIA Annual Symposium Proceedings*, pp. 361–370. eCollection 2016. PMID: 28269831

Cornet, R. and N. deKreizer. 2008. Forty years of SNOMED: A literature review. *BMC Medical Informatics and Decision Making* 8(Suppl):S2.

Fung K. W. and J. Xu. 2015. An exploration of the properties of the CORE problem list subset and how it facilitates the implementation of SNOMED CT. *Journal of the American Medical Informatics Association* 22(3):649–658. doi: 10.1093/jamia/ocu022. Epub 2015 Feb 26. PMID: 25725003.

Khorrami, F., M. Ahmadi, and A. Sheikhtaheri. 2018. Evaluation of SNOMED CT content voverage: A systematic literature review. *Studies in Health Technology and Informatics* 248:212–219. PMID: 29726439

Koopman, B., P. Bruza, L. Sitbon, and M. Lawley. 2012. Towards semantic search and inference in electronic medical records: An approach using concept-based information retrieval. *Australasian Medical Journal.* 5(9):482–488.

Lee, D., N. de Kelzer, F. Lau, and R. Cornet. 2013. Literature review of SNOMED CT use. *Journal of American Medical Informatics Association* 0:1–9.

Nandigam, H. and M. 2016 (July). Topaz. Mapping Systematized Nomenclature of Medicine--Clinical Terms (SNOME CT) to International Classification of Diseases, Tenth Revision, Clinical Modification (ICD-10-CM): Lessons learned from applying the National Library of Medicine's mappings. *Perspectives in Health Information Management.*

Rodrigues J. M., D. Robinson, V. Della Mea, J. Campbell, A. Rector, S. Schulz, H. Brear, B., et al. 2015. Semantic alignment between ICD-11 and SNOMED CT. *Studies in Health Technology and Informatics* 216:790–794. PMID: 26262160.

Stearns, M. and J. C. Fuller. 2014. What's the difference? SNOMED CT and ICD systems are suited for different purposes. *Journal of AHIMA* 85(11):70–72.

Wei, D., H. Gu, Y. Perl, M. Halper, C. Ochs, G. Elhanan, and Y. Chen. 2015. Structural measures to track the evolution of SNOMED CT hierarchies. *Journal of Biomedical Informatics* 57:278–287. doi: 10.1016/j.jbi.2015.08.001. Epub 2015 (August 7).

7

ICD-11 Overview

Christopher G. Chute, MD, DrPH

LEARNING OBJECTIVES

- Explain the purpose and characteristics of ICD-11
- Outline the approach to developing ICD-11
- Discuss how ICD-11 may be used
- Examine the relationship ICD-11 has with other classifications, terminologies, and code sets
- Compare tools available to access and use
- Demonstrate how ICD-11 is used in an electronic environment

KEY TERMS

- Common Ontology
- Content model
- Exhaustive
- Foundation Component
- ICD-11 for Morbidity and Mortality Statistics (ICD-11-MMS)
- ICD-11-MMS Reference Guide
- Linearizations
- Mutually exclusive
- Uniform Resource Identifiers (URIs)

Introduction to ICD-11

This chapter outlines the purposes and some of the innovations of the June 2018 revision of the International Classification of Diseases, 11th Revision (ICD-11) (WHO 2018a). The shape and form of the revision has been in development for more than a decade and, with its release for implementation, it will be finalized. This chapter describes some of its distinguishing features and new innovations. While the scaffolding that supports ICD-11 is radically different from historical versions, incorporating modern computer science notions of knowledge organization and linkages, the "tabular" derivatives are familiar to users of legacy ICD revisions.

The US healthcare system adopted ICD-10-CM (the American Clinical Modification of the World Health Organization's (WHO) base International Classification of Diseases ICD-10) in October 2015. Thus, to an American audience, it may seem odd to raise the topic of ICD-11. From a global perspective, ICD-10 was released in 1990, when an expectation and pattern of decennial updates to the venerable ICD had long been established. While many commentaries on the timing of the US transition have appeared, refreshing the core ICD system as published by WHO (ICD-11) is overdue (Chute et al. 2012).

Developer

The ICD-11 development process was deliberately inclusive and broadly based. The core development group includes over a score of clinical topic advisory groups, each comprising 10 to 20 international experts in the disease or domain area. These domain groups were partnered with groups with deep coding expertise, focusing on pediatric adoptions, morbidity, mortality, and functioning issues associated with creating robust and resilient classifications. All of these teams were supported by an informatics advisory group that brought modern principles of computer science and ontology development to the ICD table, including sophisticated tooling and tracking resources, to make ICD-11 a truly 21st century information resource coupled to a correspondingly modern development process.

An extended beta phase engaged broad-based review of the draft artifact by an even wider circle of domain experts, field trials, stability analyses for longitudinal consistency, and public review and comment on an open ICD-11 browser web resource.

Purposes of the ICD

The historical application of ICD has been for the statistical tabulation of mortality and, later, morbidity. As a statistical classification, the requirement that the system be **mutually exclusive** (events cannot occur at the same time to avoid double-counting them) and **exhaustive** (every condition has a place to be coded, even if that is a residual category, such as "other specified") has defined ICD's architecture as a strict hierarchy, where every concept has one and only one parent.

Beyond these traditional roles, mutually exclusive and exhaustive classifications of disease find usefulness in clinical data aggregation for quality, research, patient safety, and reimbursement.

Historically, the ICD has not clearly defined the meaning of its rubrics, publishing little more than a title, a code, and some inclusion terms to provide scope and nuanced implications. The accompanying index does detail which terms should be explicitly coded where, though this is definition by inference. ICD-11 aspires to include clinical criteria for each rubric, in addition to formal text definitions and fully specified names. These criteria, as discussed later in the chapter, will form the basis for phenotyping logics that may ultimately inform automated classification logic and software (Jiang et al. 2015; Li et al. 2013; Mo et al. 2015; Newton et al. 2013; Pathak et al. 2013).

Content and Structure

WHO recognizes that an information artifact with the multiple use expectations of the ICD functioning in the information age must be revised within the framework of an explicit design. While ICD-11 is not software as such, it does incorporate explicit semantics, mutual exclusion, synonymy, translations, interterm relationships, and metadata. As such, it must organize this content and these connections in a consistent way. Substantial opportunities to view and use the ICD in unprecedented ways arise from this organization.

Multi-Layered Manifestation

The most dramatic innovation of ICD-11 is that it may appear to some as many classifications, though logically there will be only one ICD-11. This is because ICD-11 will have several planes of viewing and use. The shared core and conceptual heart of ICD-11 will be in the **Foundation Component**, a semantic network of all terms, meanings, and practical relationships. From the Foundation Component will derive many **linearizations**, where each linearization will resemble and act like historical tabular forms of the ICD (see figure 7.1). Finally, the **Common Ontology**, prototyped in partnership with the International Health Terminology Standards Development Organisation (now SNOMED International), the developers of SNOMED CT, promises a semantic scaffolding shared between ICD-11 and SNOMED CT, from which all foundation layer entities can be defined. Common ontology is discussed further in the Relationships section of this chapter.

The Foundation Component

The Foundation Component is a semantic network, meaning it allows terms within it to have an arbitrary and nonexclusive number of parents and relationships. Gastric cancer can remain under

FIGURE 7.1. ICD-11 components

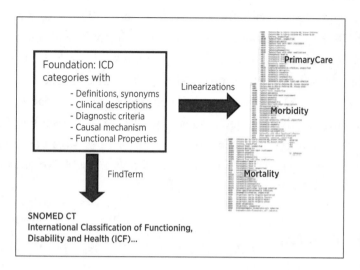

Source: Üstün 2011.

cancer, but it can also be under GI diseases, since both assignments are true. The Foundation Component is not mutually exclusive because of its multiple parents. Further, the Foundation Component has no residual categories, such as "Other" or "Unspecified," so it is also not exhaustive; those properties are ceded to the derivative linearizations from the Foundation Component. The Foundation Component can have children that go arbitrarily deep, since the identifiers for each entry are meaningless when formed as **Uniform Resource Identifiers (URIs)** rather than hierarchical codes (W3C 2001). This identifier is a unique character string for each entity. Each entry in the Foundation Component has an information structure embodying the content model described below, including synonyms and preferred terms. More importantly, the Foundation Component also contains the logic as to how any term mapping into the Foundation Component could be reduced into each of the ICD-11 linearizations. Thus, an immediate secondary use of the Foundation Component is as an index to any of its derivative linearizations, since all of the synonyms, child terms, and synonyms of those child terms are organized within the Foundation Component, enabling the mapping of any entry into its appropriate linearized "code."

The Foundation Component forms the core of ICD-11. It enables all derivative linearizations to be semantically mapped between and among each other through the relationships and logic contained within the Foundation Layer.

The Linearizations

Because virtually all common use cases of the ICD require the mutually exclusive and exhaustive properties of a statistical classification, ICD-11 explicitly supports the generation and curation of such derivatives from the Foundation Component. The most important is **ICD-11 for Morbidity and Mortality Statistics (ICD-11-MMS),** which will effectively look and act very similarly to ICD-10 with substantial content updating. ICD-11-MMS is the classification that replaces WHO's ICD-10. However, the structure of ICD-11 allows for an arbitrary number of linearizations, such as primary care, verbal autopsy, decision support, quality- and safety-oriented, specialized reimbursement, subspecialty extensions, or research classifications. Because all of these would derive from a common Foundation Component, they retain the capacity to participate in cross mappings between and among these linearizations that algorithmically derive from the Foundation Component. These cross mappings allow for international comparisons.

An important attribute of linearizations, by definition, is that each rubric has one and only one parent, selected from the possibly multiple options in the Foundation Component. The previous example of gastric cancer would require that the linearization opt for Cancer or GI Diseases as the parent of this term; it cannot be both. A design decision within ICD-11 asserts that the historically assigned parent (in this case, cancer) would be the specified parent in the morbidity linearization, unless there is compelling new or under-recognized scientific evidence to justify changing a linearization parent. In this way, linearizations preserve the property of mutual exclusivity. The logic for specifying which parent is relevant for which rubric in which linearization is maintained as part of the Foundation Component, though it is humanly vetted.

Correspondingly, all linearizations contain residual categories to preserve the exhaustiveness property. These categories are algorithmically created for the MMS from the Foundation, with the implication that these residual categories cannot contain children. An example of a residual category is other specified sleep-wake disorders.

The Content Model

Among the earliest innovations of the ICD-11 revision was achieving consensus on what an ICD-11 information model would include. Historically, little attention was given to the attributes of an ICD rubric, which raised the potential for confusion and inconsistency. Some codes were fully specified (meaning they made unambiguous sense as terms out of their hierarchical context), while others were hopelessly underspecified (for example, "Other," begging the question "other what?" absent the term being seen in its hierarchical context). The explicit information model for each rubric is called a **content model** (see figure 7.2), and briefly includes these attributes:

- A fully specified, unambiguous, context-free version of the concept name
- A context-free or meaningless identifier in the form of a URI
- A language-specific preferred term, which is typically shorter than the fully-specified name
- Common synonyms and variations of the term, which would subsume the historical inclusion terms

- An enumeration of all the parents for any term in the Foundation Layer, and of which parent is selected for each linearization in which a term participates
- The term "type" among disease, syndrome, or health condition, among others
- A concise and structured definition of the term
- A longer textual description of the term, which may include non-definitional features
- Exclusion terms, though only relevant to elements defined using query expressions in the Foundation Layer
- Some inclusion terms, drawn from synonyms or children, which may exemplify paradigmatically the rubric's use
- Relevant or valid body system, structures, or anatomical locations
- Etiologic factors, including genomic causes, external agents, or preconditions
- Temporal properties, including acuity or age group restrictions
- Measures and valid characterization of severity, such as extent, degree, or stage
- Functional impacts of the specific condition
- Special considerations: for example, gender or age restrictions, if any.
- Diagnostic criteria, stratified by levels of technology (experimental at this time)

FIGURE 7.2. Content model

THE CONTENT MODEL

Any Category in ICD is represented by:

1. ICD Concept Title
 1.1. Fully Specified Name

2. Classification Properties
 2.1. Parents
 2.2. Type
 2.3. Use and Linearization(s)

3. Textual Definition(s)

4. Terms
 4.1. Base Index Terms
 4.2. Inclusion Terms
 4.3. Exclusion

5. Body Structure Description
 5.1. Body System(s)
 5.2. Body Part(s) [Anatomical Site(s)]
 5.3. Morphological Properties

6. Manifestation Properties
 6.1. Signs & Symptoms
 6.2. Investigation findings

7. Causal Properties
 7.1. Etiology Type
 7.2. Causal Properties - Agents
 7.3. Causal Properties - Causal Mechanisms
 7.4. Genomic Linkages
 7.5. Risk Factors

8. Temporal Properties
 8.1. Age of Occurrence & Occurrence Frequency
 8.2. Development Course/Stage

9. Severity of Subtypes Properties

10. Functioning Properties
 10.1. Impact on Activities and Participation
 10.2. Contextual factors
 10.3. Body function

11. Specific Condition Properties
 11.1. Biological Sex
 11.2. Life-Cycle Properties

12. Treatment Properties

13. Diagnostic Criteria

Black already exists in ICD-10 either explicity or implicitly. Content model specifies them in a more systematic way. Blue are new – they exit in some specialty adaptations already such as oncology, mental health, neurology, dermatology.

Source: Üstün 2011.

The initial releases of the ICD are unlikely to have all attributes of all rubrics fully populated; this process will evolve with the maintenance and update of ICD-11. Nevertheless, on initial publication, fully specified names, preferred names, descriptions, and relationships are expected to be complete.

Identifiers and Codes

No taxonomy can function as a generalizable and referenceable classification absent the deployment of consistent identifiers or codes. This has been a historical problem for the ICD, which in many instances has reused codes within a classification, if only to make room for new codes. Good terminology practices have long argued that codes should never be reused, and furthermore should be "meaningless" or free from hierarchical context (Chute et al. 1998). ICD-11 follows these precepts in the Foundation Component but relaxes them in the linearizations. Thus, all codes found in linearizations will have at least two kinds of identifiers.

Meaningless Identifiers

All Foundation Component rubrics will receive a permanent, globally unique identifier, manifest as a World Wide Web Consortium (W3C)-conformant URI. The unique identifier is the standard identifier for ICD entities. An example would be:

http://id.who.int/icd/entity/1480627948

This is the foundation URI for pneumonia due to Streptococcus pneumoniae. It is comprised of a fixed prefix and an arbitrary 32-bit integer, serially generated. The fixed prefix is http://id.who.int/icd/entity/ which is a namespace created by WHO for the ICD schema. Note that this looks and preferably acts like a Uniform Resource Locator. Semantic Web tooling would expect a terminology reference to return useful content, such as the text string associated with a code (this is not the case with ICD URIs at the time of this writing). More complex specifications, such as language, can be included in such a service call, which begins to specify a well-behaved Representational State Transfer (REST) terminology service (beyond the scope of this chapter) (Jiang et al. 2012).

Meaningful Linearization Codes

Each linearization will also have a more traditional hierarchical code associated with each element of the linearization; these will look more familiar to ICD users, although they may involve more characters. The ICD-11-MMS will have an up to seven-digit alphanumeric code derived from mostly base 34 numbers (numbers 0 to 9 and capital letters except O and I to avoid ambiguity with the numbers 0 and 1). Some digits may be base 10, to break up the letters, and the second digit may be base 24 (letters only) to visually distinguish the code from all ICD codes. The decimal place is after the fourth digit, though this is really only a visual aid to interpretation and has no content meaning. An example of the ICD-11-MMS code for the URI above for pneumonia due to Streptococcus pneumoniae would be:

CA40.07 Pneumonia due to Streptococcus pneumoniae

As such, there is potentially a vast coding space; though in MMS, only the first six digits can be used for coding (see Post-Coordination, later in this chapter). Thus MMS could accommodate $34^5 \times 24$ rubrics, just over 1 billion unique codes. The availability of such a vast number of unique codes makes it improbable that reuse of codes will be necessary due to space limitations.

Principles and Guidelines

To assist in the proper use of the mortality and morbidity linearization, WHO published the **ICD-11-MMS Reference Guide**. This guide provides material such as explanation of terms and rules to assist in the correct classification of its content. It contains three parts—An Introduction to ICD-11, Using ICD-11, and New in ICD-11—and can be accessed from the ICD-11 website (WHO n.d.). What follows is an example of the guidance that is available.

Post-Coordination

The creation of a classification is always a balance between maintaining a reasonably sized body of content and being able simultaneously to capture codes and concepts at a level of detail to satisfy demanding users. The traditional model of expanding content is to make additional children with increasing levels of detail and granularity; however, this leads to a combinatorial explosion, as seen with the 500+ modes of bicycle accidents in ICD-10. To avoid this, while supporting expressivity, ICD-11 expands upon the post-coordination that already exists, albeit sparingly, in ICD-10. Post-coordination is where the specification of more than one code for a specific condition is required. ICD-11 allows and, in some cases, requires post-coordination.

For example, it is possible to add detail to most disease codes in the MMS that might include laterality, severity, specific detailed anatomy, or acuity. Additionally, one may use an extension to represent diagnosis code descriptors such as "present on admission" or as the main condition for the episode. Thirteen axes of post-coordination content are included in the "X Chapter" of ICD-11-MMS.

Achieving such arbitrary linkages requires some kind of grammar to associate related descriptors to their codes. While many are possible and potentially envisioned, the present mechanism is a concatenation of modifiers separated by slashes between stem codes and the use of an ampersand (&) before X-chapter modifiers and qualifiers. This syntax comes at the cost of expanding the number of characters to fully capture a post-coordinated code.

An interesting implication of engaging post-coordination is that the number of "root codes," or base codes, that exist in the final morbidity linearization is considerably smaller than the number in ICD-10, since much of the complexity and detail of ICD-10 is rendered as post-coordinated expressions. Nevertheless, as a rule of thumb, if a pre-coordinated term existed in ICD-10 at the three-digit level or above, it was retained as a pre-coordinated term in ICD-11 even if it could be rendered as a post-coordinated expression.

Finally, it is clear that not all modifiers are appropriate for all codes, and some codes will restrict the values permitted. For example, cancers might limit modifiers to specific stage codes. There is also the problem of post-coordinating an expression for which a pre-coordinated code already exists and must be the preferred form to maintain mutually exclusive coding. To address all these circumstances, sanctioning rules, which specify and in many cases can correct incorrect or non-allowable post-coordinated expressions, are embedded. Much of the detail for these sanctioning rules will be derived from the appropriate metadata in the content model of the Foundation Component.

Process for Revision and Updates

Refinement of the content model within the Foundation Component is expected to continue indefinitely, substantially improving the usability and generalizability of the family of linearizations anticipated. This implies that new linearizations are also anticipated as use cases demand them. The structure of ICD-11 allows for an arbitrary number of linearizations, such as primary care, verbal autopsy, decision support, quality- and safety-oriented, specialized reimbursement, sub-specialty extensions, or research classifications. It is expected that future national adaptations will be simply more specific linearizations, although WHO will require that they ultimately derive from the Foundation Component.

The Foundation Component, therefore, can and will be updated frequently, possibly as often as daily. However, the derivative linearizations will be much more stable. Furthermore, these linearizations will be versioned, so that a particular country or use case, such as mortality, may choose to use a specified linearization version for many years before updating.

WHO has established an ICD maintenance process for the MMS along with an online platform for individuals to submit their proposals and review and comment on those submitted by others. There are several proposal types, including add new entity, content enhancement, and structural change. The update cycle determined to keep stability for mortality and allow quicker updates for morbidity use is (WHO 2018b):

- Updates that impact on international reporting (the 4- and 5-digit structure of the stem codes) will be published every five years.

- Updates at a more detailed level can be published at annual rates and, pending the needs of clinical modifications, also twice a year.
- Additions to the index can be done on an ongoing basis.
- Mortality and morbidity rules will be updated in a 10-year cycle.

A number of scientific and classification experts are involved in review of the submissions. This includes the mortality reference group (MRG) or morbidity reference group (MbRG), a medical scientific advisory committee (MSAC), and a classification and statistics advisory committee (CSAC).

Relationship with Other Terminologies, Classification Systems, and Code Sets

ICD-11 has an inherent relationship with previous versions of ICD as well as the International Classification of Functioning, Disability, and Health (ICF), International Classification of Health Interventions (ICHI), and International Classification of Diseases for Oncology. In addition, work has been done to form a close relationship with SNOMED CT.

The Common Ontology

To establish a logically coherent, ontological basis for ICD-11, WHO and the International Health Terminology Standards Development Organisation (IHTSDO) prototyped a subset of SNOMED CT that could serve as the shared semantic scaffolding of ICD-11 (Rodrigues et al. 2015). In this common ontology framework, both ICD and SNOMED CT would share the same entities with the same relations (Rodrigues et al. 2013) (see figure 7.3). The prototype was developed for the cardiovascular chapter of ICD-11 (Rodrigues et al. 2014). The Common Ontology is not completed, and work is continuing on the core ICD-11 Foundation and the MMS, which was released in June 2018. The Common Ontology enables algorithmic term matching, between and among linearizations of the Foundation, which can include legacy revisions such as ICD-10 and the many national modifications (Schultz et al. 2017). While incomplete, the Common Ontology has already pioneered advances in linking classifications and ontologies (Schultz et al. 2014).

Not all terms in the Foundation Component can or will be part of the common ontology. For example, ICD terms that involve exclusions, such as "Hypertension," which excludes hypertension of pregnancy (Preeclampsia), cannot be easily expressed in SNOMED CT, or for that matter in most description logic-based ontologies. To address this, such terms will be constructed as logical queries, using a machine-interpretable rendering of a set-theory query syntax, which will specify something like "All Hypertension *minus* Preeclampsia." In this way, all Foundation Component rubrics can be expressed as either full-rank common ontology elements or set-based

FIGURE 7.3. ICD-10 common ontology

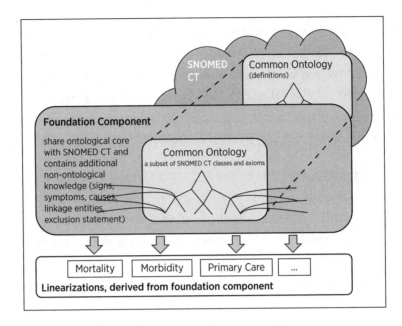

Source: Campbell et al., 2013, 9.

query expressions comprised of common ontology elements. Either way, these are fully computable renderings of a concept space.

Tools to Access and Use

The use of classifications and terminologies in the information age will be accompanied by a user expectation of machine assistance in the coding process. The Foundation Component comprises in one way the complete, machine-processable index to all ICD-11 content. It forms the basis for computer search, subsumption, and cross-linearization mapping. WHO anticipates an ecosystem of tools and applications that can and will leverage the detail and structure of the Foundation Component to assist coding. These will likely range from sophisticated Natural Language Processing algorithms to smartphone apps that can cheaply and easily exercise sanctioning rules using REST Web services remotely. The ecosystem of computer-assisted browsers and sophisticated coding tools developed by WHO is accessible from the ICD-11 website (see [WHO n.d.] in the resource list at the end of this chapter).

The most interesting new resource for the machine-assisted application of ICD coding is the Application Programming Interface (API). It provides a rich suite of programming tools leveraging indices, spell correction, synonym mapping, the sanctioning rules for post-coordination, translations, and algorithmic mapping of text strings to optimal codes. This API suite can enable the development of purpose-specific coding apps and tools on a wide range of computers, tablets, and handheld devices.

Adoption and Use Cases

The official release of the implementation version of ICD-11-MMS occurred June 2018. The final version will be submitted for approval by the World Health Assembly, the governing body of WHO, in the spring of 2019 and will go into effect on January 1, 2022. Individual WHO Member states are evaluating this official release to begin preparations for implementation. Countries planning to produce national modifications must establish contractual arrangements with WHO and follow the rules below when doing so (WHO 2018b):

- Modifications will be agreed on by the ICD-11 maintenance bodies before they are implemented nationally.
- Modifications are only added below the level of coding depth that is specified in the Tabular List for Morbidity and Mortality Statistics and should not conflict with the foundation.
- All national modifications will consider if suitable additional detail exists already in the foundation.
- If a change is performed to the international version, the respective national modification must be adapted as soon as possible.

This chapter was modified from a previous version that had been jointly authored with Bedirhan Üstün, MD. Dr. Üstün was Coordinator for Classifications and Terminology at WHO at the time.

CHECK YOUR UNDERSTANDING

1. The common ontology provides a semantic framework shared between:
   a. ICD-11 and ICD-10
   b. ICD-11 and the mortality linearization
   c. ICD-11 and SNOMED CT
   d. ICD-11 and the morbidity linearization

2. True or false? The Foundation Component is a semantic network of all terms, meanings, and practical relationships in ICD-11.
   a. True
   b. False

3. In which chapter(s) of ICD-11 are the axes for post-coordination found?

   a. X
   b. Y
   c. Z
   d. X and Y

4. Which characteristic will ICD-11 employ to address the combinatorial explosion seen in ICD-10?

   a. Pre-coordination
   b. NEC
   c. NOS
   d. Post-coordination

5. The semantic core of ICD-11 is known as:

   a. Common ontology
   b. Foundation Component
   c. Core model
   d. SNOMED CT

REVIEW

1. True or false? Linearizations are used to derive the Foundation Component.

   a. True
   b. False

2. An important attribute of _____ is that each rubric has one and only one parent, selected from the possibly multiple options in the Foundation Component.

   a. Linearizations
   b. Synonyms
   c. Child terms
   d. Parent terms

3. Which of the following is not an attribute of the content model?

   a. A fully specified, unambiguous, context-free version of the concept name
   b. A longer textual description of the term, which may include non-definitional features
   c. A concise and structured definition of the term
   d. A meaningful unique identifier in the form of a code

4. True or false? Post-coordinating an expression is the preferred form over an already existing pre-coordinated code.

    a. True
    b. False

5. Fill in the blank. WHO will require that national adaptations of ICD-11 be derived from the _____.

6. True or false? The MMS linearization will contain residual categories such as Unspecified and Other.

    a. True
    b. False

7. ICD-11-MMS index additions will be updated

    a. Every five years
    b. On an ongoing basis
    c. Semiannually
    d. Once stable, never

8. Codes found in linearizations will have which kind of identifier(s)?

    a. Meaningful identifiers and meaningless linearization codes
    b. Meaningful identifiers
    c. Meaningless identifiers and meaningful linearization codes
    d. Meaningless identifiers and meaningless modifier codes

9. ICD-11 Indices will be machine-derivable from the:

    a. Common ontology
    b. Core model
    c. Linearizations
    d. Foundation Component

10. True or false? ICD-11 will allow the specification of more than one code for a specific condition.

    a. True
    b. False

References

Campbell, J. R., C. G. Chute, V. Della Mea, M. Harry, J. Millar, A. Rector, J. M. Rodrigues, S. Schulz, H. Solbrig, K. Spackman, and B. Ustün. 2013. "A Common Ontology for ICD 11 and SNOMED CT." Presented at WHO

Family of International Classifications Network Annual Meeting, Beijing, China, October 2013. http://www.who.int/classifications/whofic2013c300.pdf.

Chute, C. G., S. M. Hugg, J. A. Ferguson, J. M. Walker, and J. D. Halamka. 2012. There are important reasons for delaying implementation of the new ICD-10 coding system. *Health Affairs* 31(4):836–842.

Chute, C. G., S. P. Cohn, and J. R. Campbell. 1998. A framework for comprehensive health terminology systems in the United States: Development guidelines, criteria for selection, and public policy implications. ANSI Healthcare Informatics Standards Board Vocabulary Working Group and the Computer-Based Patient Records Institute Working Group on Codes and Structures. *JAMIA* 5(6):503–510.

Jiang, G., H. R. Solbrig, and C. G. Chute. 2012. Building standardized semantic web RESTful services to support ICD-11 revision. http://ceur-ws.org/Vol-952/paper_24.pdf.

Jiang, G., H. R. Solbrig, R. Kiefer, L. V. Rasmussen, H. Mo, P. Speltz, W. K. Thompson, J. C. Denny, C. G. Chute, and J. Pathak. 2015. A standards-based semantic metadata repository to support EHR-driven phenotype authoring and execution. *Studies in Health Technology and Informatics* 216:1098.

Li, D., G. Simon, C. G. Chute, and L. Pathak. 2013. Using association rule mining for phenotype extraction from electronic health records. *AMIA Joint Summits on Translational Science Proceedings* 2013:142–146.

Mo, H., W. K. Thompson, L. V. Rasmussen, J. A. Pacheco, G. Jiang, R. Kiefer, Q. Zhu, J. Xu, E. Montague, D. S. Carrell, T. Lingren, F. D. Mentch, Y. Ni, F. H. Wehbe, P. L. Peissig, G. Tromp, E. B. Larson, C. G. Chute, J. Pathak, J. C. Denny, P. Speltz, A. N. Kho, G. P. Jarvik, C. A. Bejan, M. S. Williams, K. Borthwick, T. E. Kitchner, D. M. Roden, and P. A. Harris. 2015. Desiderata for computable representations of electronic health records-driven phenotype algorithms. *JAMIA* 22(6):1220–1230.

Newton, K. M., P. L. Peissig, A. N. Kho, S. J. Bielinski, R. L. Berg, V. Choudhary, M. Basford, C. G. Chute, I. J. Kullo, R. Li, J. A. Pacheco, L. V. Rasmussen, L. Spangler, and J. C. Denny. 2013. Validation of electronic medical record-based phenotyping algorithms: results and lessons learned from the eMERGE network. *JAMIA* 20(e1):e147–154.

Pathak, J., K. R. Bailey, C. E. Beebe, S. Bethard, D. C. Carrell, P. J. Chen, D. Dligach, C. M. Endle, L. A. Hart, P. J. Haug, S. M. Huff, V. C. Kaggal, D. Li, H. Liu, K. Marchant, J. Masanz, T. Miller, T. A. Oniki, M. Palmer, K. J. Peterson, S. Rea, G. K. Savova, C. R. Stanci, S. Sohn, H. R. Solbrig, D. B. Suesse, C. Tao, D. P. Taylor, L. Westberg, S. Wu, N. Zhou, and C. G. Chute. 2013. Normalization and standardization of electronic health records for high-throughput phenotyping: the SHARPn consortium. *JAMIA* 20(e2):e341–348.

Rodrigues, J. M., S. Schulz, A. Rector, K. Spackman, B. Üstün, C. G. Chute, V. Della Mea, J. Millar, and K. B. Persson. 2013. Sharing ontology between ICD 11 and SNOMED CT will enable seamless re-use and semantic interoperability. *Studies in Health Technology and Informatics* 192:343–346.

Rodrigues, J. M., S. Schulz, A. Rector, K. Spackman, J. Millar, J. Campbell, B. Üstün, C. G. Chute, H. Solbrig, V. Della Mea, and K. B. Persson. 2014. ICD-11 and SNOMED CT Common Ontology: circulatory system. *Studies in Health Technology and Informatics* 205:1043–1047.

Rodrigues, J. M., D. Robinson, V. Della Mea, J. Campbell, A. Rector, S. Schulz, H. Brear, B. Üstün, K. Spackman, C. G. Chute, J. Millar, H. Solbrig, and K. B. Persson. 2015. Semantic alignment between ICD-11 and SNOMED CT. *Studies in Health Technology and Informatics* 216:790–794.

Schulz, S., J. M. Rodrigues, A. Rector, K. Spackman, J. Campbell, B. Üstün, C. G. Chute, H. Solbrig, V. Della Mea, J. Millar, and K. B. Persson. 2014. What's in a class? Lessons learnt from the ICD - SNOMED CT harmonisation. *Studies in Health Technology and Informatics* 205:1038–1042.

Schulz, S., J. M. Rodrigues, A. Rector, and C. G. Chute. 2017. Interface terminologies, reference terminologies and aggregation terminologies: A strategy for better integration. *Studies in Health Technology and Informatics* 245:940–944.

Üstün, T. B. 2011. To code or not to code? AHIMA 2011 Convention. https://www.slideshare.net/ustunb/ ahima-icd10-icd11-switch-to-icd10cm-in-the-usa.

World Health Organization (WHO). 2018a. WHO releases new International Classification of Diseases (ICD 11). http://www.who.int/news-room/detail/18-06-2018-who-releases-new-international-classification-of-diseases-(icd-11).

World Health Organization (WHO). 2018b. ICD-11-MMS Reference Guide. https://icd.who.int.

World Wide Web Consortium (W3C). 2001. URIs, URLs, and URNs: Clarifications and Recommendations 1.0. http://www.w3.org/TR/uri-clarification/.

Resources

World Health Organization (WHO). n.d. ICD-11. https://icd.who.int.

8

RxNorm

Terri Meredith RPh, MSCIS

LEARNING OBJECTIVES

- Discuss the history and development of RxNorm
- Explain the components of RxNorm
- Review the process for updating RxNorm
- Apply current principles and guidelines for using RxNorm
- Summarize who has adopted RxNorm and how it may be used
- Examine the relationship RxNorm has with other classifications, terminologies, and code sets
- Compare tools available to access and use
- Explain how RxNorm is used in an electronic environment

KEY TERMS

- Atom
- Dose form
- Electronic prescribing (e-Rx)
- Normalized name
- RxNorm
- RxNorm concept unique identifier (RXCUI)
- Semantic Branded Drug (SBD)
- Semantic Clinical Drug (SCD)
- Term type (TTY)

Introduction to RxNorm

RxNorm is a vocabulary about drugs, specifically the types of medications taken by patients, prescribed by practitioners, and dispensed by pharmacists. As a controlled vocabulary, it limits itself to only this domain. But even though it is limited to a very narrow domain, it illustrates the complexity of naming and managing a controlled vocabulary used to describe medications in the real world.

RxNorm is a standardized nomenclature for clinical drugs that supports semantic inter-operation between proprietary drug terminologies and pharmacy knowledge-based systems. The RxNorm terminology enables healthcare systems using different drug compendia or knowledge-based systems to communicate using a common terminology.

History

In the late 1990s, some discussions at the HL7 Vocabulary Working Group focused on the problems of understanding medication names in various systems. Hospitals and pharmacies were using different systems. These systems were of two varieties: those developed locally for use, or those purchased from a pharmacy compendium. The pharmacy compendia would have information about drug interactions, pricing and rebates for medications, reimbursement details, contraindications for medicines, and other useful material. Those who developed their own local systems found it difficult to manage all of that related information. Furthermore, the pharmacy compendia also tracked the use of National Drug Codes (NDC), something the Food and Drug Administration (FDA) was unable to achieve. The NDC codes were valuable, as reimbursement was based on them. Chapter 4 explains the NDC codes.

It was proposed in this group that some standards be developed for communicating about drugs at the clinical level, loosely defined as that of an ingredient and a strength, or **dose form**. However, no single group or individual seemed capable of building something that all would agree on.

At this point, the National Library of Medicine (NLM), which had been party to those discussions, undertook a set of experiments in cooperation with the Veterans Administration (VA) to ascertain if there was any way to convert the drugs named in the VA's National Drug Formulary (NDF) into something that might be appropriate for use elsewhere. By a combination of methods, involving computer parsing of the names given in NDF, and by human review and approval of those names, or by human generation of names, it was deemed feasible to approach this domain using largely human review.

The key ingredient to creating those names was to create a set of rules for the names to be created, or a normalization of the names. These normalization rules provided a template for all medications to be named in a way that clinicians usually talk of them, but with a set of strictly enforced standards. The standards included the name of the ingredient or ingredients of the product, the strength and units of strength of each ingredient of the product, and the form in which the product was prepared for administration to the individual.

Having established, by the experiment with the VA, that a process of establishing a **normalized name**, or "normal form," for medications was practical, the NLM then began to add naming systems from the pharmacy knowledge-base vendors to use as the basis for a new system, RxNorm. Each of the proprietary sources agreed to allow certain pieces (but not all) of the naming information to be used. Additionally, the VA NDF and the FDA NDC code listings were added to the mix.

At the same time, the NLM and the FDA signed an agreement that the NLM would create a website to present the information usually written on the paper shipped with each box of product, known technically as the label or package insert. This website, named DailyMed (see [NLM n.d.a] in the resources at the end of the chapter), received the newly submitted labels on every drug product from the FDA, whether prescription or over-the-counter. This information was also incorporated into the names generated for RxNorm.

The Agency for Healthcare Research and Quality (AHRQ) contributed funds to both FDA and to NLM to develop the system to handle the labels electronically, and the system to create the names for RxNorm, advancing the efforts of both agencies in this arena. Thus, RxNorm was built with the support and cooperation of several federal agencies.

As the system for supporting the RxNorm editing efforts was being built, RxNorm began a practice of monthly releases. The releases were based on updates from the source vocabularies, many of which originate from pharmacy compendia such as First DataBank, Gold Standard, Micromedex, and Multum, and information gleaned from the labels for products.

Today, the RxNorm team continues the practice of monthly updates, but with weekly updates as well. These weekly updates are largely generated from data coming into DailyMed and are for newly marketed products.

Purpose

According to testimony to the National Committee on Vital and Health Statistics (NCVHS), the requirements for a drug terminology to be used as a standard in the electronic health record (EHR) are that it must be:

- Maintained by a primary code-assigning authority
- Available for use at little or no cost
- Updated frequently and promptly
- Backwardly compatible with the National Drug Code (NDC) system
- Composed of abstractions at multiple levels of granularity

Drug concepts that must be represented to support common clinical and administrative functions include the following:

- Active ingredients, important for allergy checking
- Routed generic, important for drug-drug interaction checking
- Clinical drug, important for provider order entry
- Manufactured drug, important for medication administration records at the nursing level
- Packaged product, important for interoperability with pharmacy systems (NCVHS 2004)

For example, according to McGinness et al., "the clinical drug supports the exchange of prescribing information, the ingredients can support the exchange of allergy information" (2013). In fact, the move toward adoption and implementation of standard drug terminologies is being partly driven by the interest in medication management and **electronic prescribing (e-Rx)**.

RxNorm met the NCVHS requirements and was selected as a standard for a number of clinical and administrative functions, including e-Rx. By providing normalized names and unique identifiers for clinical drugs and drug delivery devices, RxNorm allows hospitals, pharmacies, and other organizations' computer systems to communicate drug-related information efficiently and unambiguously. RxNorm achieved its originally conceived purpose of supporting semantic interoperability between multiple drug terminologies. Standards organizations that use RxNorm as a part of their electronic transactions include Health Level 7 (HL7), the National Council for Prescription Drug Programs (NCPDP), and the Centers for Medicare and Medicaid Services (CMS).

Structure and Contents

RxNorm prepares a number of different source vocabularies for inclusion in the Unified Medical Language System (UMLS). The source vocabularies are:

- Anatomical Therapeutic Chemical Classification System (ATC)
- Centers for Disease Control Vaccine Codes (CVX)
- CMS Formulary Reference File (MTHCMSFRF)
- Drug Bank
- Gold Standard Drug Database
- Medical Subject Headings (MeSH)
- Multum MediSource Lexicon
- Micromedex Red Book
- FDA Structured Product Labels (SPL)

- FDB MedKnowledge (formerly NDDF Plus)
- Relationships
- United States Pharmacopeia (USP)
- US Edition of SNOMED CT (drug information)
- Veterans Health Administration National Drug File (VANDF)
  (NLM 2018a)

For RxNorm to process a drug and create RxNorm identifiers, it must have a Structured Product Label (SPL) approved and distributed by the FDA and its use cannot be considered out of scope. Radiopharmaceuticals, contrast media, food, dietary supplements, and medical devices, such as bandages and crutches, are all out of scope for making names in RxNorm, even if those names are in a source supplied to the RxNorm staff. However, those out-of-scope names are simply passed through to the UMLS, and not included in any of the processes that produce RxNorm. In the case of one source, SNOMED CT, only the drug-related portion of the source vocabulary is processed in RxNorm, and most of it enters the UMLS without any handling in RxNorm.

RxNorm contains the names of prescription and over-the-counter drugs available in the US. It includes generic and branded names for the following:

> Clinical drugs are pharmaceutical products given to (or taken by) a patient with therapeutic intent, specified as ingredient(s), strength(s), and a dose form. Ciprofloxacin 250 MG Oral Tablet [Cipro] is a **Semantic Branded Drug (SBD)** and Ciprofloxacin 250 MG Oral Tablet is a **Semantic Clinical Drug (SCD)**. The SCD is the generic name for the SBD.
>
> Drug packs are medications supplied in packaging that contain multiple drugs, or drugs designed to be administered in a specified sequence. An example for birth control pills is {7 (Ethinyl Estradiol 0.035 MG / Norethindrone 0.5 MG Oral Tablet) / 7 (Ethinyl Estradiol 0.035 MG / Norethindrone 0.75 MG Oral Tablet) / 7 (Ethinyl Estradiol 0.035 MG / Norethindrone 1 MG Oral Tablet) / 7 (Inert Ingredients 1 MG Oral Tablet)} Pack (NLM 2018c).

Principles and Guidelines

Drug names from many data sources are received by NLM where they undergo analysis and are processed and output into RxNorm files in a standard format. While the complete process is outside the scope of this chapter, one can reasonably understand the general method by following what happens to the source data.

Here is a set of sample source data:

Naproxen Tab 250 MG

Naproxen 250 mg tablet (product)

NAPROXEN@250 mg@ORAL@TABLET

Naproxen 250 MILLIGRAM In 1 TABLET ORAL TABLET

NAPROXEN 250 MG TAB, UD [VA Product]

(NLM 2018c)

Easily observable is the fact that the sources format their drug names in many ways.

Products of Naproxen are in scope for RxNorm, so each one of these names is associated with an RxNorm normalized name and identifier. If there is no RxNorm name, then one is created. The normalized name consists of the ingredient, strength, and dose form (in that order) for a generic drug. In the example, the RxNorm normalized name is "Naproxen 250 MG Oral Tablet." The branded version of this drug uses the same format but includes the brand name in brackets at the end (such as "Naproxen 250 MG Oral Tablet [Naprosyn]").

Once it has been recognized that all the names above are for a single product, it can be given one RxNorm name. For that reason, these names are considered synonymous at this level of abstraction and brought together as a single concept. This notion is the key to understanding all of RxNorm: each RxNorm name and all its synonyms constitute a single concept.

After the concept is created, each concept receives an **RxNorm concept unique identifier (RXCUI)**. The RXCUI:

- is unique to that concept;
- is essentially the "name" of a concept that computers read and understand;
- is never deleted or reused; and
- the meanings of concepts persist from one RxNorm release to the next (NLM 2018c).

In the NLM RxNorm Overview, concepts are defined as collections of synonyms at a given level of abstraction. The documentation further states that each drug name carries additional characteristics, including source, code (the unique identifier assigned by its source), and **term type (TTY)** (NLM 2018c). NLM also assigns an RxNorm atom unique identifier (RXAUI). According to the NLM, "An **atom** is a drug name, plus these additional characteristics." A product named by First Databank, such as AZITHROMYCIN@250 mg@ORAL@CAPSULE (HARD, SOFT, ETC.) produced from three separate fields in their files, is provided an RXAUI, an RXCUI, as well as its own First Databank code. The same is true for the other sources.

NLM assigns the RXCUI 141962 to this Azithromycin concept. Each of the atoms associated with the drug names listed above receives a separate RXAUI. For the example above, the RXAUI is 2407920.

NLM includes the **relationships** that link drug names to other drug names and ingredients, as well as other information, such as NDCs, marketing categories, and pill imprint information from the source data (NLM 2018c). For each drug product thus named in RxNorm, there will be relationships to synonyms and ingredients, as well as NDC, manufacturer, and pill size attribute.

RxNorm also creates names at levels of specificity other than the fully complete drug name (ingredient, strength, and dose form) including

- ingredient
- precise ingredient
- multiple ingredients
- ingredient + strength (Semantic Clinical Drug Component)
- ingredient + dose form (Semantic Clinical Drug Form)
- ingredient + dose form group (Semantic Clinical Dose Form Group)

Creating these names allows for matching sources or uses in text of these more general names, so that one can then navigate from the less specific name to the most specific, or vice versa.

The creation of a fully specified drug name, or normal form, results in the creation of more general names (and the concepts that contain these names) if they do not already exist, along with relationships that link these concepts together (NLM 2018c). A set of concepts and relationships results in a graph. The system completes the graph computationally by creating the related drug names (and their concepts) that do not already exist and in the case of branded drugs, their generic counterparts when they do not already exist in the data (NLM 2018c).

For the fully specified name "Cetirizine hydrochloride 5 MG Oral Tablet," the system creates the following RxNorm names:

"Cetirizine hydrochloride"
"Cetirizine hydrochloride 5 MG"
"Cetirizine hydrochloride Oral Tablet" /"Cetirizine Oral Product" /"Cetirizine Pill"

RxNorm links these names using relationships. Here are a few examples:

"Cetirizine hydrochloride 5 MG Oral Tablet" *has_dose_form* "Oral Tablet"
"Cetirizine" *ingredient_of* "Cetirizine hydrochloride 5 MG"
"Cetirizine hydrochloride 5 MG Oral Tablet" *is a* "Cetirizine hydrochloride Oral Tablet"
"Cetirizine Pill" *has_ingredient* "Cetirizine"

The RxNorm graph for any drug can be researched with RxNav. RxNav is an online tool that is available for researching drugs and displaying their relationships and identifiers (see [NLM 2018b] in the references at the end of the chapter).

Figure 8.1 shows the RxNorm Graph for a cetirizine hydrochloride 5 MG Oral Tablet (brand name Zyrtec).

FIGURE 8.1. RxNorm graph for a Zyrtec 5 mg oral tablet

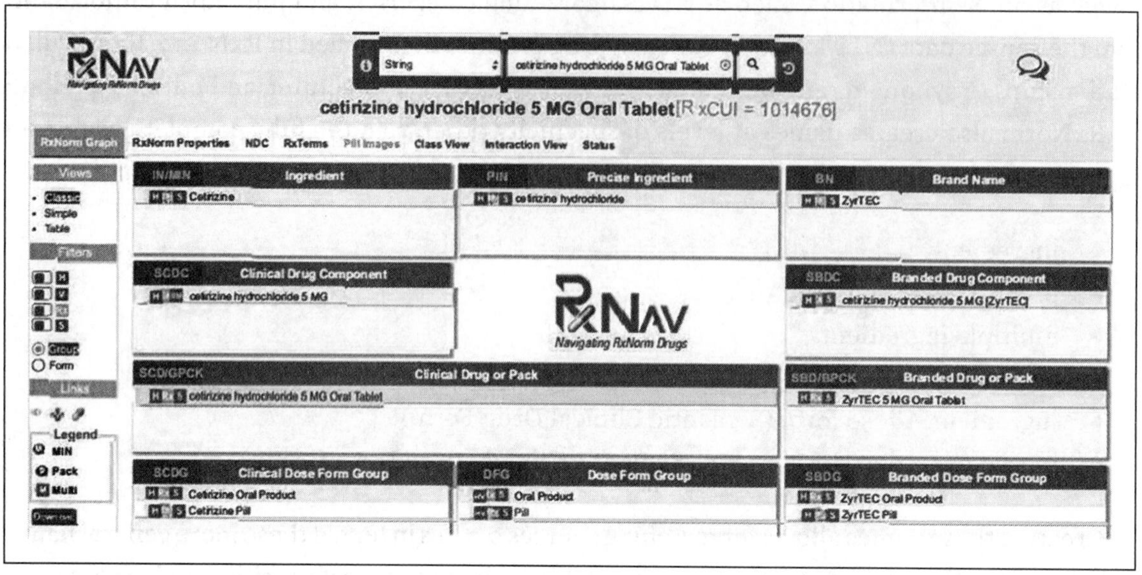

Source: NLM 2018b.

The derived normalized drug names become a terminology (NLM 2018c). The normalized names are based upon the information received from the source terminologies. The normalized drug names are referred to as SAB=RXNORM (NLM 2018c). As per NLM (see table 8.1), the SAB=RXNORM normalized name follows the pattern of the ingredient, strength, and dose form; includes the brand name for branded drugs; and includes the quantities of each drug for packs of drugs where:

- Ingredients generally use the United States Adopted Name (USAN) and most of these names are also the International Nonproprietary Names.
- Strength is based on the strength of the active ingredient(s), which may be either the precise (salt or ester) or the base ingredient of the drug. Strengths are expressed to three significant digits and use the "milli" metric system equivalents (for example milligrams, milliliters); liquids per milliliter. In the case of a powder that can be reconstituted to a range of liquid concentrations, the highest concentration in the range is used for the normalized form.
- Dose forms used in the RxNorm name are intended to represent the form in which a product is presented to the patient. While some of the dose forms have names that indicate a route, the meaning here is only that this is the form in which the product is prepared, not how it is necessarily administered. For example, an aminoglycoside like gentamycin might be prepared in a solution suitable for use in the eye but prescribed for use in the ear. Table 8.2 provides definitions and usage notes for dose forms.

TABLE 8.1. SAB=RXNORM

Drug Type/Drug Delivery Device	Pattern
Generic drugs (SCD)	Ingredient Strength Dose Form
Branded drugs (SBD)	Ingredient Strength Dose Form [Brand Name]
Generic drug packs (GPCK)	{# (Ingredient Strength Dose Form) / # (Ingredient Strength Dose Form)} Pack
Branded drug packs (BPCK)	{# (Ingredient Strength Dose Form) / # (Ingredient Strength Dose Form)} Pack [Brand Name]

Source: NLM 2018c.

TABLE 8.2. Dosage forms

Form	Definition and Usage Notes
Inhalants and Sprays	
Inhalants	
Gas for Inhalation	Gas that can be breathed into the nose or mouth
Inhalant Solution	Solution intended to be inhaled
Metered Dose Inhaler	Liquid medication delivered as a mist to be inhaled as a measured dose
Nasal Inhalant	Medication intended to be inhaled through the nose
Inhalant Powder (Powdered Dose Inhaler)	Powdered medication that is intended to be inhaled
Dry Powder Inhaler	Powdered medication inhaled as a measured dose
Spray	Substance propelled by gas(es)
Metered Dose Nasal Spray	Nasal solution intended for use in the nasal cavity delivered by a spray as a measured dose (see also Nasal Spray & Nasal Inhalant)
Mucosal Spray	Spray intended for use on the mucous membranes
Nasal Spray	Nasal solution intended for use in the nasal cavity delivered by a spray (see also Metered Dose Nasal Spray & Nasal Inhalant)
Oral Spray	Spray intended to be applied into the oral cavity
Rectal Spray	Spray intended to be used in or around the rectum
Topical Spray (Dermal Spray)	Spray intended for use on the skin
Powder Spray	Powder delivered on the skin as a spray

(continued)

TABLE 8.2. Continued

Form	Definition and Usage Notes
Liquids	
Cream	Homogenous mixture that contains two liquid phases–usually oil in water or water in oil
Ophthalmic Cream	Cream intended for use in the eye
Oral Cream	Cream intended for use on or in the mouth
Rectal Cream	Cream intended for use in or around the rectum
Topical Cream	Cream intended to be used on the skin
Augmented Topical Cream	Cream with enhanced drug delivery capability
Vaginal Cream	Cream intended for use in or around the vagina
Foam	Bubbles of gas that are introduced into a liquid
Injectable Foam	Foam intended to be injected
Oral Foam	Foam intended to be administered into the mouth
Rectal Foam	Foam intended for use in the rectum
Topical Foam	Foam intended for use on the skin
Vaginal Foam	Foam intended for use in the vagina
Liquid Cleanser	Liquid containing a detergent (see also Bar Soap)
Medicated Liquid Soap	Liquid containing a detergent and a medication
Medicated Shampoo	Medicated liquid soap intended for use on hair
Oil	Fatty liquid
Topical Oil	Oil intended to be applied on the skin
Prefilled Applicator	Medication in an applicator delivered as a single measured dose
Solution	Homogenous mixture of one or more solutes completely dissolved in a liquid solvent
Inhalant Solution	Solution intended to be inhaled
Injectable Solution	Multiple use solution or reconstituted powder intended to be injected
Auto-Injector	Single-use solution or suspension contained in a spring-loaded injection system that can be administered by activating the device, causing automatic insertion of the needle through the skin
Cartridge	Single- or multiple-use solution or a suspension contained in a vessel used with a separate reusable injection system
Injection	Single-use sterile solution, suspension, or reconstituted powder intended for parenteral use

TABLE 8.2. Continued

Form	Definition and Usage Notes
Intraperitoneal Solution	Solution intended for use in the peritoneal cavity
Jet Injector	Single-use solution or a suspension contained in a needlefree injection system
Pen Injector	Single- or multiple-use solution or suspension contained in a mechanical injection system used to administer the drug through a needle manually inserted into the skin
Prefilled Syringe	Single-use solution or suspension intended to be injected in a syringe
Irrigation Solution	Solution intended for use as a flushing or rinsing agent
Douche	Irrigation solution intended for use in the vagina
Enema (Rectal Solution; Rectal Suspension)	Irrigation solution intended to cleanse the bowel or administer diagnostic drugs
Ophthalmic Irrigation Solution	Irrigation solution intended for use in the eye
Nasal Solution (Nasal Drops; Nose Drops)	Solution intended for use on the nasal mucosa
Ophthalmic Solution (Ophthalmic Drops; Eye Drops)	Solution intended for use in the eye
Oral Solution (Oral Drops)	Solution intended to be taken by mouth. For solutions applied to the teeth, use Mouthwash
Mouthwash (Oral Rinse; Topical Dental Solution)	Oral solution intended to be used as a rinse or for irrigation. This includes oral solutions that are applied to the teeth
Mucous Membrane Topical Solution	Oral solution intended for use on the mucous membranes
Otic Solution (Otic Drops; Ear Drops)	Solution intended for use in the ear
Rectal Solution	Solution intended for use in the rectum
Topical Solution (Tincture; Liniment)	Solution intended for use on a surface (do not use for Oral Solutions)
Topical Liquefied Gas	Gas that is cooled or pressurized to its liquid form and used topically on the skin for cryotherapy or freezing skin lesions
Pack	Package that contains multiple drugs, or drugs designed to be administered in a specified sequence
Suspension	Nonhomogenous mixture of one or more substances not completely dissolved in a liquid
Injectable Suspension	Multiple-use suspension or reconstituted powder intended to be injected

(continued)

227

TABLE 8.2. Continued

Form	Definition and Usage Notes
Auto-Injector	Single-use solution or suspension contained in a spring-loaded injection system that can be administered by activating the device, causing automatic insertion of the needle through the skin
Cartridge	Single- or multiple-use solution or a suspension contained in a vessel used with a separate reusable injection system
Injection	Single-use sterile solution, suspension, or reconstituted powder intended for parenteral use
Jet Injector	Single-use solution or a suspension contained in a needlefree injection system
Pen Injector	Single- or multiple-use solution or suspension contained in a mechanical injection system used to administer the drug through a needle manually inserted into the skin
Prefilled Syringe	Single-use solution or suspension intended to be injected in a syringe
Intratracheal Suspension	Suspension intended for use in the trachea
Lotion	Viscous liquid suspension
Topical Lotion	Lotion intended for use on the skin
Augmented Topical Lotion	Lotion with enhanced drug delivery capability
Nasal Suspension (Nasal Drops; Nose Drops)	Suspension intended for use in the nose
Ophthalmic Suspension (Ophthalmic Drops; Eye Drops)	Suspension intended for use in the eye
Oral Suspension (Oral Drops)	Suspension intended to be taken by mouth
Extended Release Suspension	Suspension that allows for a timed or controlled release of the solute
Otic Suspension (Otic Drops; Ear Drops)	Suspension intended for use in the ear
Topical Suspension	Suspension intended for external application on the skin
Solid	
Bar	Block of solid material that is longer in length than width
Bar Soap	Bar intended to be used to cleanse the body
Medicated Bar Soap	Bar of soap containing medication
Capsule	Contained dosage form filled with solid or liquid ingredients that can be poured or squeezed
Oral Capsule	Capsule taken by mouth

TABLE 8.2. Continued

Form	Definition and Usage Notes
Delayed Release Oral Capsule	Solid dosage form in which the drug is enclosed within either a hard or soft soluble container made from a suitable form of gelatin, and which releases a drug (or drugs) at a time other than promptly after oral administration (enteric-coated articles are delayed release dosage forms)
Extended Release Oral Capsule	Capsule that allows medication to be released over an extended period of time at a controlled rate
Chewing Gum	Insoluble material that is chewed to release medication
Oral Flakes	Collection of small, flat, thin pieces of matter
Gel (Jelly)	Fine particles dispersed in a medium resulting in a solid substance
Nasal Gel (Nasal Jelly)	Gel intended for use on or in the nasal cavity
Oral Gel (Oral Jelly)	Gel intended for use on or in the oral cavity
Ophthalmic Gel (Ophthalmic Jelly)	Gel intended for use on or in the eye
Rectal Gel (Rectal Jelly)	Gel intended for use in or around the rectum
Topical Gel (Topical Jelly)	Gel intended for use on the skin
Augmented Topical Gel	Gel with enhanced drug delivery capability
Urethral Gel (Urethral Jelly)	Gel intended for use in the urethra
Vaginal Gel (Vaginal Jelly)	Gel intended for use in or around the vagina
Granules	Numerous particles forming a larger unit
Granules for Oral Solution	Granules to be reconstituted with solvent just before dispensing to form a solution intended to be taken by mouth
Granules for Oral Suspension	Granules to be reconstituted with diluent prior to administration to form a suspension intended to be taken by mouth
Oral Granules	Granules intended to be taken by mouth
Drug Implant	Solid form inserted into the body that releases medication over time
Intrauterine System	Drug delivery system inserted and left in the uterus to provide uniform release of drugs over several years
Oral Lozenge (Oral Troche)	Solid mass intended to be held in the mouth to allow for slow dissolution
Medicated Pad (Medicated Swab)	Non-adhesive patch used to apply medication (see also Medicated Patch and Transdermal System)
Medicated Tape	Adhesive tape used to apply medication (see also Medicated Patch and Transdermal System)

(continued)

TABLE 8.2. Continued

Form	Definition and Usage Notes
Ointment	Viscous occlusive mixture
Nasal Ointment	Ointment intended for use on or in the nose
Ophthalmic Ointment	Ointment intended for use on or in the eye
Oral Ointment	Ointment intended for use on or in the mouth
Otic Ointment	Ointment intended for use on or in the ear
Rectal Ointment	Ointment intended for use on or in the rectum
Topical Ointment	Ointment intended for use on or in the skin
Augmented Topical Ointment	Ointment with enhanced drug delivery capability
Vaginal Ointment	Ointment intended for use on or in the vagina
Oral Strip	Medicated thin strip that dissolves–intended for oral use
Buccal Film	Film that adheres to the inner lining of the cheek until dissolved
Paste	Smooth, viscous mixture of material; semisolid in nature
Oral Paste	Paste to be taken or used orally
Toothpaste	Paste intended to be used in cleaning teeth
Patch	Type of material that can be used to cover or repair an affected area
Medicated Patch	Adhesive patch that delivers medication locally to the area beneath the patch (see also Transdermal System and Medicated Tape)
Transdermal System	Adhesive patch that delivers medication at a set rate systemically over a defined period of time (see also Medicated Patch)
Oral Pellet	Small rounded body
Oral Wafer	Thin, cookie-like, baked form
Powder	Loose state of particulate matter
Inhalant Powder (Powdered Dose Inhaler)	Powdered medication that is intended to be inhaled
Nasal Powder	Powder intended for use in the nasal cavity
Oral Powder	Powder given orally, often sprinkled on or mixed with food. Not for powders mixed with liquids
Powder for Nasal Solution	Powder which, upon the addition of suitable vehicles, yields a solution intended for use on the nasal mucosa
Powder for Oral Solution	Powder which, upon the addition of suitable vehicles, yields a solution intended to be taken by mouth
Powder for Oral Suspension	Powder which, upon the addition of suitable vehicles, yields a suspension intended to be taken by mouth

TABLE 8.2. Continued

Form	Definition and Usage Notes
Sublingual Powder	Powder intended for use under the tongue
Topical Powder	Powder intended for use on the outside surface of the body
Suppository	Solid drug delivery vehicle that melts at normal body temperature
Rectal Suppository	Suppository intended to be inserted into the rectum
Vaginal Suppository	Suppository intended to be inserted into the vagina
Urethral Suppository	Suppository intended to be inserted into the urethra
Tablet	Solid, compressed dosage form
Oral Tablet (Caplet)	Tablet containing medicated materials to be taken by mouth
Oral Tablet with Sensor	Tablet taken orally that digitally tracks if patients have ingested their medication
Buccal Tablet	Tablet held in the hollow pockets of the cheek until dissolved
Sustained Release Buccal Tablet	Tablet held in the hollow pockets of the cheek while the slowed delivery system allows the drug to be released over an extended period of time at a controlled rate
Chewable Tablet	Tablet taken by mouth and crushed into smaller pieces before swallowing
Delayed Release Oral Tablet	Solid dosage form which releases a drug (or drugs) at a time other than promptly after oral administration (enteric-coated articles are delayed release dosage forms)
Disintegrating Oral Tablet	Tablet dissolved in the mouth to release medication
Effervescent Oral Tablet	Solid dosage form containing mixtures of acids (e.g., citric acid, tartaric acid) and sodium bicarbonate that release carbon dioxide when dissolved in water; it is intended to be dissolved or dispersed in water before oral administration
Extended Release Oral Tablet	Tablet whose contents are slowly released over an extended period of time at a controlled rate
Sublingual Tablet	Tablet held under the tongue until dissolved
Tablet for Oral Suspension	Tablet to be reconstituted with diluent prior to administration to form a suspension intended to be taken by mouth
Vaginal Tablet	Tablet that contains medicated materials to be inserted vaginally
Topical Cake	Block of compressed or firm matter intended for use on a surface
Vaginal Film	Film that adheres to the inner lining of the vagina until dissolved
Vaginal Ring	Pliable delivery system surrounded by a polymeric membrane that provides controlled drug release to the vagina

Source: NLM 2018e.

Brand names are those as usually seen on the packaging (such as Zyrtec, Aleve, and Bicillin L-A). When the name on the packaging includes extra information that represents information beyond ingredient or strength, the extra information is removed (NLM 2018c).

SAB=RXNORM normalized drug name may include additional elements. Some specific dose forms require a quantity factor even though they are not drug packs. Examples here might be the volume of drug in a prefilled syringe, number of actuations in a metered dose inhaler, or duration of action of an extended release capsule.

SAB=RXNORM contains other descriptions for drug products that enable easier identification of a drug. This includes the TTY of SY, which is a term type used for synonyms of names, and PSN, or prescribable name. TTY=SY contains other synonymous descriptions for the RxNorm normalized term. There can be zero to many SYs for an RxNorm normalized atom. TTY=PSN contains a prescribable name, a name that clinicians can easily identify. There is only one PSN for an RxNorm normalized term.

RXCUI 731571
SBD: 4 ML penicillin G benzathine 600000 UNT/ML Prefilled Syringe [Bicillin L-A]
SY: Bicillin L-A 2,400,000 UNT per 4 ML Prefilled Syringe
SY: 4 ML PCN G benzathine 600000 UNT/ML Prefilled Syringe [Bicillin L-A]
SY: 4 ML PEN G benzathine 600000 UNT/ML Prefilled Syringe [Bicillin L-A]
PSN: BICILLIN L-A 2,400,000 UNT in 4 ML Prefilled Syringe
(NLM 2018d)

Structure of RxNorm

Term types (TTYs) indicate generic and branded names of products at different levels of specificity (NLM 2018c). Except for SY, this specificity of the term type allows easy identification of what the content of the name will include. Table 8.3 includes the full list of SAB=RXNORM term types.

As mentioned earlier, RxNorm uses relationships to link concepts that contain the same ingredient or dose form. Using these relationships, the SAB=RXNORM graph can be navigated from an ingredient to a fully specified drug and so forth. Table 8.4 lists the RxNorm relationships for TTY Semantic Clinical Drug (SCD).

Process for Revisions and Updates

The basic structure of RxNorm has changed little since it first began. Most of the changes that have taken place have been in terms of addition of new attributes, some new term types (such as the dose form groups and prescribable names), and some methods of representing history. The

TABLE 8.3. SAB=RXNORM term types

TTY	Name	Description	Example
IN	Ingredient	A compound or moiety that gives the drug its distinctive clinical properties. Ingredients generally use the United States Adopted Name (USAN).	Fluoxetine
PIN	Precise Ingredient	A specified form of the ingredient that may or may not be clinically active. Most precise ingredients are salt or isomer forms.	Fluoxetine Hydrochloride
MIN	Multiple Ingredients	Two or more ingredients appearing together in a single drug preparation, created from SCDF. In rare cases when IN/PIN or PIN/PIN combinations of the same base ingredient exist, created from SCD.	Fluoxetine / Olanzapine
DF	Dose Form	These describe the form of a medication as it is administered to the patient. For example, injectable solution rather than lyophilized powder for reconstitution.	Oral Solution
DFG	Dose Form Group	A dose form group describes a shorthand name for one of several possible dose forms, when a prescriber is not particular about the dose form. For example, pill might be used rather than oral tablet or oral capsule.	Oral Liquid
SCDC	Semantic Clinical Drug Component	Ingredient + Strength	Fluoxetine 4 MG/ML
SCDF	Semantic Clinical Drug Form	Ingredient + Dose Form	Fluoxetine Oral Solution
SCDG	Semantic Clinical Dose Form Group	Ingredient + Dose Form Group	Fluoxetine Oral Product
SCD	Semantic Clinical Drug	Ingredient + Strength + Dose Form	Fluoxetine 4 MG/ML Oral Solution
BN	Brand Name	A proprietary name for a family of products containing a specific set of active ingredient(s).	Prozac

(continued)

233

TABLE 8.3. Continued

TTY	Name	Description	Example
SBDC	Semantic Branded Drug Component	Ingredient + Strength + Brand Name	Fluoxetine 4 MG/ML [Prozac]
SBDF	Semantic Branded Drug Form	Ingredient + Dose Form + Brand Name	Fluoxetine Oral Solution [Prozac]
SBDG	Semantic Branded Dose Form Group	Ingredient + Dose Form Group + Brand Name	Prozac Pill
SBD	Semantic Branded Drug	Ingredient + Strength + Dose Form + Brand Name	Fluoxetine 4 MG/ML Oral Solution [Prozac]
SY	Synonym	Synonym of another TTY, given for clarity.	Prozac 4 MG/ML Oral Solution
TMSY	Tall Man Lettering Synonym	Tall Man Lettering synonym of another TTY, given to distinguish between commonly confused drugs.	FLUoxetine 10 MG Oral Capsule [PROzac]
PSN	Prescribable Name	A name for a product as it is usually displayed to a clinician	FLUoxetine 20 MG in 5 ML Oral Solution
BPCK	Brand Name Pack	{# (Ingredient Strength Dose Form)/# (Ingredient Strength Dose Form)} Pack [Brand Name]	{12 (Ethinyl Estradiol 0.035 MG/ Norethindrone 0.5 MG Oral Tablet)/ 9 (Ethinyl Estradiol 0.035 MG/Norethindrone 1 MG Oral Tablet)/ 7 (Inert Ingredients 1 MG Oral Tablet)} Pack [Leena 28 Day]
GPCK	Generic Pack	{# (Ingredient + Strength + Dose Form)/ # (Ingredient + Strength + Dose Form)} Pack	{11 (varenicline 0.5 MG Oral Tablet)/ 42 (varenicline 1 MG Oral Tablet)} Pack

Source: NLM 2018c.

creation of the Current Prescribable Content Subset was a new addition, without changes in structure but just providing a more compact view of a part of the data.

Updates are of two varieties. A full set of files is distributed monthly, currently the first working day on or after the first Monday in a month. Products that are thought to be off the market are marked as obsolete, but not removed from RxNorm. While there may be modest changes in how a certain name is treated, the contents of the concepts of RxNorm rarely change. Additions are most common when a new product is introduced. Each of the major drug compendia will incorporate that name into their system, and it will then make its way into RxNorm. At the same time, if a label for a new product is produced and submitted to the FDA, that information will generate data, which is then made available to RxNorm for creation of a new concept. This might happen before any of the vendors alter their systems.

TABLE 8.4. RxNorm relationships for semantic clinical drug

RXNREL RXCUI2 TTY	RELA	RXNREL RXCUI1 TTY	Example with Strings
SCD	contained_in	BPCK	'Acetaminophen 500 MG Oral Tablet' contained_in '{24 (Acetaminophen 500 MG / Diphenhydramine Hydrochloride 25 MG Oral Tablet [Tylenol PM]) / 50 (Acetaminophen 500 MG Oral Tablet [Tylenol]) } Pack [Tylenol Extra Strength Day and Night Pack]'
SCD	has_dose_form	DF	'Acetaminophen 325 MG Oral Tablet' has_dose_form 'Oral Tablet'
SCD	contained_in	GPCK	'Acetaminophen 500 MG Oral Tablet' contained_in '{24 (Acetaminophen 500 MG / Diphenhydramine Hydrochloride 25 MG Oral Tablet) / 50 (Acetaminophen 500 MG Oral Tablet) } Pack'
SCD	has_ingredients	MIN	'Acetaminophen 325 MG / Diphenhydramine Hydrochloride 50 MG Oral Tablet' has_ingredients 'Acetaminophen / Diphenhydramine'
SCD	has_tradename	SBD	'Acetaminophen 325 MG Oral Tablet' has_tradename 'Acetaminophen 325 MG Oral Tablet [Tylenol]'
SCD	quantified_form_of	SCD	'8 HR Acetaminophen 650 MG Extended Release Tablet' quantified_form_of 'Acetaminophen 650 MG Extended Release Tablet'
SCD	has_quantified_form	SCD	'Acetaminophen 650 MG Extended Release Tablet' has_quantified_form '8 HR Acetaminophen 650 MG Extended Release Tablet'
SCD	consists_of	SCDC	'Acetaminophen 325 MG Oral Tablet' consists_of 'Acetaminophen 325 MG'
SCD	isa	SCDF	'Acetaminophen 325 MG Oral Tablet' isa 'Acetaminophen Oral Tablet'
SCD	isa	SCDG	'Acetaminophen 325 MG Oral Tablet' isa 'Acetaminophen Pills'

Source: NLM 2018f.

A weekly update is released regularly, currently every Wednesday. It consists only of new material that has become available through the process involving DailyMed. It may have RXCUIs in it that are new, or those that already exist but a new name from DailyMed or new attributes from DailyMed (for example, a new NDC code) have been added to the concept or to MTHSPL (the source name given to DailyMed).

With each full release, a set of release notes is issued with the files. These notes will indicate any changes in structure or content of the files and should be reviewed before trying to use the new files.

Relationship with Other Terminologies, Classification Systems, and Code Sets

RxNorm is the terminology that joins many sources of drug information to a common identifier. The list of sources map to a concept that is contained in RxNorm to an external code set. The most common mappings are from generic product to Semantic Clinical Drug (SCD) or Generic Drug Pack (GPCK) and brand product to Semantic Branded Drug (SBD), but some sources, including ingredients (IN or PIN) dose forms (DF), brand names (BN), National Drug Codes (NDC), and Medicare billing codes (HCPCS), have additional information that can be mapped in RxNorm. Some mappings, such as HCPCS codes, are indirectly contained in RxNorm and use additional external information to define them. Table 8.5 lists mapping in RxNorm.

Tools to Access and Use

RxNorm data can be accessed in several ways. The most common way is that the data is downloaded as a file and that data is used within a proprietary application to provide a common identifier for a drug product. The reason for this is that RxNorm contains large volumes of data and usually only a small subset is needed for recording in the patient health record, e-prescribing, formulary, and medication history. The RxNorm Full Monthly Release contains information from sources that require a license agreement to use their proprietary codes and relationships to external sources, such as HCPCS (NLM 2018g). The RxNorm Current Prescribable Content:

- is an approximation of the prescription drugs currently marketed in the US
- includes some frequently prescribed over-the-counter drugs
- includes only the active RxNorm names, codes (RXCUIs), attributes, and relationships, as well as the FDA structured product label drugs and ingredients
- does not include data from any of the other RxNorm data providers, such as First DataBank, Micromedex, or the Veterans Administration
- is in the public domain and requires no license
  (NLM 2018h)

RxNorm provides an Application Programming Interface (API) as a web service to automate the retrieval of the RxNorm dataset for electronic records. This API can be used as a Simple Object Access Protocol (SOAP) or a Representational State Transfer (REST)ful service. See [NLM n.d.b.] in the resources at the end of the chapter.

The best depiction of RxNorm with a graphic user interface is RxNav. This web application allows lookup of drugs or ingredients with their relationships to each other, therapeutic classification, and other information (see [NLM 2018b] in the references at the end of this chapter).

TABLE 8.5. Mappings in RxNorm

SOURCE	BN	CLASS	DF	IN/PIN	NDC	SBD/BPCK	SCD/GPCK
Anatomical Therapeutic Chemical Classification System (ATC)		X					
Centers for Disease Control Vaccine Codes (CVX)					X	X	X
CMS Formulary Reference File (MTHCMSFRF)					X	X	X
Drug Bank				X			
Gold Standard Drug Database (GS)					X	X	X
Medical Subject Headings (MeSH) maps ingredients to IN or PIN				X			
Multum MediSource Lexicon	X			X	X	X	X
Micromedex Red Book					X	X	X
FDA Structured Product Labels (SPL)			X	X (UNII)	X	X	X
FDBMedKnowledge (formerly NDDF Plus)			X		X		X
United States Pharmacopeia (USP)				X			X
US Edition of SNOMED CT (drug information)							X
Veterans Health Administration National Drug File (VANDF)							X

Source: NLM 2018g.

Adoption and Use Cases

While the RxNorm system was originally intended for use in supporting interoperability during e-prescribing and formulary management, it became apparent that the normalized names used in the creation of the system, which we know here as RxNorm, have other uses. As a set of standardized names covering all prescription medications in the US, it can be used for communication between hospital, pharmacy, and other organizations' computer systems, for order entry and analytics, and for managing a medication list. The names that fully describe a product, with term types SCD, semantic branded drug (SBD), generic pack (GPCK), and branded name pack (BPCK), are designated in the Meaningful Use (MU) Stage II requirements for communication to other systems.

For example, the common set of MU data types, or elements for which certification is required across several certification criteria, was created by the Office of the National Coordinator. The Common Clinical Data Set (CCDS), formally referred to as the Common MU Data Set, is used by inpatient and ambulatory care providers in information exchange. The CCDS means data is expressed according to the specified standard terminology in any instance where that data element is indicated. For medications and medication allergies, RxNorm was the named standard in the Common MU Data Set and continues in the CCDS. The Medicare EHR Incentive Program, more frequently known as MU, is now a part of the Promoting Interoperability Programs (CMS 2018).

In addition, e-Rx via certified EHR technology is a requirement for eligible professionals to receive reimbursement under the Medicare and Medicaid EHR Incentive Programs.

RxNorm is also the terminology the Pharmacist Collaborative Value Set Committee is using in the development of an allergy value set for submission to the Value Set Authority Center for incorporation into MU requirements (PHITC 2018). This work is expected to lead to improved accuracy and usefulness of medication allergy information in the provision of patient care (ACCP 2018).

Other common users of RxNorm include CMS, which uses it in its Formulary Reference File, and the Observational Health Data Sciences and Informatics research group's use in the analysis of prescription data (NCVHS 2017).

Use Case One: Supporting Interoperability and Long-term Data Collection

Supporting semantic interoperability implies that from a name in any given vocabulary included in the system, one should be able to successfully identify, without human intervention, the corresponding name or names in another vocabulary. The entire structure of RxNorm is built to support exactly that identification.

Such functionality was tested by the Clinical Health Data Repository (CHDR) group, which was attempting to translate medication records from the Department of Defense record system to that of the Veterans Administration. Using an early version of RxNorm, a 74 percent success rate was achieved (Warnekar et al. 2007). Given the newness of the program during that attempt, one could safely predict much better results would be found with a later, more seasoned version.

Another conceivable use is in long-term summarization of medication data over time. In various records systems, the data may be stored at various levels of abstraction using different vocabularies. By using RxNorm, data originally derived from different vocabularies can be aggregated over multiple levels of abstraction. This might make long-term collection of data about medication exposure over time, and even, in some cases, total dose exposure to a given medication, possible. These types of historical or epidemiologic questions may become quite important as more and more clinical data, especially medication data, is recorded electronically.

Use Case Two: Transmitting Prescriptions Electronically and Order Entry

The National Council Prescription Drug Programs has established a standard for transmitting prescriptions electronically. While that standard requires much more than the name of the product, the standard accommodates the RxNorm names as the names of the prescribed products.

Some systems have adopted the use of the RxNorm names for order entry. The dose form group names were specifically added to facilitate this process, as providers often are not particular about specifying a precise form. For example, a provider may not care if the patient is given a tablet or a capsule. Synonyms and Prescribable Names, which often express names in a more recognizable format than that of the formal normalized names, also facilitate this process.

CHECK YOUR UNDERSTANDING

1. Which of the following is included in the normalized name of a clinical drug in RxNorm? (Mark all that apply.)

    a. Ingredient
    b. Strength
    c. Dose form
    d. Route

2. RxNorm serves as a means of preparing which source vocabularies for inclusion in the UMLS? (Mark all that apply.)

    a. DrugBank
    b. Multum
    c. Micromedex
    d. First DataBank
    e. Gold Standard

3. Each RxNorm name and its synonyms constitute a:

    a. Branded version of the drug
    b. Single concept

c. Generic version of the drug

d. Term type

4. True or false? RxNorm uses term types to indicate generic and branded names of products at different levels of specificity.

a. True

b. False

5. Which one of the following is *not* included in RxNorm?

a. Prescription drugs in the US

b. Over-the-counter drugs available in the US

c. Generic drugs

d. Dietary supplements

REVIEW

1. True or false? Naproxen 250 MG Oral Tablet [Naprosyn] is an example of a normalized name for a generic drug.

a. True

b. False

2. True or false? Dose forms used in the RxNorm name always represent the form in which the manufacturer supplied it.

a. True

b. False

3. The full set of files updating RxNorm are released:

a. Weekly

b. Monthly

c. Quarterly

d. Yearly

4. True or false? RXCUIs are deleted from one RxNorm release to the next.

a. True

b. False

5. Which RxNorm web program presents a graphic view of a drug?

   a. RxNorm Application Programming Interface
   b. RxNav
   c. DailyMed
   d. RxNorm APIs

6. In RxNorm, the semantic clinical drug is which of the following?

   a. Ingredient + strength + dose form
   b. Ingredient + dose form
   c. Ingredient + strength + brand name
   d. Ingredient + dose form + brand name

7. Who held the meeting that resulted in the development of RxNorm?

   a. HL7
   b. NLM
   c. CDC
   d. FDA

8. True or false? Reimbursement of drugs is based on RxNorm codes.

   a. True
   b. False

9. Weekly updates to RxNorm are to account for:

   a. New products
   b. NDF updates
   c. NDC updates
   d. Discontinued products

10. True or false? RxNorm contains the names of prescription and over-the-counter drugs.

   a. True
   b. False

References

American College of Clinical Pharmacy (ACCP). 2018. Call for participants: RxNorm classification system. http://www.accp.com/announcements/rxnorm.aspx.

Centers for Medicare and Medicaid Services (CMS). 2018. "Electronic Public Health Reporting." Presented at the ONC Annual Meeting, Washington DC, November 30, 2018.

McGinness, D., J. Bronnert, C. Masarie, and F. Naeymi-Rad. 2013. RxNorm's drug interface terminology supports interoperability. *Journal of AHIMA* 84(2):44–47.

National Committee on Vital and Health Statistics (NCVHS). 2017. Clinical terminology standards required for US health data exchange: SNOMED CT, LOINC, RxNorm. https://ncvhs.hhs.gov/wp-content/uploads/2017/06/Day1-Humphreys-SNM-LOINC-RXN-002.pdf.

National Committee on Vital and Health Statistics (NCVHS). 2004. September 2, 2004 Letter to the Secretary – First Set of Recommendations on E-Prescribing Standards. https://ncvhs.hhs.gov/rrp/september-2-2004-letter-to-the-secretary-first-set-of-recommendations-on-e-prescribing-standards/.

National Library of Medicine (NLM). 2018a. RxNorm technical documentation. https://www.nlm.nih.gov/research/umls/rxnorm/docs/2018/rxnorm_doco_full_2018-1.html.

National Library of Medicine (NLM). 2018b. RxNav, Version:04-Sep-2018. https://mor.nlm.nih.gov/RxNav/#.

National Library of Medicine (NLM). 2018c. RxNorm overview. https://www.nlm.nih.gov/research/umls/rxnorm/overview.html.

National Library of Medicine (NLM). 2018d. "Label: Bicillin L-A- penicillin g benzathine injection, suspension." https://dailymed.nlm.nih.gov/dailymed/drugInfo.cfm?setid=012d46f1-d0a0-4676-a879-cd320297ab16.

National Library of Medicine (NLM). 2018e. Appendix 2 – RxNorm dose forms (TTY=DF) with definitions. https://www.nlm.nih.gov/research/umls/rxnorm/docs/2018/appendix2.html.

National Library of Medicine (NLM). 2018f. Appendix 1– RxNorm relationships (RELA). https://www.nlm.nih.gov/research/umls/rxnorm/docs/2018/appendix1.html.

National Library of Medicine (NLM). 2018g. RxNorm full monthly release. https://www.nlm.nih.gov/research/umls/rxnorm/docs/rxnormfiles.html.

National Library of Medicine (NLM). 2018h. RxNorm current prescribable content. https://www.nlm.nih.gov/research/umls/rxnorm/docs/rxnormfiles.html.

Pharmacy Health Information Technology Collaborative (PHITC). 2018. Workgroups and Committees. http://www.pharmacyhit.org/index.php/workgroups-and-committees.

Warnekar, P. P., O. Bouhaddou, F. Parrish, N. Do, J. Kilbourne, S. H. Brown, and M. J. Lincoln. 2007. Use of RxNorm to exchange codified drug allergy information between Department of Veterans Affairs (VA) and Department of Defense (DoD). *AMIA Annual Symposium Proceedings*; 781–785. Published online 2007 with PMCID:PMC2655912.

Resources

Nelson, S. J., K. Zeng, J. Kilbourne, T. Powell, and R. Moore. 2011. Normalized names for clinical drugs—RxNorm at 6 years. *Journal of the American Medical Informatics Association* 18(4):441–448.

National Library of Medicine. n.d.a. DailyMed. https://dailymed.nlm.nih.gov/dailymed/.

National Library of Medicine. n.d.b. RxNorm API. https://rxnav.nlm.nih.gov/RxNormAPIs.html#.

9

Diagnostic and Statistical Manual of Mental Disorders (DSM)

Michael B. First, MD

LEARNING OBJECTIVES

- Discuss the development and purpose of *Diagnostic and Statistical Manual of Mental Disorders* (DSM)
- Identify the party responsible for developing and updating DSM
- Differentiate the types of information in DSM
- Categorize the different users of DSM
- Examine the relationship DSM has with other classifications, terminologies, and code sets
- Compare tools available to access and use
- Understand how DSM is used in an electronic environment

KEY TERMS

- American Psychiatric Association (APA)
- Descriptive text
- *Diagnostic and Statistical Manual of Mental Disorders*, Fifth Edition (DSM-5)
- Diagnostic criteria
- *International Classification of Diseases, Tenth Revision, Clinical Modification* (ICD-10-CM)
- *International Classification of Diseases, Eleventh Revision* (ICD-11)

Introduction to DSM-5

Diagnostic and Statistical Manual of Mental Disorders, **Fifth Edition (DSM-5)** is the standard classification of mental disorders used by mental health and medical professionals throughout the US. DSM-5 contains names and *International Classification of Diseases, Tenth Revision, Clinical Modification* **(ICD-10-CM)** codes for mental disorders, criteria for making specific diagnoses, assessment measures, and other helpful text for clinicians. DSM-5 is used across all types of healthcare settings and strives to meet the needs of various diverse populations. Moreover, it has been translated into numerous foreign languages. This chapter discusses the developer, history, purpose, principles, maintenance, and adoption including use cases of DSM-5. The most up-to-date information on DSM-5, including updates to the DSM-5 criteria and ICD-10-CM codes, can be found at the **American Psychiatric Association (APA)** website (see [APA 2018a] in the reference list at the end of this chapter).

Developer

The APA develops and publishes *Diagnostic and Statistical Manual of Mental Disorders* (DSM). The APA is a medical specialty society consisting of more than 37,800 member physicians in the US and abroad. The first edition, DSM-I, was published in 1952. There have been six updates since then, the most recent being DSM-5, published in 2013. The APA owns and holds the copyright to DSM.

History of DSM

The history of DSM is intertwined with several other national efforts to classify mental disorders over the past 170 years. This history has been summarized by the APA (2013a; 2013b). In 1840, the US census began collecting statistics regarding the mental illness of insanity. Forty years later, the US census expanded its statistical collecting to include mania, melancholia, monomania, paresis, dementia, dipsomania, and epilepsy. By the end of the 1800s, inpatient mental health facilities began developing their own unique diagnostic classification systems for statistical information.

In 1917, the American Medico-Psychological Association (today named the APA) and the National Committee for Mental Hygiene developed a standard classification consisting of 21 groups of "mental diseases" for use by US institutional facilities. By 1935, the revised APA classification list was incorporated into the second edition of the American Medical Association's Standard Classified Nomenclature of Diseases.

Psychiatric classification systems developed before World War II were mainly for use in psychiatric hospitals and did not meet the needs of other healthcare settings. During World War II, the US Army developed a classification system to assist in reporting diagnoses of its servicemen and veterans. This classification system, called Medical 203, was later modified by the Veterans Administration (VA).

In 1948, the World Health Organization (WHO) included, for the first time, a section on mental disorders in the sixth revision of the *International Classification of Diseases, Injuries, and Causes of Death* (ICD-6). The ICD-6 section was influenced by the VA modification of Medical 203. Unfortunately, ICD-6 did not meet all the needs of the psychiatric profession, which led to

TABLE 9.1. History of the DSM

Version	Year	Description
DSM-I	1952	The APA developed and published the first official DSM edition, based on ICD-6. The classification organized mental disorders around presumed pathogenic processes called "reactions," based on prevailing psychobiological theories. DSM-I included a glossary of definitions for the mental categories and was recognized as the first classification system for mental disorders to focus on clinical utility.
DSM-II	1968	Developed at the same time as ICD-8, this edition was similar to DSM-I. It continued the use of the glossary of definitions but dropped the term "reaction." The psychodynamic concept of neurosis was retained however.
DSM-III	1980	The third edition of the DSM represented a major shift in the diagnosis of mental disorders and significantly facilitated clinical practice and empirical research. DSM-III included explicit diagnostic criteria for each mental disorder and a multiaxial assessment method. A descriptive atheoretical approach was incorporated rather than categorizing disorders based on presumed underlying causes. DSM-III was accepted on an international level and provided a common language for mental health professionals. ICD-9 was published in 1975.
DSM-III-R	1987	This revision primarily addressed inconsistencies in the DSM-III.
DSM-IV	1994	Much of the five-year DSM-IV development project involved evaluations of research evidence through literature reviews, data analysis, and field trials. Numerous incremental changes were made to the classification, to the diagnostic criteria sets, and to the descriptive text. Through a close working relationship with WHO, the differences between DSM-IV and ICD-10 which was published in 1992, were minimized. ICD-9-CM, which initially went into effect in 1979, remained the official coding system in use in the US.
DSM-IV-TR (Text Revision)	2000	The DSM-IV-TR edition focused on updating the descriptive text. Only a small number of criteria sets were revised to correct errors identified in previous editions. Some diagnostic codes were revised to reflect updates to the ICD-9-CM coding system.
DSM-5	2013	DSM-5 revisions included new disorders and criteria sets, removal of the multiaxial approach to documenting diagnoses, a new diagnostic chapter structure, and the introduction of dimensional assessments of symptoms and disability. Both ICD-9-CM and ICD-10-CM codes were originally listed in DSM-5 because its May 2013 publication date predated the anticipated October 1, 2015, adoption of ICD-10-CM in the US. Efforts were also made between the APA and the WHO to harmonize the development of DSM-5 and ICD-11.

development of *Diagnostic and Statistical Manual: Mental Disorders* (DSM-I), released in 1952. Table 9.1 summarizes the history of DSM since then.

Purpose

According to the APA, the primary purpose of DSM-5 is "to assist trained clinicians in the diagnosis of their patients' mental disorders as part of a case formulation assessment that leads to a fully informed treatment plan for each individual" (APA 2013b, 19).

Clinical Users of DSM-5

DSM-5 is an authoritative guide used by mental health professionals such as practicing psychiatrists, clinical psychologists, and clinical social workers. It is also used by other medical professionals, including nurses and non-psychiatrist physicians. The manual provides these clinicians with common language and standards to assist in making psychiatric diagnoses. It does not include guidance on treatment of patients with these diagnoses. The DSM manual includes an important statement that cautions: "**Diagnostic criteria** are offered as guidelines for making diagnoses, and their use should be informed by clinical judgment" (APA 2013b, 21).

Forensic Users of DSM-5

DSM-5 can be a valuable diagnostic tool for professionals who conduct forensic evaluations for legal issues, including civil, criminal, and correctional matters. It is also used for legislation and government regulations. However, the APA includes the following cautionary information regarding the use of the DSM in a forensic context:

> When DSM-5 categories, criteria, and textual descriptions are employed for forensic purposes, there is a significant risk that diagnostic information will be misused or misunderstood. These dangers arise because of the imperfect fit between the questions of ultimate concern to the law and the information contained in a clinical diagnosis. In most situations, the clinical diagnosis of a DSM-5 mental disorder such as intellectual disability (intellectual developmental disorder), schizophrenia, major neurocognitive disorder, gambling disorder, or pedophilic disorder does not imply that an individual with such a condition meets legal criteria for the presence of a mental disorder or a specified legal standard (for example, for competence, criminal responsibility, or disability). For the latter, additional information is usually required beyond that contained in the DSM-5 diagnosis, which might include information about the individual's functional impairments and how these impairments affect the particular abilities in question (APA 2013b, 25).

Information Management Users of DSM-5

The ICD-9-CM and ICD-10-CM diagnostic codes are incorporated into the DSM-5 system. The diagnoses in DSM-5 all have been assigned valid codes according to the ICD-10-CM coding classification that is the official code set under the Centers for Medicare and Medicaid Services (CMS) Administrative Simplification provision of the Health Insurance Portability and Accountability Act of 1996 (HIPAA). ICD-10-CM codes are used to report public health statistics and are required under payer policies. The version of DSM-5 published in 2013 included both ICD-9-CM along with the corresponding ICD-10-CM codes to facilitate the transition from ICD-9-CM to ICD-10-CM in 2015. Future printings will include only ICD-10-CM codes.

Content

DSM-5 is divided into three sections. Section I includes a chapter describing the DSM-5 revision process and important conceptual changes to the manual, including integration of dimensional assessments; enhanced age-, culture- and gender-related material; the introduction of "other specified" and "unspecified" diagnostic categories; removal of the multiaxial system; and the use of online supplemental material. The second chapter in Section I, titled "Use of the Manual," provides user instructions on clinical case formulation and essential elements of a diagnosis. This chapter also provides instructions and introductory information related to the diagnostic criteria. The final chapter explains the Cautionary Statement for Forensic Use of DSM-5.

Section II of DSM-5 contains the diagnostic criteria, ICD-10-CM codes, and **descriptive text** for mental disorders. Descriptive text is narrative content, such as diagnostic chapter introductory sections and informative material following the diagnostic criteria, that help support diagnosis. Also included are chapters on medication-induced disorders and other adverse effects of medication, as well as other conditions that may be a focus of clinical attention.

Finally, Section III includes several dimensional assessment measures that may enhance diagnosis, treatment planning, and monitoring treatment response, but are not required for clinical use. Among the assessment measures included in the manual is a patient-completed "Level 1" measure of cross-cutting symptoms that briefly reviews problems that might be seen with any mental disorder, including depression, anxiety, sleep disturbance, and substance use. A second, more detailed set of "Level 2" dimensional measures can also be completed to obtain further information on potentially problematic symptom domains. These Level 2 questionnaires are not included in DSM-5 but are available for downloading (see [APA 2018b] in the reference list at the end of this chapter). A third type of dimensional assessment concerns measures to rate the severity of a given diagnosis. Many, but not all, of the mental disorders in DSM-5 include corresponding diagnosis-specific severity scales, also available for downloading. The last type of dimensional assessment introduced in DSM-5 is the World Health Organization Disability Assessment Schedule 2.0 (WHODAS 2.0), which is discussed later in this chapter (see Removal of the DSM-IV Multiaxial System).

DSM-5 Classification and Corresponding ICD-10-CM Codes

The DSM-5 Classification includes a listing of all the mental disorders, their corresponding ICD-10-CM diagnostic codes, subtypes, specifiers, and coding notes that are unique to the DSM-5 system. The ICD-10-CM coding classification system represents all diseases across all of medicine; however, the DSM mainly uses codes from Chapter 5 (Mental, Behavioral and Neurodevelopmental Disorders). Some mental disorder codes are taken from other chapters, such as the Sleep-Wake disorders, some of which have codes from Chapter 6 (Diseases of the Nervous System). Although for the most part there is a one-to-one correspondence between the mental disorders in ICD-10-CM Chapter 5 and those in DSM-5, there are a number of instances where the disorders do not precisely line up. This is because the mental disorder chapter in ICD-10-CM was developed while the diagnostic classification in effect was DSM-IV. Thus, the ICD-10-CM structure more closely follows DSM-IV than DSM-5. This is most evident in the fact that some of the ICD-10-CM fifth digit codes corresponding to DSM-IV diagnostic specifiers that were eliminated from DSM-5 do not appear among the ICD-10-CM codes listed in the DSM-5 classification. For example, the Schizophrenia category in DSM-IV included five subtypes which are reflected in the ICD-10-CM codes for Schizophrenia: F20.0 paranoid type, F20.1 disorganized type, F20.2 catatonic type, F20.3 undifferentiated type, and F20.5 residual type. Since these five subtypes were removed from DSM-5 (in favor of an optional dimensional symptom rating scale), these ICD-10-CM diagnostic codes are not included in DSM-5. Instead, the DSM-5 classification has assigned F20.9 to the DSM-5 diagnosis of Schizophrenia. Similarly, the lack of alignment between some DSM-IV disorders and their DSM-5 counterparts has resulted in several different DSM-5 diagnoses sharing the same ICD-10-CM code. For example, the DSM-IV category of Alcohol Dependence was divided into Moderate Alcohol Use Disorder and Severe Alcohol Use Disorder in DSM-5. Thus, both Moderate Alcohol Use Disorder and Severe Alcohol Use Disorder share the ICD-10-CM code corresponding to Alcohol Dependence in ICD-10-CM (that is, F10.20).

DSM-5 includes ICD-10-CM diagnostic codes in several places, including:

- In the DSM-5 Classification (that is, the overall listing of disorders and diagnostic codes in the beginning of the DSM-5)
- As part of the descriptive text section for each mental disorder
- In the diagnostic criteria for each disorder
- In the appendices as separate alphabetic and numeric listings of DSM-5 diagnoses and ICD-10-CM codes

Removal of the DSM-IV Multiaxial System

The DSM-IV manual recommended that each patient be assessed using a five-level "multiaxial" system. The multiaxial assessment was an innovative feature first incorporated into the third edition of DSM in 1980. However, DSM-5 eliminated the multiaxial system for several reasons. The placement of certain disorders, such as personality disorders and mental retardation, on Axis II rather than Axis I was originally implemented to generate much-needed clinical and research attention to those disorders, which is no longer necessary. It also implied a hierarchy among disorders such that Axis II mental disorders were considered less serious or important than Axis I disorders. The separation of mental disorders on Axes I and II from other medical disorders on Axis III also implied a separation that is arbitrary and unnecessary. Additionally, clinicians often did not use the multiaxial system consistently. Removal of the system makes DSM-5 more consistent with international classifications and other medical specialties. Table 9.2 shows a comparison of the DSM-IV multiaxial approach with DSM-5's non-axial approach.

In DSM-5, all mental and non-psychiatric medical disorders are recorded in a list. Clinicians should note the name of the disorder as well as the appropriate ICD-10-CM code. Other reasons for the clinical visit or other conditions that are a focus of assessment or treatment (for example, ICD-10-CM T codes for neglect or abuse) may also be included in this list.

TABLE 9.2. Comparison of the DSM-IV multiaxial assessment system and the DSM-5 non-axial approach

DSM-IV Multiaxial Assessment	DSM-5 Non-axial Approach
Axis I: Clinical Disorders and Other Conditions That May Be a Focus of Clinical Attention	All mental disorders are listed, with the primary diagnosis or reason for visit listed first.
Axis II: Personality Disorders and Mental Retardation	Personality disorders and intellectual disability (formerly mental retardation) are listed with all other mental disorders. There is no longer a requirement to separate them in another axis.
Axis III: General Medical Conditions	Other medical conditions are listed after the mental disorder diagnoses, except when the other medical condition is considered to be causing the mental disorder. In such cases, following the ICD-10-CM coding convention, the medical condition is listed first, followed by the mental disorder.
Axis IV: Psychosocial and Environmental Problems	Psychosocial and environmental problems are listed, along with their respective Z code, if they are a reason for visit or a focus of treatment. Psychosocial and environmental problems that are important for understanding the patient but are not a reason for visit or focus of treatment are not coded, but can be recorded in the medical record.
Axis V: Global Assessment of Functioning (GAF)	Instead of a global assessment of "functioning," assessments of the patient's symptom or disorder severity and level of disability should be documented. Clinicians have flexibility in how to accomplish this. The DSM-5 contains optional assessments of symptom and disorder severity in Section III and online. The World Health Organization Disability Assessment Schedule (WHODAS 2.0) is also included in DSM-5 as an optional measure.

While Axes IV and V have been deleted in DSM-5, clinicians are still encouraged to record this information in the medical record. A listing of psychosocial and environmental problems that may affect an individual's diagnosis, treatment, or prognosis can be found in a chapter of conditions in Section II entitled, "Other Conditions That May Be a Focus of Clinical Attention." These conditions replace Axis IV in DSM-5. Finally, the Global Assessment of Functioning (GAF) Scale contained in DSM-IV's Axis V is no longer recommended. The GAF conflated the assessment of disability with assessment of symptom severity and potential for self-harm into a single scale, which also required training for best results. As a result, the GAF was determined to be a problematic, often unreliable scale. To assess disability, DSM-5 encourages (but does not require) clinicians to use the World Health Organization Disability Assessment Schedule version 2.0 (WHODAS 2.0), which was developed to be used with patients who have any health condition and has been shown to be a reliable and valid measure. Section III includes a print version of the WHODAS 2.0, but it is also freely available online (see [APA 2018c] in the reference list at the end of this chapter). There are also online measures of symptom severity in DSM-5. For the assessment of danger to self, the APA develops Clinical Practice Guidelines that can support clinician decision-making (see [APA 2018d] in the reference list at the end of this chapter).

DSM-5 Diagnostic Criteria and Descriptive Text

The DSM-5 system organizes mental disorders into 20 chapters. There are two additional sections titled Medication-Induced Movement Disorders and Other Adverse Effects of Medication, and Other Conditions That May Be a Focus of Clinical Attention.

The 20 diagnostic chapters include:

- Neurodevelopmental Disorders
- Schizophrenia Spectrum and Other Psychotic Disorders
- Bipolar and Related Disorders
- Depressive Disorders
- Anxiety Disorders
- Obsessive-Compulsive and Related Disorders
- Trauma- and Stressor-Related Disorders
- Dissociative Disorders
- Somatic Symptom and Related Disorders
- Feeding and Eating Disorders
- Elimination Disorders
- Sleep-Wake Disorders
- Sexual Dysfunctions
- Gender Dysphoria

- Disruptive, Impulse-Control, and Conduct Disorders
- Substance-Related and Addictive Disorders
- Neurocognitive Disorders
- Personality Disorders
- Paraphilic Disorders
- Other Mental Disorders

FIGURE 9.1. Excerpt of a mental disorder illustrating diagnostic criteria

Panic Disorder F41.0

Diagnostic Criteria

A. Recurrent unexpected panic attacks. A panic attack is an abrupt surge of intense fear or intense discomfort that reaches a peak within minutes, and during which time four (or more) of the following symptoms occur:

Note: The abrupt surge can occur from a calm state or an anxious state.

1. Palpitations, pounding heart, or accelerated heart rate
2. Sweating
3. Trembling or shaking
4. Sensations of shortness of breath or smothering
5. Feelings of choking
6. Chest pain or discomfort
7. Nausea or abdominal distress
8. Feeling dizzy, unsteady, light-headed, or faint
9. Chills or heat sensations
10. Paresthesias (numbness or tingling sensations)
11. Derealization (feelings of unreality) or depersonalization (being detached from oneself)
12. Fear of losing control or "going crazy"
13. Fear of dying

Note: Culture-specific symptoms (e.g., tinnitus, neck soreness, headache, uncontrollable screaming or crying) may be seen. Such symptoms should not count as one of the four required symptoms.

B. At least one of the attacks has been followed by 1 month (or more) of one or both of the following:

1. Persistent concern or worry about additional panic attacks or their consequences (e.g., losing control, having a heart attack, "going crazy")
2. A significant maladaptive change in behavior related to the attacks (e.g., behaviors designed to avoid having panic attacks, such as avoidance of exercise or unfamiliar situations)

C. The disturbance is not attributable to the physiological effects of a substance (e.g., a drug of abuse, a medication) or another medical condition (e.g., hyperthyroidism, cardiopulmonary disorders).

D. The disturbance is not better explained by another mental disorder (e.g., the panic attacks do not occur only in response to feared social situations, as in social anxiety disorder; in response to circumscribed phobic objects or situations, as in specific phobia; in response to obsessions, as in obsessive-compulsive disorder; in response to reminders of traumatic events, as in posttraumatic stress disorder; or in response to separation from attachment figures, as in separation anxiety disorder).

Within each of the 20 diagnostic chapters are listed specified mental disorders. For each mental disorder, a set of detailed diagnostic criteria is provided (see figure 9.1). The diagnostic criteria indicate symptoms that must be present, often with frequency, duration, and age of onset specification. Other criteria might require the clinician to rule out certain conditions that could better account for the clinical presentation. As previously noted, users of DSM find the diagnostic criteria particularly useful because they provide a summarized description of each disorder. Also, use of the diagnostic criteria has been shown to increase diagnostic reliability.

The DSM-5 descriptive text that accompanies each mental disorder is included under the following headings:

- Subtypes and Specifiers
- Recording Procedures
- Diagnostic Features
- Associated Features Supporting Diagnosis
- Prevalence
- Development and Course
- Risk and Prognostic Factors
- Culture-Related Diagnostic Issues
- Gender-Related Diagnostic Issues
- Diagnostic Markers
- Differential Diagnosis
- Comorbidity
- Relationship to Other Classifications

The appendices in DSM-5 include the following:

- Highlights of Changes from DSM-IV to DSM-5
- Glossary of Technical Terms
- Glossary of Cultural Concepts of Distress
- Alphabetical Listing of DSM-5 Diagnoses and Codes
- Numerical Listing of DSM-5 Diagnoses and Codes (ICD-9-CM)
- Numerical Listing of DSM-5 Diagnoses and Codes (ICD-10-CM)
- DSM-5 Advisors and Other Contributors

Principles and Guidelines

General coding and reporting guidelines for DSM-5 are found at the front of the manual. DSM-5 also contains recording notes that alert clinicians when a specific ordering of disorders is needed (for example, to list a medical condition before the mental disorder that it is causing).

ICD-10-CM Diagnostic Codes

Each diagnosis listed in DSM-5 is assigned a valid ICD-10-CM code, in most cases taken from Chapter 5 of ICD-10-CM. For DSM-5 diagnoses in which codes are not straightforward, coding notes are included in the criteria sets to explain coding procedures. An example of this is the ICD-10-CM coding for DSM-5 substance- or medication-induced mental disorders in which the ICD-10-CM code is determined according to types of symptoms induced by the substance or medication (for example, psychotic disorder, anxiety disorder, delirium), the class of substance, whether a comorbid substance use disorder is present, and, if present, the severity of the substance use disorder. Figure 9.2 shows an example of a coding note that pertains to a substance- or medication-induced psychotic disorder. Instructions to clinicians on how to record a diagnosis in the medical record may also be given in the coding note or in a separate text section called Recording Procedures (see figure 9.3).

The developers of DSM-IV and ICD-10 worked together to harmonize the two systems which resulted in ICD-10 Chapter 5, Mental and Behavioral Disorders (F01–F99), remaining more compatible with DSM-IV than with the new DSM-5 in terms of terminology and structure. For example, DSM-5 gave new names to some disorders, such as intellectual disability replacing mental retardation. Also, DSM-5 introduced totally new disorders, which were not included in the initial October 1, 2015 version of ICD-10-CM because of the "freeze" on the addition of new codes that was originally imposed on ICD-10-CM. Although such diagnoses were originally assigned "other" codes in the initial printing of DSM-5, they have been assigned new codes in subsequent versions of ICD-10-CM at the request of the APA. For example, there was no ICD-10-CM disorder corresponding to the newly added DSM-5 diagnosis of disruptive mood dysregulation disorder, so that was originally assigned the ICD-10-CM code F34.8 (Other persistent mood disorder). Subsequently, the APA requested a new ICD-10-CM code for disruptive mood dysregulation disorder, requiring that F34.8 be expanded to F34.81 for disruptive mood dysregulation disorder and F34.89 for Other specified persistent mood disorders. APA continues

FIGURE 9.2. Example of coding note

> **Coding Note**
>
> Coding note: Include the name of the other medical condition in the name of the mental disorder (e.g., 293.81 [F06.2] psychotic disorder due to malignant lung neoplasm, with delusions). The other medical condition should be coded and listed separately immediately before the psychotic disorder due to the medical condition (e.g., 162.9 [C34.90] malignant lung neoplasm; 293.81 [F06.2] psychotic disorder due to malignant lung neoplasm, with delusions).

Source: DSM-5, page 115. Reprinted courtesy of the American Psychiatric Association.

FIGURE 9.3. Example of recording procedures

Recording Procedures.

ICD-10-CM. The name of the substance/medication-induced psychotic disorder begins with the specific substance (e.g., cocaine, dexamethasone) that is presumed to be causing the delusions or hallucinations. The diagnostic code is selected from the table included in the criteria set, which is based on the drug class and presence or absence of a comorbid substance use disorder. For substances that do not fit into any of the classes (e.g., dexamethasone), the code for "other substance" with no comorbid substance use should be used; and in cases in which a substance is judged to be an etiological factor but the specific class of substance is unknown, the category "unknown substance" with no comorbid substance use should be used. When recording the name of the disorder, the comorbid substance use disorder (if any) is listed first, followed by the word "with," followed by the name of the substance-induced psychotic disorder, followed by the specification of onset (i.e., onset during intoxication, onset during withdrawal). For example, in the case of delusions occurring during intoxication in a man with a severe cocaine use disorder, the diagnosis is F14.259 severe cocaine use disorder with cocaine-induced psychotic disorder, with onset during intoxication. A separate diagnosis of the comorbid severe cocaine use disorder is not given. If the substance-induced psychotic disorder occurs without a comorbid substance use disorder (e.g., after a one-time heavy use of the substance), no accompanying substance use disorder is noted (e.g., F16.959 phencyclidine-induced psychotic disorder, with onset during intoxication). When more than one substance is judged to play a significant role in the development of psychotic symptoms, each should be listed separately (e.g., F12.259 severe cannabis use disorder with cannabis-induced psychotic disorder, with onset during intoxication; F16.159 mild phencyclidine use disorder with phencyclidine-induced psychotic disorder, with onset during intoxication).

Source: DSM-5, page 112. Reprinted courtesy of the American Psychiatric Association.

to work with the developers of ICD-10-CM, particularly the National Center for Health Statistics (NCHS), to request coding changes to increase its compatibility with DSM-5.

Subtypes and Specifiers

The DSM-5 subtypes and specifiers provide additional details about a particular disorder such as course (for example, alcohol use disorder, in sustained remission), severity (for example, anorexia nervosa, severe), and symptomatic features (for example, schizoaffective disorder, bipolar type, conversion disorder with paralysis). DSM-5 defines subtypes as "mutually exclusive and jointly exhaustive phenomenological subgroupings within a diagnosis [that] are indicated by the instruction 'specify whether' in the criteria set" (APA 2013b, 21). Specifiers are not necessarily mutually exclusive or jointly exhaustive, and therefore more than one can be applied to a disorder if appropriate. Specifiers are indicated by the instruction "specify" or "specify if" in the criteria set.

A minority of the subtypes and specifiers are indicated by the use of a specific ICD-10-CM code (for example, F50.01 for Anorexia nervosa, restricting type and F50.02 for Anorexia nervosa, binge-eating/purging type). Most subtypes and specifiers do not have specific ICD-10-CM codes associated with them and are noted by including the applicable subtype or specifier after the name of the disorder (for example, F40.10 Social Anxiety Disorder, performance only). Some disorders employ a combination of specifiers that are reflected in the choice of ICD-10-CM code and uncoded specifiers that are recorded after the name of the disorder and the coded specifiers. As can be seen in figure 9.4, the diagnostic code for Major Depressive Disorder depends on two coded specifiers: whether there is only a single depressive episode (in which case the first three characters are F32) or recurrent episodes (in which case the first

FIGURE 9.4. Coding and recording procedures for Major Depressive Disorder

Coding and Recording Procedures

The diagnostic code for major depressive disorder is based on whether this is a single or recurrent episode, current severity, presence of psychotic features, and remission status. Current severity and psychotic features are only indicated if full criteria are currently met for a major depressive episode. Remission specifiers are only indicated if the full criteria are not currently met for a major depressive episode. Codes are as follows:

Severity/course specifier	Single episode	Recurrent episode
Mild	F32.0	F33.0
Moderate	F32.1	F33.1
Severe	F32.2	F33.2
With psychotic features	F32.3	F33.3
In partial remission	F32.4	F33.41
In full remission	F32.5	F33.42
Unspecified	F32.9	F33.9

In recording the name of a diagnosis, terms should be listed in the following order: major depressive disorder, single or recurrent episode, severity/psychotic/remission specifiers, followed by as many of the following specifiers without codes that apply to the current episode.

Specify:
 With anxious distress (p. 184).
 With mixed features (pp. 184–185).
 With melancholic features (p. 185).
 With atypical features (pp. 185–186).
 With mood-congruent psychotic features (p. 186).
 With mood-incongruent psychotic features (p. 186).
 With catatonia (p. 186). Coding note: Use additional code 293.89 (F06.1).
 With peripartum onset (pp. 186–187).
 With seasonal pattern (recurrent episode only) (pp. 187–188).

Source: DSM-5, page 162. Reprinted courtesy of the American Psychiatric Association.

three characters are F33). The fourth digit depends on the applicable severity/course specifier. The remaining applicable specifiers are uncoded and, if applicable, are listed after the severity/course specifiers. Thus, a case of recurrent Major Depressive Disorder occurring in a seasonal pattern, with a current episode of moderate severity, that is characterized by anxious distress, would be recorded as follows: F33.1 major depressive disorder, recurrent, moderate, with anxious distress, with seasonal pattern. Note that the anxious distress and seasonal pattern specifiers are listed at the end because their presence does not affect the diagnostic code.

Sequencing Diagnoses

The guidelines contained in DSM note that the principal diagnosis (in an inpatient setting) or the reason for visit (outpatient settings) is indicated by listing that diagnosis first. Remaining disorders, including mental and non-mental medical disorders, are listed next and sequenced according to the amount of clinical attention and treatment given to each disorder. One exception to this guideline is the case whether a medical condition is determined to be the cause of the symptoms of the mental disorder (for example, hypothyroidism causing a depressive disorder). In such cases, ICD coding rules require the medical condition be listed first, followed by the mental disorder (for example, E03.9 hypothyroidism; F06.31 Depressive disorder due to hypothyroidism). If a medical condition is present but is either unrelated to the primary mental disorder or of an uncertain relationship to the primary mental disorder, the mental disorder is listed first, followed by the medical condition.

Other Specified and Unspecified Diagnoses

The category "Other specified [diagnostic class] disorder" is used in clinical scenarios where the symptomatic presentation does not meet criteria for any of the specific disorders in the indicated diagnostic class and the clinician chooses to indicate the reason that the presentation does not meet the diagnostic criteria. This may be because the patient's clinical presentation is below the required symptomatic threshold, or the clinician has assigned a specific diagnosis that is not included as an official category in DSM-5. For example, for a patient who has a clinically significant depressive disorder that has lasted four weeks but has only three of the required nine symptoms for a major depressive episode, the clinician would record, "other specified depressive disorder, depressive episode with insufficient number of symptoms." An example of a presentation that is not included in DSM-5 as an official category is night eating syndrome, which would be recorded as "other specified feeding or eating disorder, night eating syndrome."

The category "Unspecified [diagnostic class] disorder" is given in clinical scenarios where the symptomatic presentation does not meet criteria for any of the specific disorders in the indicated diagnostic class and the clinician chooses not to specify the reason that the criteria are not met. This includes presentation in which there is insufficient information to make a diagnosis beyond the level of the diagnostic class, which may occur in situations where acute patient management considerations must take precedence over a full diagnostic workup, or in situations where it is not yet known whether the patient's clinical presentation is caused by a substance, another medical condition, or neither of these factors. For example, a patient in an emergency room setting with psychotic symptoms and agitation might be given a diagnosis of unspecified schizophrenia spectrum or other psychotic disorder until substances and other medical conditions can be ruled out and a more definitive diagnosis made. In hopefully rare situations, a clinician may record a vague diagnosis that cannot be coded more specifically. For example, a diagnosis that is recorded only as "depression" should be coded as unspecified depressive disorder.

Provisional Diagnosis

The term *provisional* can be listed after the diagnosis when there is a strong presumption that the full criteria will ultimately be met for a disorder but not enough information is available to make a firm diagnosis, such as in situations in which the differential diagnosis depends exclusively on the duration of illness. For example, a diagnosis of schizophreniform disorder requires that the duration of psychotic symptoms be at least one month but less than six months. Although a diagnosis of schizophreniform disorder applies to a patient who has been psychotic for three months, this diagnosis must be considered to be provisional at the time of the diagnostic evaluation since it is not yet known whether the symptoms will remit within the required six-month window. Once the symptoms persist beyond the six-month window, the diagnosis is changed from a provisional schizophreniform to schizophrenia, in which the duration is six months or longer.

Relationship with Other Terminologies, Classification Systems, and Code Sets

As explained previously, DSM-5 has a direct relationship with ICD-10-CM. Formal efforts were made by APA and WHO during the development of DSM-5 and the Mental, Behavioral, and Neurodevelopmental disorders chapter in the *International Classification of Diseases, Eleventh Revision* (ICD-11) to harmonize the two classification systems as much as possible. Accordingly, with some exceptions, the overall chapter structure is shared between the classifications, and the definitions of the majority of mental disorders are largely the same. Some notable differences include diagnoses like schizophrenia, in which DSM-5 requires a minimum duration of six months whereas ICD-11 allows the diagnosis to be made over only one month of symptoms. Moreover, there are a number of mental disorders that are included in one system and not the other. For example, prolonged grief disorder (a condition characterized by the persistence of an intense grief reaction for an abnormally long period of time) is included in ICD-11 but not DSM-5, and disruptive mood dysregulation disorder (characterized by recurrent severe temper outbursts associated with a persistently irritable or angry mood) is included in DSM-5 but not ICD-11. Although the DSM-5 manual includes sleep-wake disorders, sexual dysfunctions, and gender dysphoria, these conditions are no longer included in the Mental, Behavioral, and Neurodevelopmental disorders chapter in ICD-11 but instead are included in separate chapters (Sleep-Wake Disorders and Disorders Related to Sexual Health). Although DSM-5 was adopted for use shortly after its publication in 2013, the adoption date of ICD-11 is up to individual countries. It is anticipated that adoption of ICD-11 in the US for coding and reporting purposes will not occur for a number of years.

Additionally, a majority of DSM-5 terms (particularly those that were in prior editions of the DSM) have been included in SNOMED CT. Efforts are being made to systematically revise the psychiatric terminology in SNOMED CT so that it is better aligned with DSM-5.

Tools to Access and Use

A mobile app is available for DSM-5, providing users with full offline access to all of the criteria sets as well as online access to supporting videos, commentary, and resources. Moreover, the complete DSM-5 text (as well as the text for two books that may enhance the use of the DSM-5: the *DSM-5 Handbook of Differential Diagnosis* and *DSM-5 Clinical Cases*) is available on the APA's website Psychiatry online, a virtual library that provides psychiatrists and mental health professionals with key resources for diagnosis, treatment, research, and professional development. (See [PsychiatryOnline 2018] in the reference list at the end of this chapter.) The version of DSM-5 that is accessible via PsychiatryOnline has two unique features that are not available in print copies of DSM-5. It is the only version of DSM-5 that includes in-line references (along with a reference list at the end of each chapter), and it is the only version that is continuously updated as changes are made by the APA to the criteria, text, and diagnostic codes. Text that has been updated is highlighted in yellow; clicking on the text causes a pop-up window to appear that indicates the original text along with the date that the change became effective.

Adoption and Use Cases

DSM-5 was published in May 2013 for immediate use. It was published with both ICD-9-CM and ICD-10-CM codes assigned to each DSM-5 disorder to facilitate its use for reporting purposes during the transition from ICD-9-CM to ICD-10-CM in October 2015.

Psychiatrists may use an electronic health record (EHR) to capture patient health information and practice management software (PMS) for scheduling, billing, or other administrative tasks. Some EHRs include PMS functionality. Web and mobile applications for these software applications are offered by vendors. Disorder-specific templates that include DSM-5 criteria to assist in documentation may be available. The billing module within the PMS provides access to ICD-10-CM.

Use Case One: Establishing a Diagnosis

It is important to remember that DSM-5 diagnostic criteria and text are just one part of the clinical case formulation. Clinicians should always consider information gathered during clinical interview, relevant contextual factors (such as those included in the "Other Conditions That May Be a Focus of Clinical Attention" chapter), and clinical judgment in developing a case conceptualization. The clinician first considers whether the patient's symptom presentation meets the diagnostic criteria for any of the mental disorders in Section II. In making a diagnosis, it is suggested, though not required, that the clinician first administer the Level 1 (and, if appropriate, Level 2) cross-cutting dimensional assessment measure as well as the WHODAS 2.0 disability scale prior to conducting the clinical interview. Responses to these measures can inform what questions are asked during interview and potential diagnoses to consider.

Narrative text that accompanies diagnostic criteria also can be used to inform diagnosis (such as use of the Differential Diagnosis section to rule in or rule out a given disorder). If, during the clinical interview, the clinician determines that diagnostic threshold for a disorder is met, he or she should then consider whether the patient's symptoms can be further described through the use of subtypes or specifiers. Next, it is suggested, though not required, that the clinician administer available diagnostic-specific severity measures, which help establish baseline clinical status and can be useful in tracking changes in symptom severity over time in response to treatment. The clinician should then apply the appropriate ICD-10-CM codes, following the relevant instructions as provided in the coding and recording procedures section of the diagnostic text. Problems and other circumstances that may affect the patient's care, which are listed in the Other Conditions That May Be A Focus of Clinical Attention, should also be recorded as appropriate. Lastly, the clinician should develop a treatment plan and approach to monitoring outcomes.

Use Case Two: Reporting Diagnosis for Payment

DSM-5 Section II contains a wealth of information, including diagnostic criteria, specifiers, subtypes, and ICD-10-CM Z codes for other relevant clinical factors. Not all of this information can or should be coded, depending on the specifics of the relevant ICD codes and the circumstances of the individual patient.

For example, a patient presents for evaluation and possible treatment reporting an inability to discard newspapers, shopping bags, empty food containers, old mail, and old clothing such that her apartment has over the years become significantly over-cluttered and identified by her landlord as a safety hazard. She states that she cannot bear to throw these items away because she may need them in the future, and that it is better to reuse items rather than contribute to the pollution caused by landfills. She believes that her landlord is exaggerating the condition of her apartment and trying to evict her so that he can charge a higher rent to the next tenant. A discussion with a concerned family member confirms the landlord's assessment, with additional information that family members' efforts to clean out the apartment have ended with the patient highly anxious and crying uncontrollably. Further evaluation reveals that she has no other mental disorder, and no substance or medication use. The patient is overweight but has no other medical conditions.

The patient's symptoms meet the criteria for hoarding disorder (persistent difficulty with discarding possessions due to a perceived need to save the items and to distress associated with discarding them, all of which results in the accumulation of possessions that congest and clutter active living areas and that causes clinically significant distress or impairment in functioning). The specifier "with poor insight" applies to the presentation since the individual is mostly convinced that her hoarding-related beliefs and behaviors are not problematic despite evidence to the contrary. The clinician should list first the diagnosis "hoarding disorder with poor insight" as the primary reason for the visit, preceded by the appropriate ICD-10-CM code (F42.3). Note that the presence of the poor insight specifier has no impact on the diagnostic code: hoarding disorder is given the same code regardless of which insight specifier (that is, "with good or fair insight," "with poor insight," or "with absent insight/delusional beliefs") is assigned. Immediate treatment plans for this patient include ensuring the patient's safety and housing status, which will involve interaction with the landlord. Therefore, to help explain the treatment, "discord with landlord" should be listed after the reason for the visit, with ICD-10-CM code Z59.2.

The treatment plan does not include addressing the patient's weight at this point, so it does not need to be coded for reimbursement. Although it is not immediately relevant to treatment needs and a focus of intervention, it is an important contextual factor that may eventually impact treatment planning, so the overweight condition should also be recorded in the health record. It may be that the patient's weight is relevant to her self-esteem, mood, and interpersonal relationships, any of which may affect her ability to engage in behavior change and develop more adaptive coping skills. As such, her progress in therapy may eventually come to a halt until her weight can be addressed. The likelihood of her making healthy lifestyle changes to reduce her weight is low given the restrictiveness of her living environment. Once the patient's home is stabilized and in safer condition, treatment may then be able to focus on such issues related to weight management.

CHECK YOUR UNDERSTANDING

1. Which of the following is true regarding DSM-5 specifiers?

   a. They are mutually exclusive.

   b. More than one can be applied to a disorder.

c. They are jointly exhaustive.

d. They are indicated by the instruction 'specify whether'.

2. The "other specified" diagnosis is to be used in each of the following diagnostic scenarios *except*:

a. The patient's clinical presentation is below the required symptom threshold.

b. The clinician has assigned a specific diagnosis that is not included as an official category in DSM-5.

c. There is insufficient information to make a diagnosis beyond the level of diagnostic class.

d. The clinician wishes to indicate the specific reason why the presentation does not meet diagnostic criteria.

3. Which of the following DSM editions first incorporated clear diagnostic criteria, a multiaxial system for classification, and descriptive text for each disorder?

a. DSM-I

b. DSM-II

c. DSM-III

d. DSM-IV

4. Each DSM-5 mental disorder includes:

a. Proposed ICD-11 code

b. Detailed diagnostic criteria

c. Multiaxial breakdown

d. Glossary

5. True or false? Each DSM-5 diagnosis has been assigned a unique ICD-10-CM code.

a. True

b. False

REVIEW

1. True or false? A Glossary of Cultural Concepts of Distress is found in one of the DSM-5 appendices.

a. True

b. False

2. An individual's level of disability:

   a. Is best documented using the DSM-5 GAF Scale
   b. Can be assessed through the WHODAS 2.0
   c. Is a required part of documenting a diagnosis
   d. Is reported on Axis V

3. True or false? DSM-5 removed the multiaxial approach because its original intent and purposes are no longer relevant and necessary.

   a. True
   b. False

4. The DSM-5 benefits which type of professional?

   a. Practicing psychiatrists
   b. Clinical psychologists
   c. Clinical social workers
   d. All of the above

5. True or false? Medical conditions are only listed when there is a direct physiological relationship between the medical condition and the mental disorder.

   a. True
   b. False

6. Which of the following organizations is responsible for development of DSM?

   a. World Health Organization (WHO)
   b. American Psychiatric Association (APA)
   c. American Psychological Association
   d. American Medico-Psychological Association

7. True or false? One of the purposes of DSM-5 is to provide clinicians with treatment guidelines for patients with mental disorders.

   a. True
   b. False

8. DSM may be used in which of the following areas?

   a. Forensic evaluations
   b. Education
   c. Clinical care
   d. All of the above

9. True or false? DSM-5 includes a set of print and electronic assessment measures, which are suggested but not required for use in clinical care, including making a diagnosis, planning treatment, or monitoring treatment response.

   a. True
   b. False

10. True or false? The only exception to the DSM coding guideline requiring the principal diagnosis to be listed first is when a medical condition is determined to be the cause of the symptoms, in which case the medical condition is listed first.

    a. True
    b. False

References

American Psychiatric Association (APA). 2018a. *Diagnostic and Statistical Manual of Mental Disorders (DSM-5)*. http://www.dsm5.org/.

American Psychiatric Association (APA). 2018b. DSM-5 Educational Resources. Online Assessment Measures. https://www.psychiatry.org/psychiatrists/practice/dsm/educational-resources.

American Psychiatric Association (APA). 2018c. Online Assessment Measures. Disability Measures. https://www.psychiatry.org/psychiatrists/practice/dsm/educational-resources/assessment-measures.

American Psychiatric Association (APA). 2018d. Clinical Practice Guidelines. https://www.psychiatry.org/psychiatrists/practice/clinical-practice-guidelines.

American Psychiatric Association (APA). 2013a. DSM: History of the Manual. http://www.psychiatry.org/practice/dsm/dsm-history-of-the-manual.

American Psychiatric Association (APA). 2013b. *Diagnostic and Statistical Manual of Mental Disorders, 5th Edition*. Arlington, VA: APA.

PsychiatryOnline. 2018. https://www.psychiatryonline.org/.

10

Logical Observation Identifiers, Names, and Codes (LOINC)

Daniel J. Vreeman, PT, DPT, MS, FACMI

LEARNING OBJECTIVES

- Explain the purpose and function of LOINC
- Discuss the approach to developing LOINC
- Identify who has adopted LOINC
- Examine the relationship between LOINC with other classifications, terminologies, and code sets
- Compare tools available to access and use
- Understand how LOINC is used in an electronic environment

KEY TERMS

- Fully specified name (FSN)
- Health Level Seven (HL7)
- Logical Observation Identifiers, Names, and Codes (LOINC)
- LOINC Committee
- Regenstrief Institute, Inc.
- Regenstrief LOINC Mapping Assistant (RELMA)
- Semantic data model

Introduction to LOINC

A comprehensive electronic health record (EHR) system must coalesce data from many producing sources. Both within and among institutions, the disparate source systems often store data with local, idiosyncratic codes to identify clinical observations and measurements. In order to understand and process incoming data, receiving systems are forced to either use the producers' codes or map them to a code system they understand. This problem is pervasive across many important types of clinical data, such as laboratory tests, radiology procedures, nursing assessments, document titles, physical measures, patient-reported outcomes, and more. As the number of interacting systems increases, the integration effort becomes hugely burdensome and poses a major barrier to interoperability.

The **Logical Observation Identifiers, Names, and Codes (LOINC)** standard provides a set of universal identifiers for health measurements, observations, and documents. LOINC is an openly developed terminology that can serve as the global lingua franca for information exchange between electronic systems (Forrey et al. 1996). Health information technology (IT) systems use LOINC to seamlessly process data for many purposes, including clinical care, quality assessment, public health, and research purposes.

History

LOINC is developed by the **Regenstrief Institute, Inc.,** a nonprofit biomedical informatics and healthcare research organization associated with Indiana University. Led by biomedical informatics pioneer Clem McDonald, MD, Regenstrief initiated the LOINC effort in 1994 by organizing a voluntary group of experts to form the **LOINC Committee.** The LOINC Committee developed a system of universal identifiers for observations being communicated electronically from data producers like clinical laboratories to downstream receiving systems, such as those in hospitals, physician offices, payers, and public health departments.

There are several reasons why the LOINC Committee focused on standardizing observation identifiers (Huff et al. 1998). By 1994, many electronic systems were beginning to send clinical information as discrete results using messaging standards such as **Health Level Seven (HL7)** or ASTM 1238. Inside these messages, laboratories and clinical systems used local, idiosyncratic names and codes to identify the test being reported. Installing a new system or connecting to a new interface meant investing large resources in mapping the codes between every participating system. Having a universal standard would allow each system in an exchange to only map their local terms to the standard. Existing terminologies were not granular enough, focused on coding for billing rather than clinical results delivery, or did not fit with the messaging models being used. Because such a standard did not exist and would be immediately useful, the LOINC Committee embarked on creating a terminology with the appropriate level of granularity for defining the names of observations used in laboratory and clinical information systems.

Developer

Regenstrief Institute, Inc. is the overall steward and developer of LOINC. The investigators at Regenstrief seek to integrate research discovery, technological advances, and systems improvement into healthcare.

Over the past four decades, Regenstrief's biomedical informaticians have pioneered many information solutions to improve health. They developed and iteratively improved the Regenstrief Medical Record System (RMRS), one of the largest and most advanced EHR systems (McDonald et al. 1999). Along the way, Regenstrief's informaticians have published more controlled trials evaluating the impact of health information technology on quality, efficiency, and costs of care than any other research center in the US (Chaudhry et al. 2006). Building on the successes of the RMRS, Regenstrief's informaticians developed the Indiana Network for Patient Care (INPC), the largest inter-organizational clinical data repository in the country, which is now operated by the Indiana Health Information Exchange (McDonald et al. 2005). The INPC's rich repository has been leveraged for a wide range of observational studies, health services research, and comparative effectiveness research (Dixon et al. 2016). In 2004, investigators at Regenstrief began collaboratively building an open source EHR platform called OpenMRS. OpenMRS was created specifically to address healthcare and management in developing countries, has been adopted widely throughout the world and is now propelled by a large community of developers and implementers (Tierney et al. 2010). (See [OpenMRS n.d.] in the resource list at the end of this chapter.) More recently, Regenstrief has been cultivating a community of practice called OpenHIE, focused on open collaborative development and support of country-driven, large-scale health information sharing architectures (see [OpenHIE n.d.] in the resource list at the end of this chapter).

Throughout its history of building and studying clinical information systems, Regenstrief's informaticians have been leaders in developing and using biomedical informatics standards. Regenstrief investigators organized the first medical informatics standards effort in 1984, wrote the ASTM and HL7 chapters for orders and observation reporting, and were the lead authors of the HL7 Version 3 Reference Information Model, and the HL7 Version 3 Data Types, and the proposed HIPAA claims attachments documents. In addition, they have developed the Unified Code for Units of Measure, a standard for unambiguously representing units of measure in electronic communications (see [UCUM n.d.] in the resource list at the end of this chapter).

Regenstrief serves as the standards development organization (SDO), overall steward, and owner of LOINC. The LOINC team at Regenstrief maintains the LOINC database and supporting documentation, processes submissions and edits to the content, develops and curates accessory content (descriptions, hierarchies, other attributes, and so on), develops tools for implementers, and coordinates LOINC releases. In addition, Regenstrief continues to cultivate the LOINC community worldwide.

The Regenstrief Institute has received financial support to develop LOINC from the US National Library of Medicine and other National Institutes of Health and US federal agencies, several non-profit foundations, industry, and other sources, including contributions from the LOINC user community (see [LOINC 2018a] in the resource list at the end of this chapter).

LOINC Committee

Composed of volunteers from academia, industry, and government, the LOINC Committee serves as the main advisory body for LOINC. Individual members may also take the lead on the development of naming rules and LOINC names for new subject matter and serve as content experts to answer questions that come up with new submissions.

The LOINC Committee is comprised of three composite committees. The Laboratory LOINC Committee focuses on content representing observations, measures, documents (and other collections thereof) made on specimens. The Clinical LOINC Committee focuses on content representing observations, measures, documents (and other collections thereof) made on patients, populations, devices, and other units of analysis. The LOINC/RadLex Committee oversees the development, use, and modification of the LOINC/RSNA Radiology Playbook, a unified terminology model for radiology orders and results (Vreeman et al. 2018).

Approach to Development

Regenstrief Institute and the LOINC Committee have intentionally shaped LOINC development to be empirical, nimble, and open (Huff et al. 1998). Since its inception, new content in LOINC has been added in response to requirements of adopters around the world. Because of this approach, the concepts in LOINC were not created de novo. Rather, they first existed as local terms in a live clinical system. When developing naming conventions for a new domain, LOINC's typical approach is to examine the existing system master files and example report messages to ensure that the modeling approach reflects real world usage.

At its inception, the LOINC Committee was deliberately organized outside of existing standards development groups to ensure LOINC could always be freely distributed. In addition, many other kinds of standards are developed with formal balloting procedures that limit revisions to every two to five years. LOINC needed to respond more quickly to the rapidly evolving field, and so developed its own process for adding content and publishing releases.

Regenstrief seeks to iteratively improve how it develops and delivers data standards. It takes an open approach to developing LOINC, striving to understand community needs, seeking feedback continually, and keeping barriers to participation low. Modeling issues are investigated thoroughly, and decisions are based on consensus expert knowledge and best-available data. At the same time, Regenstrief places a high value on practical solutions, not letting "theoretically perfect" encumber the process or prevent LOINC from being used in the field.

LOINC is copyrighted by the Regenstrief Institute to protect its integrity and prevent multiple variations, but it is made available worldwide at no cost under an open license (see

[LOINC 2018b] in the resource list at the end of this chapter). The LOINC license permits use, copying, and distribution of the standard for both commercial and non-commercial purposes. These terms of use mean that LOINC can be incorporated into EHRs or laboratory information systems, the codes sent in clinical messages, and many other uses all without payment of royalties. The primary restriction the license imposes is that it forbids using LOINC to develop or promulgate a different standard vocabulary for orders or observations. LOINC's unrestrictive terms of use are designed to result in a low barrier to widespread adoption. More information about Regenstrief's approach to licensing LOINC is available online (Vreeman n.d.).

Purpose

LOINC's primary role is to provide identifiers and names for observations (McDonald et al. 2003). Here we use "observation" as a general term. In some domains, these items may be referred to as tests, variables, data elements, and so on.

Within and among health IT systems, observations are communicated with format that has two key structural elements. The first element identifies *what the observation is*; for example, diastolic blood pressure, prothrombin time, or blood type. The second element carries *the result value of the observation*; for example 90 (mmHg), 10.5 (seconds), or O Positive. When used together, these two elements carry an instance of a person's specific test result.

In human communication you might consider this model like questions and answers. The first element of the structure (the observation) is the question, and the second element (the observation value) is the answer. For example, the question might be: *How much does this patient weigh?* The answer might be *65 kg.*

LOINC provides a code (29463-7) and formal name (Body weight:Mass:Pt:^Patient:Qn) for observations such as these. When the observation value is reported as a quantity, no coding system is needed for the answer (except for identifying its associated units of measure). On the other hand, ordinal or nominal observation values would benefit from being identified with a standard code. The choice of which coding system to use for observation values depends on the domain. One might use COSMIC to report a somatic DNA sequence variant, RxNorm to report the name of medication, or SNOMED CT to report the name of a bacteria (Bamford et al. 2004; Liu et al. 2005; Wang et al. 2002).

Content

In June 2018, Regenstrief Institute released version 2.64 of LOINC containing names and codes for 87,863 laboratory and clinical variables. This latest release was the 61st edition of the vocabulary. The overall growth of LOINC content since its first release is shown in figure 10.1. LOINC has two major categories of content: Laboratory and Clinical.

FIGURE 10.1. Number of LOINC terms per release

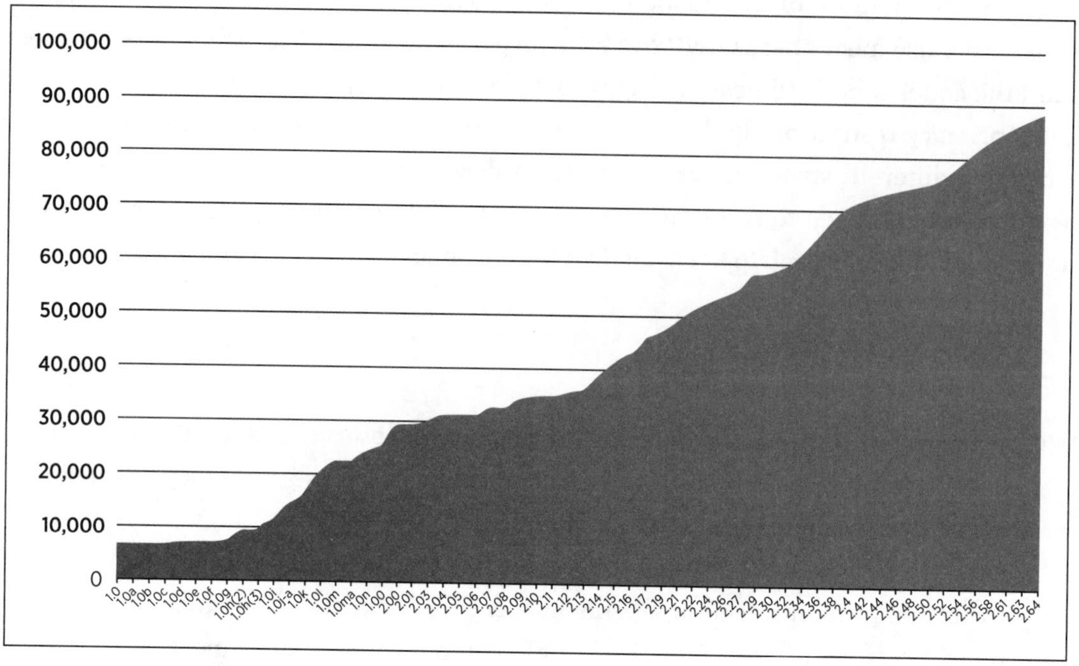

Source: Reprinted courtesy of Regenstrief Institute, Inc.

Laboratory

The laboratory section of LOINC covers the domains of clinical laboratory testing, including chemistry, urinalysis, hematology, serology, microbiology (including parasitology and virology), toxicology, and molecular genetics. Of the more than 87,000 terms in LOINC version 2.64, about 62 percent are laboratory terms. At its start, LOINC initially focused on developing codes for single test observations. Over time, LOINC has continued to expand coverage not only for single tests, but also for collections of observations referred to generically as panels. LOINC version 2.64 contains about 1,200 laboratory panels, including many common order panels, such as arterial blood gases, electrolytes, urinalysis, complete blood count, and differential.

Clinical

The overall domain scope of clinical LOINC is extremely broad. Some of the sections of terms include:

- Anthropometric measures
- Cardiac ultrasound
- Clinical documents and sections
- Colonoscopy/endoscopy reports

- Discharge summaries
- EKG
- Emergency medicine variables
- Fluid intake/output
- Hemodynamic measurements
- History and physical exam findings
- Obstetrical ultrasound
- Ophthalmology measurements
- Pathology findings
- Patient assessment instruments (for example, survey instruments)
- Radiology report titles
- Respiratory therapy
- Tumor registry
- Vital signs

Because of recent growth, the relative proportion of clinical versus laboratory content in LOINC has shifted. In 2003 (version 2.10), clinical terms accounted for about 21 percent of the content in LOINC, whereas today (version 2.64) they account for 38 percent (Vreeman 2018).

Within this broad scope of domains, special effort has been devoted to defining naming conventions and building new content in nursing, radiology report titles, clinical document names and sections, and patient assessment instruments.

Nursing

Nursing content is one of the domains with a special focus in Clinical LOINC (Matney et al. 2003). The Clinical LOINC Committee has organized a nursing subcommittee whose mission is to facilitate the development and use of LOINC codes for observations used during key stages of the nursing process, including assessments, goals, and outcomes. By doing so, the subcommittee will help meet the needs for administrative, research, and quality measurement initiatives related to nursing care.

Members of the nursing subcommittee have collaborated with many partners to expand the nursing content represented in LOINC. Some examples include skin and wound assessments, pain assessments, physiological assessments, and care planning concepts (Matney et al. 2003; Matney et al. 2016; Tilley and Matney 2005). In addition to clinical content of relevance to nursing, LOINC also contains terms to represent the Nursing Management Minimum Data Set. This collection contains a set of essential standardized management data useful to support nursing management and administrative decisions for quality improvement (Subramanian et al. 2008; Westra et al. 2010).

Radiology

LOINC has iteratively defined a detailed set of naming conventions for radiology studies that were first published in 2000. LOINC creates terms for radiology studies that are defined at the level of granularity typically used for ordering and reporting results. For example, "CT Head without and with IV contrast" and "XR Knee Merchants view."

From 2013 to 2017, Regenstrief partnered with the Radiological Society of North America (RSNA) to create a unified terminology standard for radiology procedures that builds on the strengths of LOINC and the RadLex Playbook, a terminology developed by the RSNA (Vreeman et al. 2018; Wang et al. 2017). This collaboration produced the LOINC/RSNA Radiology Playbook, a complete resource of standardized imaging procedure codes and a significant advancement for interoperability. The LOINC/RSNA Radiology Playbook is jointly governed by the two organizations through the newly established LOINC/RadLex Committee. All of the existing LOINC content has been transformed into the unified model, which uses LOINC codes as the primary concept identifier and contains links to detailed radiology-specific attributes that are expressed as LOINC Parts mapped to RadLex concepts.

The current LOINC release (version 2.64) contains more than 5,800 terms for radiology procedures. Two early evaluations in independent systems found that LOINC provides terms for around 90 percent of diagnostic radiology terms found in hospital radiology systems (Vreeman and McDonald 2005, 2006). An evaluation currently underway has demonstrated that for computed tomography terms, LOINC's content type and token coverage was very high (greater than 90%) for these terms in a regional health information exchange (Peng et al. 2019).

Document Titles

Over time, LOINC has also developed a comprehensive framework for representing document and section titles. This work has created an ontology of names for clinical notes (such as Discharge Summary and Progress Note) and other documents, called the LOINC Document Ontology. These terms are designed for use within healthcare institutions, in clinical document repositories, and in exchange between organizations. Regenstrief has developed a specialized release artifact called the LOINC Document Ontology File that contains all of the LOINC terms in the ontology linked to their specialized metadata attributes that are expressed as LOINC Parts. The current release (version 2.64) contains about 2,700 LOINC terms in the Document Ontology, and this domain has remained an active area of development since its inception around 2000.

Organizations that have implemented and analyzed LOINC's approach in this area have generated numerous scientific publications (Chen et al. 2010; Dugas et al. 2009; Frazier et al. 2001; Hyun and Bakken 2006; Hyun et al. 2006; Hyun et al. 2009; Li et al. 2011; Shapiro et al. 2005). LOINC document terms have been adopted as the standard coding for documents within HL7's Clinical Document Architecture (CDA) standard (Dolin et al. 2006). A detailed implementation guide describing how to implement the LOINC Document Ontology to facilitate queries and retrieval of documents by clinicians or clinical and administrative staff was developed by the U.S. Department of Defense and U.S. Department of Veterans Affairs and published by HL7 (HL7 International 2015a).

Patient Assessment Instruments

LOINC has also developed a formal model for representing standardized patient assessment instruments, patient reported outcomes, and other sets of clinical data variables (Hyun and Bakken 2006; Vreeman et al. 2010; White and Hauan 2002). Representing this content has led to three major enhancements to the LOINC content representation, including 1) an extended set of attributes for LOINC observation terms, 2) a detailed model for representing the collection of observation values allowed as responses to a particular question, and 3) the capability of representing certain attributes of LOINC terms in the context of the particular panels in which they appear.

Some of the context-specific attributes that were added include skip logic, form coding instructions, question text and source fields, and inline-displayed images that are essential references for answering a particular question. The detailed structure for linking the parent-child relationships of panels and the context-specific attributes are represented in the LOINC Panels and Forms File. The connection between LOINC observation terms and structured lists of answers that are allowed as observation values are represented in the LOINC Answer File. The LOINC Answer File includes coded value sets (LOINC Answer Lists) containing coded LOINC Answers, score values for answers that are used in summary calculations, and the binding that links a question term to an answer list (such as Example, Preferred, or Normative).

The current LOINC release contains more than 16,000 non-laboratory terms represented in this detailed panel structure. Some examples of the content include all of the variables from the Patient Reported Outcomes Measurement Information System (PROMIS®), Adverse Childhood Experience (ACE), Patient Activity Scale (PAS), American National Adult Reading Test (AmNART), Patient Health Questionnaire-9 (PHQ-9), Morse Fall Scale, and a very large set of measurements for use in genome-wide association studies called Phenotypes and Exposures (PhenX) (Pan et al. 2012). In addition, through a collaboration with the Centers for Medicare and Medicaid Services (CMS), LOINC has represented the four major clinical assessments that are required for use in post-acute care settings.

Structure

LOINC has been developed as a structured medical vocabulary with a **semantic data model (SDM)**, a description of how vocabulary items can be combined to make a valid representation of medical information (Huff et al. 1998). A LOINC term corresponds to a single kind of observation, measurement, or test result. It signifies a concept whose meaning applies to all tests with clinically equivalent results.

Each term in LOINC is assigned a unique permanent identifier, the LOINC code, that serves as its computer processable representation. LOINC codes themselves have no embedded meaning; they are sequentially assigned, unique numbers that include a MOD10 check digit as a hyphen-separated suffix. Applications can use the check digit to detect common typographic errors when LOINC codes are entered manually.

LOINC Naming Conventions

Each LOINC term is provided with several names that give a human-readable text rendering of the concept. Presently, LOINC publishes four main names: the fully specified name (FSN), long

TABLE 10.1. Example laboratory LOINC terms with their LOINC names

LOINC Code	Fully Specified Name	Long Common Name	Short Name	Display Name
2951-2	Sodium:SCnc:Pt:Ser/Plas:Qn:	Sodium [Moles/volume] in Serum or Plasma	Sodium SerPl-sCnc	Sodium molar conc
21525-1	Sodium:SCnc:24H:Urine:Qn:	Sodium [Moles/volume] in 24 hour Urine	Sodium 24h Ur-sCnc	Sodium molar conc (24H U)
4544-3	Hematocrit:VFr:Pt:Bld:Qn:Automated count	Hematocrit [Volume Fraction] of Blood by Automated count	Hct VFr Bld Auto	Hematocrit Auto Volume Fraction (Bld)
1514-9	Glucose^2H post 100 g glucose PO:MCnc:Pt:Ser/Plas:Qn:	Glucose [Mass/volume] in Serum or Plasma --2 hours post 100 g glucose PO	Glucose 2h p 100 g Glc PO SerPl-mCnc	Glucose 2 hours p 100 g glucose PO mass conc
21662-2	CYP2D6 gene.c.2637delA:PrThr:Pt:Bld/ Tiss:Ord:Molgen	CYP2D6 gene c.2637delA [Presence] in Blood or Tissue by Molecular genetics method	CYP2D6 c.2637delA Bld/T QI	CYP2D6 gene c.2637delA Molgen QI (Bld/Tiss)
81151-3	Dengue virus 1+2+3+4 5' UTR RNA:PrThr:Pt:CSF:Ord:Probe.amp.tar	Dengue virus 1+2+3+4 5' UTR RNA [Presence] in Cerebral spinal fluid by NAA with probe detection	DENV 1+2+3+4 5' UTR RNA CSF QI NAA+probe	Dengue virus 1+2+3+4 5' UTR RNA NAA+probe QI (CSF)

Source: Regenstrief Institute, Inc. 2018.

common name, short name, and display name. The display name is the newest addition, and at the time of this writing is considered "Alpha" status. The *LOINC Users' Guide* is the definitive source describing the LOINC naming conventions (McDonald et al. 2018).

Examples of LOINC terms and their names are given for laboratory LOINC codes in table 10.1 and for clinical LOINC codes in table 10.2.

FULLY SPECIFIED NAME

The primary name for a LOINC term is called the **fully specified name (FSN)**, and it models the semantic structure of precoordinated expressions using a multiaxial representational approach. The separate attributes of the FSN are designed for distinguishing the key features

TABLE 10.2. Example clinical LOINC terms with their LOINC names

LOINC Code	Fully Specified Name	Long Common Name	Short Name*	Display Name†
8480-6	Intravascular systolic:Pres:Pt:Arterial system:Qn:	Systolic blood pressure	BP sys	-
8301-4	Body height:Len:Pt:^Patient:Qn:Estimated	Body height Estimated	Body height Est	-
28655-9	Discharge summary note :Find:Pt:{Setting}:Doc:Physician attending	Physician attending Discharge summary	MD Attend Discharge sum	-
38214-3	Pain severity:Score:Pt:^Patient:Qn:Reported. visual analog score	Pain severity [Score] Visual analog score	Pain severity Score VAS	-
30612-6	Multisection^WO & W contrast IV:Find:Pt:Abdomen>Liver:Doc:CT	CT Liver WO and W contrast IV	CT Liver WO+W contr IV	-
76513-1	How hard is it for you to pay for the very basics like food, housing, medical care, and heating:Find:Pt:^Patient:Ord:CARDIA	How hard is it for you to pay for the very basics like food, housing, medical care, and heating [CARDIA]	-	-
55411-3	Exercise duration:Time:Pt:^Patient:Qn:	Exercise duration	Exercise duration	-

* LOINC terms in the Survey Instrument Class do not have Short Names.

† Display Name is not yet created for any Clinical LOINC terms.

Source: Regenstrief Institute, Inc. 2018.

of measurements and observations. As such, they are key for matching local terms to the appropriate LOINC term (Vreeman 2016).

Each LOINC FSN includes as many as six main axes that are called parts:

- Component (analyte): The substance or entity that is measured, evaluated, or observed. Examples include glucose, sodium, systolic blood pressure, and pain onset.
- Kind of property: The characteristic or attribute of the component that is measured, evaluated, or observed. Examples include length, volume, time stamp, mass, ratio, number, and temperature.
- Time aspect: The interval of time over which the observation or measurement was made. Examples include "point in time" and "over a 24-hour time period."
- System: The system (context) or specimen type upon which the observation was made. Examples include urine, serum, fetus, patient (person), and family.
- Type of scale: The scale of the measure. Examples include quantitative (a true numeric measurement), ordinal (a ranked set of options), nominal (for example, Escherichia coli, Staphylococcus aureus), and document (for example, a provider's discharge summary).
- Type of method: The procedure used to make the measurement or observation. Method is only specified when different methodologies would significantly change the interpretation of the result. Method is the only axis that is optional.

In general, the FSN uses official scientific names in the Component but uses abbreviations for the Property and System (as described in the *LOINC Users' Guide*). As a result, some FSNs appear unfamiliar to clinicians. For example, the FSN for the common INR test is "Coagulation tissue factor induced.INR:RelTime:Pt:PPP:Qn:Coag."

LONG COMMON NAME

The Long Common Name is designed to be a fully spelled out and human readable name for a LOINC term. Some of the important conventions used in the Long Common Name include using common names for things like allergens in the Component, transforming the somewhat cryptic Property abbreviations like "MCnc" into more understandable phrases such as "Mass/volume," and omitting the default timing of "Pt" (point in time).

In general, the Long Common Name is the recommended name to include in any data dictionary of LOINC terms and in exchange structures transmitting clinical data coded with LOINC. The Long Common Name offers several advantages for these purposes, including that they are more human friendly, contain fewer instances of "reserved characters," and are populated for all LOINC terms.

SHORT NAME

The Short Name is designed to accommodate situations and systems with extreme character limits, such as older laboratory information systems or column headers on clinical reports. Regenstrief sets a target limit of 40 characters when creating Short Names. To achieve this limit, the Short Name makes extensive use of acronyms and abbreviations. In contrast to the FSN, character case matters in the Short Name.

There are a couple of important caveats to note about the Short Name. First, for terms that measure multiple analytes, it is nearly impossible to create a meaningful name with so few characters. Second, not all LOINC terms have a Short Name. And third, not all Short Names are unique. As a result, the Short Name cannot be used as a key in any database containing LOINC terms.

DISPLAY NAME

Even after creation of the Long Common Name in 2009, LOINC users have continued to make requests for simpler display names for use in user interfaces. Over many years of discussions and proposals, it became clear that mostly what users wished for are for names that leave out some of the defining attributes of the term (such as Property, Scale, and "default" specimens in the System) because they are unfamiliar to clinicians. This is problematic across all of LOINC because it would create ambiguous and duplicate names. In general, users were expected to link their own local preferred names to LOINC terms for use in reports and displays because those ambiguities created by names omitting these attributes could be resolved within a given local system context.

As of the LOINC version 2.64 release (June 2018), Regenstrief began to publish a new set of names that were developed as a prototype (labeled "Alpha" status) for more user-friendly names. Like the Long Common Name and the Short Name, the new Display Names are created algorithmically from the manually crafted display text for each Part that is specifically honed for these new names. The Display Names are created by a different set of algorithmic rules that operate with a published set of "defaults" that omit certain Parts from the name. For example, in the System, both Ser/Plas and ^Patient are implied (omitted), and any other System is included in parentheses at the end of the name. For terms with a Scale of Quantitative, the Scale is omitted. Regenstrief anticipates evolving the naming rules used to create the Display Names over time with feedback from the user community. Presently, they are only generated for laboratory terms, but Regenstrief anticipates expanding to cover more clinical terms in the future.

Principles and Guidelines

By design, LOINC terms were meant for use in the context of clinical data exchange formats like HL7 Version 2 messages, Clinical Document Architecture XML documents, or the newer FHIR resources. These structures have designated fields for specific kinds of information, and thus the LOINC name is not intended to capture all possible information about the testing procedure or the result—only enough to unambiguously identify it. For example, several things are specifically excluded from the name: the testing instrument and protocol, testing priority (such as STAT), sample volume, testing location, and the actual result value (such as 120 mmHg). All of these other aspects can be communicated in specific parts of the exchange format.

Distinct LOINC terms are created for each specimen for which a test kit has been calibrated. So, if an instrument or kit produces one value for each specimen and the test is recommended for use on two specimens, then two LOINC terms are created. An example would be one for whole blood and another for cerebrospinal fluid. If two or more results per specimen are reported (for example, a control value or a total and a percentage), two or more LOINC terms are needed per supported specimen. However, LOINC concepts are not unique per test manufacturer.

As noted above, the method axis is an optional element of the FSN. The method axis is used only when the method distinction makes an important difference in the clinical interpretation of the result. This matters primarily when the other five name axes do not sufficiently distinguish measurements that have important differences in the reference range, sensitivity, or specificity. Whether or not method is specified in the FSN is guided by pragmatics and follows the conventions seen in typical local test names. For this reason, the method is specified at a relatively general level. In molecular genetics for example, LOINC distinguishes target amplification followed by probe-based detection (Probe.amp.tar) in the Method, but not each specific technique (such as PCR, transcription mediated amplification, hybridization protection assay, strand displacement amplification) because the methods do not produce significantly different results. Furthermore, detailed information about the testing procedure can be sent in other parts of an observation message.

LOINC codes themselves have no embedded meaning; they are sequentially assigned, unique numbers that include a MOD10 check digit as a hyphen-separated suffix. Applications can use the check digit to detect common typographic errors when LOINC codes are entered manually. LOINC codes are never deleted from the database. If a term happens to be an error or duplicate, it is flagged in the database as "deprecated."

Process for Revision and Updates

Because of its commitment to open development, the LOINC effort has always welcomed suggestions for additions or revisions to the content and has kept its committee meetings open to the public. Now, after reaching a certain state of maturity, the vast majority of new term additions come at the request of end users. Developing content based on end-user requests has helped LOINC stay nimble in adding content to emerging and immediately relevant domains. In 2013, nearly 3,000 new term requests were submitted to Regenstrief. By 2017, the number of requested terms grew to more than 7,500. In the period from 2013 to 2017, about 200 organizations have requested new LOINC terms (Vreeman 2018).

Historically, most requests for new terms have come from data producers (such as clinical laboratories) or receivers (such as downstream provider systems). Increasingly, more in vitro diagnostic (IVD) testing companies are requesting new terms for the tests they manufacture. The major benefit of IVD vendors identifying which LOINC terms are relevant for their tests is it will greatly improve the efficiency and consistency with which laboratories can deploy standard terminology in their information systems.

Regenstrief provides high transparency into the submission process. Current statistics, including turnaround time, and historical trends of new term requests are published online (see [LOINC 2018c] in the resource list at the end of this chapter). The entire queue of term requests and their current status is also published publicly and updated each day (see [LOINC 2018d] in the resource list at the end of this chapter). Once a requested term has passed the multilevel quality assurance process and is slated for publication in the next LOINC release, it is published on a special "Prerelease" page of the LOINC website for informational purposes (see [LOINC 2018e] in the resource list at the end of this chapter).

Overall, Regenstrief follows sound terminology development practices in managing LOINC (Cimino 1998). For example, LOINC terms are never deleted from the database. If a term happens to be an error or duplicate, it is flagged in the database as "deprecated."

New releases of the standard are published twice yearly (in June and December), though occasionally interim releases are published in response to emergent needs. With each release, a file identifying the changes between versions and several other kinds of accessory files are also distributed. Each release artifact is distributed with a detailed ReadMe file that provides usage notes and a Release Notes file that describes key changes over time.

Relationship with Other Terminologies, Classifications, and Code Sets

As an openly developed standard, Regenstrief is committed to working with others who have similar goals of building seamless networks of health systems and data. Some of the key relationships LOINC has with other terminologies, classifications, and code sets are described below.

Diagnostic Imaging

As previously discussed in this chapter, Regenstrief collaborates with the RSNA to produce a unified terminology for radiology procedures, the LOINC/RSNA Radiology Playbook (Vreeman et al. 2018). In addition, the DICOM part 20 standard for sending Imaging Reports using HL7 Clinical Document Architecture (DICOM Standards Committee 2019) requires a LOINC code for labeling the imaging procedure report, as does the Diagnostic Imaging Report template in HL7's Consolidated CDA standard (HL7 International 2015b). The ImagingStudy resource of the FHIR standard now references the LOINC/RSNA Radiology Playbook as the set of procedure codes to use.

SNOMED International

In July 2013, the Regenstrief Institute and SNOMED International (formerly, the International Health Terminology Standards Development Organisation) formed a long-term collaborative relationship with the objective of developing coded content to support order entry and result reporting by linking their respective terminologies: LOINC and SNOMED CT (Regenstrief Institute, Inc. n.d.).

In this agreement, both organizations endorsed this statement that illustrates how LOINC and SNOMED CT work effectively together: "LOINC provides codes that represent the names of information items, such as questions, and SNOMED CT provides codes that may represent nominal and ordinal values, or answers, for these named information items." They also committed to working together to minimize duplicate work, create semantic links between their respective terminologies, and deliver consistent guidelines on effective ways to use LOINC and SNOMED CT together.

Under the agreement, the organizations identified key domain areas for collaboration and progressed four primary activities:

- Existing SNOMED CT concepts that are subtypes of Observable Entity or Evaluation Procedure will be mapped to LOINC Terms.
- The LOINC Parts used by LOINC terms will be mapped to SNOMED CT concepts.
- LOINC Terms that are not already represented by SNOMED CT concepts will be associated with post-coordinated expressions.
- Where appropriate, the LOINC Answer values associated with LOINC terms for ordinal or nominal observables will be mapped to SNOMED CT concept names and codes.

The approach outlined in this agreement means that new SNOMED CT observable entity concepts will not be added routinely to the terminology. Rather, each LOINC observable will be represented as "SNOMED CT Expression," which means a structured combination of one or more SNOMED CT concept Identifiers used to express an instance of a clinical idea. This method prevents SNOMED CT from having to assign a duplicate identifier for every concept that exists in LOINC, yet provides a bridge from the LOINC concept into the semantic relationships that are defined within SNOMED CT.

IEEE Standards Association (IEEE-SA)

The Institute of Electrical and Electronics Engineers (IEEE) Standards Association (IEEE-SA) and Regenstrief Institute, Inc. are working together to bridge the gap between healthcare devices and EHRs. IEEE-SA is a global standardization body within IEEE that is dedicated to creating consensus-based technology standards, including the IEEE device nomenclature, a unified, consensus-based terminology across device manufacturers. In 2015, Regenstrief and IEEE-SA signed a Memorandum of Understanding (MOU) that enables a map between LOINC and the IEEE 11073™ family of standards for medical device communication.

This collaboration has produced the LOINC/IEEE Medical Device Code Mapping Table file, which is updated and published with each LOINC release. The current version contains mappings between more than 600 LOINC terms and concepts from the IEEE 11073™10101 Standard for Health informatics - Point-of-care medical device communication - Nomenclature and 10101a Nomenclature Amendment. The table contains mappings for variables produced by ventilators, anesthesia gas machines, invasive blood pressure monitoring, and EKG devices. This collaboration remains a work in progress, with the anticipated outcome being that the mappings enable information from a variety of devices to flow into and integrate in EHRs so that the data are interpretable, actionable, and accessible for many purposes.

Unified Code for Units of Measure (UCUM)

The Unified Code for Units of Measure (UCUM) is a code system for unambiguously communicating units of measure in electronic exchanges and systems (see [UCUM n.d.] in the resource list at the end of this chapter). UCUM is also developed and maintained by the Regenstrief Institute, Inc. and made available at no cost worldwide. UCUM has been adopted internationally by many organizations, including HL7, IEEE, DICOM, and others. LOINC has adopted UCUM as its preferred representation of units of measure.

LOINC terms are not differentiated by specific reporting units of measure, but the LOINC Property defines a scope of allowable units. For example, the LOINC terms with a Property of Mass Concentration could be reported with any unit of measure that represents a mass per volume, such as mg/dL, g/L, and so on. Within the LOINC Table, Regenstrief provides example units of measure expressed as UCUM codes for most quantitative terms. These example units of measure are helpful as a cross-reference when mapping to local terms to LOINC terms. In addition, Regenstrief publishes a list of UCUM codes for commonly used units of measure on the LOINC website (see [LOINC 2018f] in the resource list at the end of this chapter).

Tools to Access and Use

LOINC is distributed and made freely available from its website (see [LOINC 2018g] in the resource list at the end of this chapter). In addition, there are a number of other resources available to access and use LOINC, some of which are described next.

Documentation

The LOINC User's Guide is the definitive document about LOINC. It describes the naming conventions and policies in detail and is updated with each LOINC release. A detailed User's Manual is also available for the **Regenstrief LOINC Mapping Assistant (RELMA)**, a desktop software application that provides tools for browsing LOINC and mapping local terms to LOINC terms. When a new LOINC version is published, Regenstrief also issues a detailed news release on the LOINC website that highlights key updates, additions, and announcements of future changes. Each specific artifact in the LOINC release also contains a Release Notes file that highlights version to version changes. Additional resources can be found on the LOINC website.

Accessory Files

Regenstrief has developed a suite of accessory files that contain specialized representations of LOINC content. These accessory files are published as part of each LOINC release. A summary of the main files is given in table 10.3.

Regenstrief also distributes a set of files for LOINC implementers that focuses on the most commonly used terms. Vreeman et al. (2007) observed that a relatively small subset of laboratory test codes account for the vast majority of the result volume seen in a typical healthcare system; as few as 80 codes account for 80 percent of the volume. Motivated by these findings, the Regenstrief Institute and the National Library of Medicine (NLM) developed a list of the most commonly reported LOINC codes. This list was derived from a large nationally representative data set and covers 98 percent of the result volume from three large institutions that had mapped all of their local laboratory codes to LOINC. Through collaborations with the NLM and other stakeholders, Regenstrief also publishes a list of common order codes covering greater than 95 percent of lab test orders in the US. This list could serve as a good starter set for use in computerized order entry systems.

Regenstrief develops two main applications for LOINC users. RELMA provides tools for browsing LOINC and mapping local terms to LOINC terms. Regenstrief also produces an online search program (see [LOINC 2018h] in the resource list at the end of this chapter). Regenstrief recently made a large portion of the LOINC content available via a terminology services application programming interface (API) that conforms to the FHIR standard specification (HL7 International n.d.). A detailed description of the LOINC content available through this API

TABLE 10.3. Accessory files in the LOINC release distribution

Accessory File	Description
LOINC Part File	LOINC Parts and their connections to current LOINC terms, as well as mappings from LOINC Parts to external vocabularies.
LOINC Answer File	LOINC Answer Lists and their connections to current LOINC terms, including the detailed enumeration of answers and related metadata.
LOINC Display Name File	LOINC Display Names for LOINC terms.
LOINC Linguistic Variants	Linguistic variant translations of LOINC terms. Each linguistic variant translation set is identified by its ISO language and country codes.
LOINC Panels and Forms File	Specialized export of the LOINC panels, including parent-child relationships and context-specific attributes of LOINC terms.
LOINC Multiaxial Hierarchy File	A computable representation that logically organizes all LOINC terms based on a combination of their FSN attributes.
LOINC Group File	A computable representation that groups together LOINC codes that could be treated as equivalent for a particular purpose such as display on a clinical flowsheet or retrieving data for quality measurement.
LOINC Document Ontology File	Specialized export of all terms in the LOINC Document Ontology, including the attribute values identified by LOINC Parts from each axis of the Document Ontology model.
LOINC/RSNA Radiology Playbook File	Specialized export of all terms in the LOINC/RSNA Radiology Playbook, including the attribute values identified by LOINC Parts from each axis of the radiology model, mappings from LOINC Parts to RadLex clinical terms, and mappings from LOINC terms to the historical procedure codes in the RadLex Playbook.
LOINC/IEEE Medical Device Code Mapping Table	A mapping from LOINC terms to terms in the IEEE EMB/11073 standard. This file is the product of a collaboration between Regenstrief and the IEEE-SA.
LOINC/SNOMED CT Expression Association and Map Sets File	A collection of LOINC terms linked to SNOMED CT expressions, mappings of LOINC Parts to SNOMED CT concepts, and other artifacts. This file is the product of a collaboration between Regenstrief and SNOMED International.

Source: Regenstrief Institute, Inc.

is available from the LOINC website (see [LOINC 2018i] in the resource list at the end of this chapter). All of these resources are made available free for use worldwide.

LOINC Table

The main artifact of the LOINC distribution is the LOINC Table, which is available in several file formats. Each record in the LOINC Table identifies a unique clinical observation and contains the LOINC code, the formal six-part FSN, other names and synonyms, and many other accessory attributes. Regenstrief publishes both a full edition with more than 45 fields and a core edition that is limited to the subset of fields that are both crucial for defining each LOINC term and whose structure is anticipated to be stable over the long run. The full table specifications are given in Appendix A of the *LOINC Users' Guide*.

RELMA

RELMA is a Microsoft Windows desktop program that contains tools for both browsing the LOINC database and mapping local observation codes to LOINC. Like LOINC, RELMA is also available at no cost. Users can import a set of local terms for mapping with a text file of their system's master test catalog. The ability to accurately map to LOINC depends on having sufficient information about the tests of interest. In general, the more information that is available, the better and faster the mapping process will be.

RELMA's primary interface allows searching and mapping on a term-by-term basis. RELMA contains many features for narrowing searches to find the most appropriate LOINC code, including a set of hierarchies that organize the LOINC concepts. A screenshot of the RELMA search interface is shown in figure 10.2.

FIGURE 10.2. Main search screen interface of the Regenstrief LOINC Mapping Assistant (RELMA) program, version 6.23

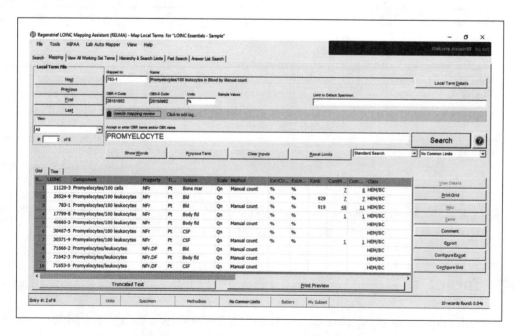

Source: Reprinted courtesy of Regenstrief Institute, Inc.

In addition to term-by-term searching, RELMA contains an additional program called Intelligent Mapper that automatically generates a ranked list of candidate LOINC codes for each local term in a set. Several studies have formally evaluated Intelligent Mapper's performance in mapping local radiology terms to LOINC and have demonstrated high accuracy (Vreeman and McDonald 2005, 2006). Propelled by a recent study demonstrating good mapping performance using techniques that operated on a large corpus of existing mappings, a new feature was added that connects RELMA to a growing community repository of local terms to LOINC mappings (Fidahussein and Vreeman 2013). When information about other institutions' mappings were made available (aggregate counts as well as the actual local term names), users agreed that it was useful and informed their mapping of local terms to LOINC (Dixon et al. 2015; Vreeman et al. 2015).

As users map to LOINC, they will occasionally encounter terms in their local catalog for which no suitable LOINC code exists. RELMA contains a set of tools for proposing additions to the LOINC database. RELMA will create a file of these new term requests that can be sent to Regenstrief for consideration. For most laboratory tests and basic clinical measurements, the tools in RELMA are a very straightforward way to make a submission. For collections of terms, complex patient assessment instruments, or other specialized content, one of the approved LOINC submission templates will be more efficient than using RELMA (see [LOINC 2018j] in the resource list at the end of this chapter).

Adoption

LOINC has been adopted in many contexts around the world. There are now more than 65,000 registered users from 172 countries, with a current growth rate of about 16,500 new users per year. LOINC is used by international e-health projects, national health programs, large health-care systems, health IT vendors, professional societies, insurance companies, research projects, large technology companies like Apple, Google, and IBM, as well as many other initiatives. LOINC has been adopted as a national standard in about 35 countries. The following contains a brief summary of LOINC adoption within the US.

United States Federal Initiatives

Federal regulations in the US now mandate the use of LOINC codes through various incentive programs now known as the Promoting Interoperability Programs. These programs (and the Meaningful Use program that preceded it) provide incentives to eligible hospitals and providers who use certified EHRs that meet specific requirements for functionality and interoperability. The current specifications require use of LOINC in various contexts, such as reporting laboratory results and vital signs (specified in the Common Clinical Data Set), exchanging patient summaries at transitions of care, using and exchanging social, psychological, and behavioral data, and reporting results to cancer registries and public health agencies.

LOINC is required by CMS for electronic quality measure reporting across many domains of content, including laboratory and non-laboratory diagnostic tests, patient preferences, functional status, and more. In addition, as part of its response to the Improving Medicare Post-Acute Care Transformation Act, CMS has adopted LOINC for the patient assessment instruments that are required in post-acute care settings and has contracted with Regenstrief to coordinate the LOINC representation of these instruments with CMS's regular update process.

The U.S. Food and Drug Administration (FDA) has recognized LOINC in its Data Standards Catalog (FDA n.d.). The FDA uses LOINC to organize the contents of Structured Product Labeling and will require the submission of laboratory data in regulated studies to be coded with LOINC beginning in 2020. Recently the FDA issued guidance that encouraged and clarified the important role that manufacturers of IVD tests can play by identifying the LOINC codes appropriate for their tests (FDA 2018).

The Centers for Disease Control and Prevention (CDC) has an overarching Public Health Information Network initiative with many programs that implement LOINC (CDC n.d.). Examples of these national programs include reporting by ambulatory providers to central cancer registries, electronic laboratory reporting to public health, syndromic surveillance, National Healthcare Safety Network (NHSN) healthcare-associated infection, reporting vital statistics, early hearing detection and intervention, and more.

Other federal initiatives have adopted LOINC as well. The Office of the National Coordinator for Health IT (ONC) publishes an Interoperability Standards Advisory that lists LOINC for many interoperability needs, including functional status, laboratory tests, imaging diagnostics, nursing observations, vital signs, and social determinants of health (ONC n.d.).

The National Cancer Institute has included LOINC in its cancer Biomedical Informatics Grid infrastructure after it passed a rigorous evaluation process (Cimino et al. 2009). LOINC is also included in the National Library of Medicine's (NLM's) Unified Medical Language System Metathesaurus. The NLM and Health Resources and Services Administration jointly developed a Newborn Screening Coding and Terminology Guide that uses LOINC for identifying newborn screening test results (NLM n.d.). Additionally, the HHS Office of Population Affairs has recently developed an interoperable, standards-based reporting system for collecting data elements in their Family Planning Annual Report from Title X family planning clinics (U.S. Office of Population Affairs n.d.). The data elements in this reporting system have been represented in LOINC.

One final example is the National Institute of Diabetes and Digestive and Kidney Diseases' (NIDDK's) development of a chronic kidney disease care plan (NIDDK n.d.). Working with Regenstrief, the NIDDK identified a set of data elements and LOINC terms that are recommended for inclusion in an electronic chronic kidney disease care plan.

Private Sector

In the private sector, large laboratories, insurance companies, professional societies, instrument manufacturers, and clinical decision-making applications use LOINC to accelerate data sharing, aggregation, and processing.

Most of the largest commercial laboratories (such as ARUP Laboratories, LabCorp, Mayo Medical Laboratories) have all adopted LOINC and have been longstanding participants in the Laboratory LOINC Committee. They make the mappings from their internal codes to LOINC codes available on their websites, and many also will deliver LOINC terms in their outbound electronic results messages. Healthcare provider organizations (such as Intermountain Health Care, Geisinger Health Systems, Kaiser Permanente, and Veterans Administration) have adopted LOINC as one of their standard code systems. Use of LOINC by many provider organizations was partly motivated by federal incentive programs. It was also supported by the EHR vendor community, which has enabled this functionality as part of becoming tested and certified by the ONC Health IT Certification program. In addition, the large-scale research networks that healthcare organizations participate in, including PCORnet, OHDSI, and the FDA's Mini-Sentinel initiative, have all adopted LOINC as part of their common data models for aggregating information across institutions.

Many applications and processes to improve healthcare quality are now leveraging standardized data with LOINC. As mentioned previously, the CMS quality measurement program defines tests and observations in their measure rules in relation to concepts from vocabulary standards, including LOINC. The Electronic Quality Measures endorsed by the National Quality Forum use LOINC codes to identify tests used in the quality measures. For example, the Healthcare Effectiveness Data and Information Set (HEDIS) is a tool used by more than 90 percent of US health plans to measure performance on important dimensions of care and service. HEDIS uses LOINC extensively in its measure definitions, and coordinates measure updates with new LOINC releases. Furthermore, LOINC has also been incorporated into many clinical decision support applications and is the second most frequently used code system in studies evaluating such systems (Ahmadian et al. 2011).

Because of its relevance and coverage of nursing content, LOINC has been recognized by the American Nurses Association (ANA) as one of the terminologies supporting nursing practice (ANA 2006). Both the ANA and the American Academy of Nursing (AAN) have strong position statements endorsing and recommending the use of LOINC for identifying nursing assessments and outcomes in cross-organizational exchanges. In 2013, LOINC also became a member of the Alliance for Nursing Informatics, which has made repeated policy comments about the use of LOINC for coding nursing assessments and outcomes (Alliance for Nursing Informatics n.d.).

The collaboration with the RSNA has produced a rich set of radiology content (Vreeman et al. 2018).

Recognizing the value of standardized, aggregate, and interoperable data, the American Physical Therapy Association developed the specification of their national physical therapy outcomes registry by linking all the data elements to LOINC terms (APTA 2016). Innovative applications are using LOINC too. For example, MedlinePlus Connect links patient portals and EHRs to consumer health information and can return information about laboratory tests when the requesting system identifies the test by its LOINC code.

Industry

A commercial ecosystem is also growing around LOINC, with many health information technology vendors adopting LOINC in their products. In part due to the certification criteria for EHRs, nearly all commercial systems (and other open source systems like OpenMRS) have support for LOINC. Most major laboratory information system vendors do as well. A growing number of vendors in the IVD testing industry have been linking their internal codes to LOINC codes. An industry consortium, called the IVD Industry Connectivity Consortium (IICC), with participation from all the major testing vendors has developed the LIVD specification for publishing and exchanging the specific LOINC codes that are relevant for a vendor's test or instrument (IVD Industry Connectivity Consortium n.d.).

Many of the largest consumer technology companies have incorporated LOINC into their products as well. With the release of the Health app in iOS 11.3, Apple enabled functionality for consumers to aggregate their health records from multiple institutions right to their mobile device. Apple recently delivered a Health Records API for software developers and researchers to interact with that health record data (Apple, Inc. 2018). Within the Health App, Apple uses the LOINC Long Common Name as the display text for laboratory test results. IBM's healthcare tools, such as Watson Care Manager, IBM® Integration Bus Healthcare Pack, IBM Unified Data Model for Healthcare, and the like, also make use of LOINC codes for validation, aggregation, and data analysis. Similarly, Google has built various tools for processing and transforming healthcare data, especially leveraging the FHIR standard that typically includes LOINC codes for observations.

There are many "calculator" apps that determine various risk scores, such as the ACC/AHA Guideline on the Assessment of Cardiovascular Risk, based on LOINC-coded laboratory data. An online application to share and manage clinical data from patients with degenerative and vascular diseases of the macula illustrates an innovative ophthalmology platform that leverages LOINC for clinical observations (Bonetto et al. 2016).

Use Cases

To illustrate how LOINC might be used operationally within clinical information systems, consider the following two use cases: electronic laboratory test reporting in a health information exchange and execution of an electronic clinical quality measure. Quality measurement is used as an illustrative example of the many possible secondary uses of standardized clinical data.

Use Case One: Electronic Laboratory Reporting

Consider the case of a primary care provider who wants her EHR to plot Hemoglobin A1C (or any other test) results for a particular patient on a longitudinal flowsheet, regardless of where the test was performed. Fortunately, her practice's EHR is connected to a regional health information exchange, like the INPC, that manages connections to all of the laboratories in the community where her patients usually have their tests performed.

After the laboratory performs the test, the laboratory information system packages the result to be sent electronically to the ordering provider via the health information exchange. Internally, the laboratory system identifies this test with the pneumonic code "A1" and has the display name of "Hgb A1c." The laboratory has mapped all of its test codes to LOINC, and thus this test is linked to LOINC code "4548-4," which has the short display name of "Hgb A1c MFr Bld" and the long display name of "Hemoglobin A1c/Hemoglobin.total in Blood." The laboratory sends the result using an HL7 version 2 message and places both its internal code and the LOINC code in the part of the message (OBX-3) that identifies this observation. An annotated example of what such a message might look like is given in figure 10.3.

The value of LOINC becomes clearer when the amount of variation that exists among institutions, even within the same community, is considered. Table 10.4 gives a sample of the idiosyncratic representations of this same test across 12 different institutions. Multiply this variation across the 2,000 to 3,000 tests in a typical laboratory catalog and the magnitude of the problem for data aggregators becomes clear. Yet, when the provider receives Hemoglobin A1C results from these 12 institutions and they are each mapped to LOINC, her EHR must only understand the LOINC code as being the universal identifier for this test. It then becomes possible to appropriately aggregate and trend the results over time.

FIGURE 10.3. Example HL7 Version 2 message containing a Hemoglobin A1c test result. The light blue-colored portion identifies a local coding, the blue portion identifies a coding with LOINC

```
MSH|...
PID|...
PV1|...
ORC|...
OBR|1|...
OBX|1|NM|A1^Hgb A1c^MyLab^4548-4^Hgb A1c MFr Bld^LN||6.7|%^%^UCUM|...
```

Source: Regenstrief Institute, Inc.

TABLE 10.4. Example test codes and names from different local laboratories for a hemoglobin A1C test that could all be mapped to LOINC code 4548-4 "Hemoglobin A1c/Hemoglobin.total in Blood"

Test Code	Test Name
A1	Hgb A1c
A1CHB	Hemoglobin A1c
HGBA1C	A1C
A1C	Haemoglobin A1c
GHB	Glycosylated Hb
HBA1C	Hemoglobin A1c Ratio
1695	Glycohemoglobin (GHb), Total
64239	Hb A1c Diabetic Assessment
918 d%A1c	% Hemoglobin A1c ~ Whole Blood
994321	Hgb Glycosylated
31222	HgbA1C % Ser EIA
LB67994325	Glycos Hgb A-1%

Source: Regenstrief Institute, Inc.

Use Case Two: Executing an Electronic Clinical Quality Measure

Consider that the primary care provider is participating in a value-based payment program that monitors how well she is performing against certain best practice benchmarks. One of the quality measurements assesses how many of her patients 18 to 75 years of age with diabetes have a Hemoglobin A1C greater than nine percent. With higher A1C values indicating poorly controlled diabetes, the provider wants a very low percentage of her patients with diabetes to fall into this category. The EHR in her office practice can help her monitor this quality measure by executing a relatively simple query to calculate the result. In fact, the vendor of this EHR pre-programmed the system with this rule since it is one of the benchmarks in the Promoting Interoperability program. So, the provider can execute it with a push of a button. Or, better yet, it is part of a regular report card used in his performance improvement reviews.

Yet, the query to evaluate this quality measure is only simple if the EHR knows exactly what to look for when the rule says "Hemoglobin A1C" test result. The vendor that sold the practice the EHR would have no way of knowing all 12 internal codes from the laboratories the provider receives results from. It can, however, build the query based on the universal identifier: the LOINC code 4548-4. There are electronic definitions of the quality measures used in the Promoting Interoperability program available from the National Quality Forum. When the measure definitions list the appropriate codes from standard vocabularies like LOINC, implementing them in clinical systems becomes much more feasible. Thus, if all of the laboratory data the practice receives is mapped to LOINC, it becomes very easy for the system to automatically calculate this measure of care quality. Such tools are extraordinarily helpful to the provider in monitoring whether her patients are keeping their diabetes under control.

CHECK YOUR UNDERSTANDING

1. The developer of the Logical Observation Identifiers, Names, and Codes (LOINC) system is:

    a. College of American Pathologists
    b. Centers for Medicare and Medicaid Services (CMS)
    c. Regenstrief Institute, Inc.
    d. American Clinical Laboratory Association

2. True or false? LOINC has been named in the Promoting Interoperability rules as a standard for more than one domain.

    a. True
    b. False

3. Which of the following is NOT a Part (axis) in the LOINC fully specified name?

    a. Time aspect
    b. Kind of property
    c. Type of method
    d. Type of test

4. Which LOINC Part (axis) is optional in the LOINC fully specified name?

    a. Type of method
    b. Kind of property
    c. Component
    d. Type of scale

5. A program for mapping local files to LOINC is:

    a. LOINC database
    b. Regenstrief LOINC Mapping Assistant (RELMA)
    c. HL7
    d. Regenstrief Medical Records System (RMRS)

REVIEW

1. True or false? LOINC provides a standard set of universal names and codes for identifying health measurements, observations, and documents.

   a. True
   b. False

2. The LOINC development process can be characterized as:

   a. Empirical, nimble, proprietary
   b. Empirical, nimble, open
   c. Ontological, nimble, balloted
   d. Ontological, bureaucratic, proprietary

3. Which of the following is an important factor in LOINC's widespread global adoption?

   a. All modern clinical laboratories now use LOINC as their internal test identifier.
   b. LOINC is included in all electronic health record systems.
   c. LOINC is used many international clinical quality measures.
   d. LOINC has an open and efficient process that has enabled many language translations.

4. LOINC contains names and codes for which kinds of variables?

   a. Laboratory and Pathology
   b. Laboratory and Clinical
   c. Clinical diseases
   d. Clinical and Pathology

5. Fill in the blank. Nursing content is found in the _____ section of LOINC.

6. True or false? LOINC is available at no cost under an open license.

   a. True
   b. False

7. The characteristic or attribute of the component that is measured, evaluated, or observed is which Part (axis) of the LOINC fully specified name?

   a. Type of scale
   b. Type of method
   c. Kind of property
   d. Component

8. Go to the main LOINC website at https://loinc.org/ and navigate to the Downloads section. Which Accessory File might you want if you were interested in building a repository of clinical documents?

9. Download the current version of the LOINC User's Guide from https://loinc.org/ and review section 4.1. Which parts of the formal LOINC name correspond exactly in meaning between laboratory LOINC codes and clinical LOINC codes?

10. True or false? LOINC is required by CMS for electronic quality measure reporting across many domains of content.

   a. True
   b. False

References

Ahmadian, L., M. van Engen-Verheul, F. Bakhshi-Raiez, N. Peek, R. Cornet, and N. F. de Keizer. 2011. The role of standardized data and terminological systems in computerized clinical decision support systems: Literature review and survey. *International Journal of Medical Informatics* 80(2):81–93. https://doi.org/10.1016/j.ijmedinf.2010.11.006

Alliance for Nursing Informatics. n.d. Statements and Positions. https://www.allianceni.org/statements-positions.

American Nurses Association (ANA). 2006 (May 11). ANA Recognized Terminologies and Data Sets. http://ana.nursingworld.org/npii/terminologies.htm.

American Physical Therapy Association (APTA). 2016 (January 16). APTA Physical Therapy Outcomes Registry Data Published in Worldwide Logical Observation Identifiers Names and Codes (LOINC) Database. http://www.apta.org/Media/Releases/Association/2016/1/21/.

Apple, Inc. 2018. Apple Opens Health Records API to Developers. https://www.apple.com/newsroom/2018/06/apple-opens-health-records-api-to-developers/.

Bamford, S., E. Dawson, S. Forbes, J. Clements, R. Pettett, A. Dogan, A. Flanagan et al. 2004. The COSMIC (Catalogue of Somatic Mutations in Cancer) database and website. *British Journal of Cancer* 91(2):355–358. https://doi.org/10.1038/sj.bjc.6601894.

Bonetto, M., M. Nicolò, R. Gazzarata, P. Fraccaro, R. Rosa, D. Musetti, M. Musolino et al. 2016. I-Maculaweb: a tool to support data reuse in ophthalmology. *IEEE Journal of Translational Engineering in Health and Medicine* 4:3800110. https://doi.org/10.1109/JTEHM.2015.2513043.

Chaudhry, B., J. Wang, S. Wu, M. Maglione, W. Mojica, E. Roth, S. C. Morton et al. 2006. Systematic review: Impact of health information technology on quality, efficiency, and costs of medical care. *Annals of Internal Medicine* 144(10):742–752.

Chen, E. S., G. B. Melton, M. E. Engelstad, and I. N. Sarkar. 2010. Standardizing clinical document names using the HL7/LOINC document ontology and LOINC codes. *AMIA Annual Symposium Proceedings* 2010:101–105.

Cimino, J. J. 1998. Desiderata for controlled medical vocabularies in the twenty-first century. *Methods of Information in Medicine* 37(4–5):394–403.

Cimino, J. J., T. F. Hayamizu, O. Bodenreider, B. Davis, G. A. Stafford, and M. Ringwald. 2009. The caBIG terminology review process. *Journal of Biomedical Informatics* 42(3):571–580. https://doi.org/10.1016/j.jbi.2008.12.003.

DICOM Standards Committee. 2019. *PS3.20 Imaging Reports Using HL7 Clinical Document Architecture*. http://dicom.nema.org/medical/dicom/current/output/html/part20.html.

Dixon, B. E., J. Hook, and D. J. Vreeman. 2015. Learning from the crowd in terminology mapping: The LOINC experience. *Laboratory Medicine* 46(2):168–174. https://doi.org/10.1309/LMWJ730SVKTUBAOJ.

Dixon, B. E., E. C. Whipple, J. M. Lajiness, and M. D. Murray. 2016. Utilizing an integrated infrastructure for outcomes research: A systematic review. *Health Information and Libraries Journal* 33(1):7–32. https://doi.org/10.1111/hir.12127.

Dolin, R. H., L. Alschuler, S. Boyer, C. Beebe, F. M. Behlen, P. V. Biron, and A. Shabo Shvo. 2006. HL7 clinical document architecture, release 2. *JAMIA* 13(1):30–39. https://doi.org/10.1197/jamia.M1888.

Dugas, M., S. Thun, T. Frankewitsch, and K. U. Heitmann. 2009. LOINC codes for hospital information systems documents: A case study. *JAMIA* 16(3):400–403. https://doi.org/10.1197/jamia.M2882.

Fidahussein, M. and D. J. Vreeman. 2013. A corpus-based approach for automated LOINC mapping. *JAMIA*. https://doi.org/10.1136/amiajnl-2012-001159.

Forrey, A. W., C. J. McDonald, G. DeMoor, S. M. Huff, D. Leavelle, D. Leland, T. Fiers et al. 1996. Logical observation identifier names and codes (LOINC) database: A public use set of codes and names for electronic reporting of clinical laboratory test results. *Clinical Chemistry* 42(1):81–90.

Frazier, P., A. Rossi-Mori, R. H. Dolin, L. Alschuler, and S. M. Huff. 2001. The creation of an ontology of clinical document names. *Studies in Health Technology and Informatics* 84(Part 1):94–98.

Health Level 7 (HL7) International. 2015a. HL7 Implementation Guide: LOINC Document Ontology, Release 1. http://www.hl7.org/implement/standards/product_brief.cfm?product_id=402.

Health Level 7 (HL7) International. 2015b. C-CDA (HL7 CDA R2.1 Implementation Guide: Consolidated CDA Templates for Clinical Note - US Realm) DSTU R2—Vol. 2: Templates. http://www.hl7.org/implement/standards/product_brief.cfm?product_id=492.

Health Level 7 (HL7) International. n.d. Welcome to FHIR®. http://hl7.org/fhir/.

Huff, S. M., R. A. Rocha, C. J. McDonald, G. J. De Moor, T. Fiers, W. D. Bidgood, A. W. Forrey et al. 1998. Development of the Logical Observation Identifier Names and Codes (LOINC) vocabulary. *JAMIA* 5(3):276–292.

Hyun, S. and S. Bakken. 2006. Toward the creation of an ontology for nursing document sections: Mapping section names to the LOINC semantic model. *AMIA Annual Symposium Proceedings*: 364–368.

Hyun, S., J. S. Shapiro, G. Melton, C. Schlegel, P. D. Stetson, S. B. Johnson, and S. Bakken. 2009. Iterative evaluation of the Health Level 7—Logical Observation Identifiers Names and Codes Clinical Document Ontology for representing clinical document names: A case report. *JAMIA* 16(3):395–399. https://doi.org/10.1197/jamia.M2821.

Hyun, S., R. Ventura, S. B. Johnson, and S. Bakken. 2006. Is the Health Level 7/LOINC document ontology adequate for representing nursing documents? *Studies in Health Technology and Informatics* 122:527–531.

IVD Industry Connectivity Consortium. n.d. LIVD – Digital Format for Publication of LOINC to Vendor IVD Test Results. https://ivdconnectivity.org/livd/.

Li, L., C. P. Morrey, and D. Baorto. 2011. Cross-mapping clinical notes between hospitals: an application of the LOINC Document Ontology. *AMIA Annual Symposium Proceedings*: 777–783.

Liu, S., W. Ma, R. Moore, V. Ganesan, and S. Nelson. 2005. RxNorm: Prescription for electronic drug information exchange. *IT Professional* 7(5):17–23. https://doi.org/10.1109/MITP.2005.122

Matney, S. A., G. Dolin, L. Buhl, and A. Sheide. 2016. Communicating nursing care using the Health Level Seven Consolidated Clinical Document Architecture Release 2 Care Plan. *Computers, Informatics, Nursing: CIN* 34(3):128–136. https://doi.org/10.1097/CIN.0000000000000214

Matney, S., S. Bakken, and S. M. Huff, 2003. Representing nursing assessments in clinical information systems using the logical observation identifiers, names, and codes database. *Journal of Biomedical Informatics* 36(4–5):287–293.

McDonald, C. J., J. M. Overhage, M. Barnes, G. Schadow, L. Blevins, P. R. Dexter, B. Mamlin et al. 2005. The Indiana network for patient care: A working local health information infrastructure. An example of a working infrastructure collaboration that links data from five health systems and hundreds of millions of entries. *Health Affairs (Project Hope)* 24(5):1214–1220. https://doi.org/10.1377/hlthaff.24.5.1214

McDonald, C. J., J. M. Overhage, W. M. Tierney, P. R. Dexter, D. K. Martin, J. G. Suico, A. Zafar et al. 1999. The Regenstrief Medical Record System: A quarter century experience. *International Journal of Medical Informatics* 54(3):225–253.

McDonald, C. J., S. M. Huff, J. Deckard, S. Armson, S. Abhyankar, and D. J. Vreeman, eds. 2018. *LOINC Users' Guide* (LOINC 2.64, Users Guide 2.64). https://loinc.org/download/loinc-users-guide/.

McDonald, C. J., S. M. Huff, J. G. Suico, G. Hill, D. Leavelle, R. Aller, A. Forrey et al. 2003. LOINC, a universal standard for identifying laboratory observations: A 5-year update. *Clinical Chemistry* 49(4):624–633.

National Institute of Diabetes and Digestive and Kidney Diseases (NIDDK). n.d. Development of an Electronic CKD Care Plan. https://www.niddk.nih.gov/health-information/communication-programs/nkdep/working-groups/health-information-technology/development-electronic-ckd-care-plan.

Office of the National Coordinator for Health Information Technology (ONC). n.d. Interoperability Standards Advisory. https://www.healthit.gov/isa.

Pan, H., K. A. Tryka, D. J. Vreeman, W. Huggins, M. J. Phillips, J. P. Mehta, J. A. Phillips et al. 2012. Using PhenX measures to identify opportunities for cross-study analysis. *Human Mutation* 33(5):849–857. https://doi.org/10.1002/humu.22074.

Peng, P., A. C. Beitia, D. J. Vreeman, G. T. Loo, B. N. Delman, F. Thum, T. Lowry, & J. S. Shapiro. 2019. Mapping of HIE CT terms to LOINC: analysis of content-dependent coverage and coverage improvement through new term creation. *JAMIA* 26(1):19–27.

Regenstrief Institute, Inc. 2018. LOINC. https://search.loinc.org/searchLOINC/search.zul.

Regenstrief Institute, Inc. n.d. Regenstrief and IHTSDO Collaboration Home Page. http://loinc.org/collaboration/ihtsdo.

Shapiro, J. S., S. Bakken, S. Hyun, G. B. Melton, C. Schlegel, and S. B. Johnson. 2005. Document ontology: supporting narrative documents in electronic health records. *AMIA Annual Symposium Proceedings*:684–688.

Subramanian, A., B. Westra, S. Matney, P. S. Wilson, C. W. Delaney, S. Huff, and D. Huber. 2008. Integrating the nursing management minimum data set into the logical observation identifier names and codes system. *AMIA Annual Symposium Proceedings*: 1148.

Tierney, W. M., M. Achieng, E. Baker, A. Bell, P. Biondich, P. Braitstein, D. Kayiwa et al. 2010. Experience implementing electronic health records in three East African countries. *Studies in Health Technology and Informatics* 160(Pt 1):371–375.

Tilley, C. and S. Matney. 2005. Contributing pain assessment concepts to a controlled terminology. *AMIA Annual Symposium Proceedings*: 1137.

U.S. Centers for Disease Control and Prevention (CDC). n.d. PHIN Tools and Resources. https://www.cdc.gov/phin/.

U.S. Food and Drug Administration (FDA). 2018 (June 15). Logical Observation Identifiers Names and Codes for In Vitro Diagnostic Tests - Guidance for Industry and Food and Drug Administration Staff. https://www.fda.gov/downloads/medicaldevices/deviceregulationandguidance/guidancedocuments/ucm610636.pdf.

U.S. Food and Drug Administration (FDA). n.d. FDA Resources for Data Standards. https://www.fda.gov/ForIndustry/DataStandards/default.htm.

U.S. National Library of Medicine (NLM). n.d. Newborn Screening Coding and Terminology Guide. https://newbornscreeningcodes.nlm.nih.gov.

U.S. Office of Population Affairs. n.d. The Family Planning Annual Report and Health Information Technology (Health IT) Initiative (FPAR 2.0). https://www.hhs.gov/opa/title-x-family-planning/fp-annual-report/health-information-technology/index.html.

Vreeman, D. J. 2018. Regenstrief LOINC team internal report. Regenstrief Institute, Inc.

Vreeman, D. J. 2016. *LOINC Essentials* (1.0). Blue Sky Premise, LLC. https://danielvreeman.com/loinc-essentials.

Vreeman, D. J. n.d. Regenstrief's approach to licensing LOINC. https://danielvreeman.com/regenstriefs-approach-to-licensing-loinc/.

Vreeman, D. J., S. Abhyankar, K. C. Wang, C. Carr, B. Collins, D. L. Rubin, and C. P. Langlotz. 2018. The LOINC RSNA radiology playbook - A unified terminology for radiology procedures. *JAMIA*. https://doi.org/10.1093/jamia/ocy053.

Vreeman, D. J., J. T. Finnell, and J. M. Overhage. 2007. A rationale for parsimonious laboratory term mapping by frequency. *AMIA Annual Symposium Proceedings*: 771–775.

Vreeman, D. J., J. Hook, and B. E. Dixon. 2015. Learning from the crowd while mapping to LOINC. *JAMIA* 22(6):1205–1211. https://doi.org/10.1093/jamia/ocv098.

Vreeman, D. J. and C. J. McDonald. 2005. Automated mapping of local radiology terms to LOINC. *AMIA Annual Symposium Proceedings*, pp. 769–773. Washington, DC: AMIA.

Vreeman, D. J. and C. J. McDonald. 2006. A comparison of Intelligent Mapper and document similarity scores for mapping local radiology terms to LOINC. *AMIA Annual Symposium Proceedings*, pp. 809–813. Washington, DC: AMIA.

Vreeman, D. J., C. J. McDonald, and S. M. Huff. 2010. LOINC® - A universal catalog of individual clinical observations and uniform representation of enumerated collections. *International Journal of Functional Informatics and Personalised Medicine* 3(4):273–291. https://doi.org/10.1504/IJFIPM.2010.040211.

Vreeman, D. J., M. T. Chiaravalloti, J. Hook, and C. J. McDonald. 2012. Enabling international adoption of LOINC through translation. *Journal of Biomedical Informatics* 45(4): 667–673.

Wang, A. Y., J. H. Sable, and K. A. Spackman. 2002. The SNOMED clinical terms development process: Refinement and analysis of content. *AMIA Annual Symposium Proceedings*: 845–849.

Wang, K. C., J. B. Patel, B. Vyas, M. Toland, B. Collins, D. J. Vreeman, S. Abhyankar et al. 2017. Use of radiology procedure codes in health care: the need for standardization and structure. *Radiographics* 37(4):1099–1110. https://doi.org/10.1148/rg.2017160188.

Westra, B. L., B. L. Westra, A. Subramanian, C. M. Hart, S. A. Matney, P. S. Wilson, S. M. Huff, D. Huber et al. 2010. Achieving "meaningful use" of electronic health records through the integration of the nursing management minimum data set. *The Journal of Nursing Administration* 40(7/8):336–343. https://doi.org/10.1097/NNA.0b013e3181e93994.

White, T. M. and M. J. Hauan. 2002. Extending the LOINC conceptual schema to support standardized assessment instruments. *JAMIA* 9(6):586–599.

Resources

LOINC. 2018a. Funding support. https://loinc.org/funding-support/.

LOINC. 2018b. LOINC and RELMA license. https://loinc.org/license/.

LOINC. 2018c. Submission queue stats. https://loinc.org/submissions/stats.

LOINC. 2018d. Submission queue details. https://loinc.org/submissions/queue.

LOINC. 2018e. LOINC prerelease terms. https://loinc.org/prerelease.

LOINC. 2018f. Common UCUM units. https://loinc.org/usage/units/.

LOINC. 2018g. https://loinc.org/.

LOINC. 2018h. https://search.loinc.org.

LOINC. 2018i. LOINC FHIR terminology server. https://loinc.org/fhir/.

LOINC. 2018j. Submitting new term requests. https://loinc.org/submissions/new-terms/.

OpenHIE. n.d. https://ohie.org.

OpenMRS. n.d. https://openmrs.org/.

Unified Code for Units of Measure (UCUM). n.d. http://unitsofmeasure.org/.

11

International Classification of Functioning, Disability, and Health

Heather R. Porter, PhD, CTRS

LEARNING OBJECTIVES

- Explain the development and purpose of the International Classification of Functioning, Disability, and Health (ICF)
- Explain the components of the ICF model and how they interrelate to impact functioning and health
- Differentiate the ICF classification system components including its coding scheme, qualifier scaling, and coding rules
- Summarize the purpose of ICF core sets and the role they play in assessment
- Indicate future directions of the ICF based on its aims and applications
- Examine the relationship among ICF and other classifications, terminologies and code sets
- Compare tools available to access and use
- Understand how ICF is used in an electronic environment

KEY TERMS

- Activity
- Activity limitation
- Barrier
- Biopsychosocial Model

- Body functions
- Body structures
- Capacity
- Coding string
- Core sets
- Disability
- Environmental factors
- Facilitator
- Functioning
- Health condition
- ICF Model
- Impairment
- International Classification of Functioning, Disability, and Health (ICF)
- Medical Model
- Participation
- Participation restriction
- Performance
- Personal factors
- Social Model

Introduction to ICF

There are codes in healthcare for diseases, disorders, and illnesses (ICD-10 codes), interventions (CPT codes), and products, supplies, and equipment (HCPCS Level II codes). Although the management of such data is valuable (for example, tracking prevalence of disease and interventions, predicting mortality), it doesn't capture other essential data such as people's health, their ability to complete tasks and activities, and the things in the environment that facilitate or hinder functioning. The World Health Organization (WHO) stated that, "diagnosis alone does not predict service needed, length of hospitalization, level of care or functional outcomes. Nor is the presence of a disease or disorder an accurate predictor of receipt of disability benefits, work performance, return to work potential, or likelihood of social integration" (WHO 2002, 4).

As a result of this quandary, the International Classification of Impairments, Disabilities, and Handicaps (ICIDH) was revised into the **International Classification of Functioning, Disability, and Health (ICF)**. Over the course of 10 years, a rigorous process was undertaken by the WHO to develop the ICF, consisting of both a classification system *and* a model to reflect the holistic and systemic perspective of functioning and disability. Over 65 countries participated in its development and in more than 50 countries extensive field-testing was conducted by 1,800 experts (WHO 2001; Brundtland 2002). Finally, in 2001, the ICF was released for use, with the subsequent release of the ICF Children and Youth version in 2007.

The overall aim of the ICF is to provide a "unified and standard language and framework for the description of health and health-related states" that can be used with *all* people, not just those with disability (WHO 2007, 3). It is a model that promotes a holistic evaluation of functioning and disability, as well as a classification system of over 1,400 health-related codes. Each of these is reviewed in detail below.

Purpose

The WHO outlines four primary aims of the ICF that provide guidance for its use:

1. *To provide a scientific basis for understanding and studying health and health-related states, outcomes, and determinants.* Using the ICF throughout the world will provide a consistent, unified, and holistic approach to understanding and classifying functioning and disability. The ICF "assists professionals to look beyond their own areas of practice, communicate across disciplines, and think from a functioning perspective rather than the perspective of a health condition" (CDC n.d.).

2. *To establish a common language for describing health and health-related states in order to improve communication between different users, such as healthcare workers, researchers, policy-makers, and the public, including people with disabilities.* The language within the ICF has been carefully chosen so that it can be translated into other languages. For example, the term "ambulation" (which means "to walk") does not exist in other languages. Consequently, the simpler term of "walking" was chosen. The word "strength" also does not exist in other languages, therefore the term "muscle power" was chosen. Likewise, when consistent terminology is utilized, comparison of information is facilitated and knowledge is built, thus expediting positive change.

3. *To permit comparison of data across countries, health care disciplines, services, and time.* Using a common language (codes) and measurement (qualifiers) will allow disciplines to easily communicate, compare, and combine information. In other words, it helps in building synergy among different types of information systems such as surveys, research, and health records (CDC n.d.).

4. *To provide a systematic coding scheme for health information systems.* The ICF consists of over 1,400 codes and is part of the WHO family of international classifications, designed to complement the International Statistical Classification of Diseases and Related Health Problems (ICD-10). The combined use of the ICD-10 (disease, injury, and disorder focus) and ICF (functioning and disability focus) within health information systems "provides a more meaningful and complete picture of the health needs of people and populations" (CDC n.d.). (WHO 2001; WHO 2007).

Furthermore, the WHO identifies four primary areas for ICF application, including its use as a statistical tool for collecting and recording data (for example, in population studies and surveys or in management information systems); a research tool to measure such things as outcomes, quality of life, and environmental factors; a clinical tool for needs assessment, matching treatments with specific conditions, vocational assessment, rehabilitation, and outcome evaluation; and a social policy tool to be used in social security planning, compensation, systems, and policy design and implementation (WHO 2001; WHO 2007).

A systematic review of the application and uses of the ICF is beyond the scope of this chapter. Consequently, those seeking to understand how the ICF is applied to their specific areas of interest should conduct their own tailored searches, as the application is expansive and growing exponentially. For example, using the search terms "International Classification of Functioning, Disability, and Health" and "application" within all the databases available through Temple University with no year designation yielded 33,029 journal articles, a four-fold increase from 2015. When reducing the search by year, 246 journal articles were written in 2001; 890 were written in 2011; and 2,777 were written in 2017. Keep in mind that this is only a subset of the ICF literature. For example, when using the term "International Classification of Functioning, and Disability" only (again, within all databases available through Temple University), over 113,442 items were found, including books, journal articles, government documents, dissertations, book chapters, newspaper articles, reports, and so on.

Content

The practitioner's perspective on health and disability colors the evaluation and treatment process, of which the Medical Model has had a traditional stronghold in healthcare. The **Medical Model** follows the assumption that the medical problem resides within the individual (such as a problem in the immune system that causes multiple sclerosis). This is quite different from the **Social Model** (also known as the Minority Model or Environmental Model) where disability is viewed as a social construction, where problems lie not within the person with a disability but in the environment that fails to accommodate people with disabilities and in the negative attitudes of people without disabilities (where people with disabilities are seen as a minority group). Although the above models are seen in all segments of society and healthcare, the WHO promotes the use of a different model, called the ICF model.

The ICF Model

The **ICF model** is a nonlinear, systemic, biopsychosocial model consisting of multiple components (see figure 11.1; see definitions below). The nonlinear systemic nature of the model is reflected through the use of multidirectional arrows throughout the model. The arrows indicate that intervention in any model component can impact other components and that all components interact and affect each other. The ICF model also follows a **Biopsychosocial Model**, which is a blend of the Medical Model and Social Model. It views functioning and disability as an

FIGURE 11.1. The ICF model

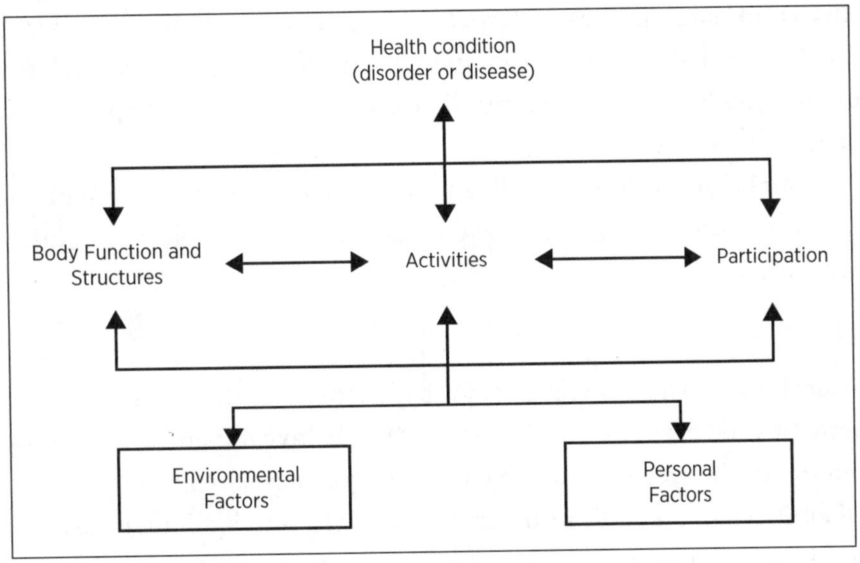

Source: International Classification of Functioning, Disability, and Health (2001). Reprinted with WHO permission.

interaction among one's biological, psychological (including thoughts, emotions, and behaviors), and social factors. The ICF model is advocated by the WHO to be used throughout the world to enhance a more holistic and unified perspective of functioning and disability. Each of the model components is defined below:

- **Health condition**: The particular disorders/diseases/injuries of the individual
- Body Structures and Functions

  - **Body structures**: Anatomical parts of the body (for example, a defect in a heart valve)
  - **Body functions**: Physiological and psychological functions of the body (for example, mental functions, sensory functions)
  - **Impairment**: Problems in body structures or functions such as a significant deviation or loss

- Activities and Participation

  - **Activity**: Execution of a task or action by an individual
  - **Participation**: Involvement in a life situation
  - **Activity limitation**: Difficulties an individual may have in executing activities
  - **Participation restriction**: Problems an individual may experience in involvement in life situations

- Contextual Factors

  - **Environmental factors**: External influences that facilitate or hinder functioning and health (for example, accessible buildings, weather); make up the physical, social, and attitudinal environment in which people live and conduct their lives

  - **Personal factors**: Internal influences that facilitate or hinder functioning and health (for example, age, gender, race, age, habits, upbringing, education, profession)

- Umbrella Terms

  - **Functioning**: An umbrella term for body structures, body functions, and activities and participation. It denotes the positive or neutral aspects of the interaction between the health condition and contextual factors.

  - **Disability**: An umbrella term for impairments, activity limitations, and participation restrictions. It denotes the negative aspects of the interaction between the health condition and contextual factors.

An important aspect of the ICF model is that it does not assume a "disablement syndrome." If an individual has a health condition, there is no assumption that she or he will have difficulties with functioning. For example, just because a person uses a wheelchair for mobility, doesn't mean that she or he can't function independently in society, whether this is with or without available resources. When scoring ICF codes, which are discussed later in this chapter, for a person who utilizes available resources, and there is no residual difficulty, the person is said to have "no difficulty." This puts an increased focus on the value of environmental factors and recognizes their impact on functioning, as well as equalizes their use across all people, not just those with disabilities.

To illustrate how these components interact, several examples are provided:

- Example #1: Mark has a complete spinal cord injury (*health condition*). He uses a wheelchair for mobility at home and in the community (*participation*). Many of the places Mark likes to go in the community are not wheelchair accessible (*environmental factors*), limiting his ability to engage in community activities (*participation*). As a result, Mark's indoor sedentary behavior increases (*participation*) and depression ensues (*body functions*).

- Example #2: Joan is a relatively healthy 40-year-old; however, she is experiencing high stress in her personal life and work life (*participation*). She is overweight and has borderline hypertension (*health condition*). She successfully learns how to handle stress through meditation, diet, and exercise (*participation*), thus reducing her risk of developing hypertension (*health condition*).

- Example #3: John is a frail older adult in poor health (*health condition*) who lives alone in the community. He contracts a bad cold (*health condition*) but does not seek medical attention because he believes that a higher power can heal him without medical intervention (*personal factor*). The cold turns into pneumonia (*health condition*) and his health further deteriorates (*health condition*).

The ICF Classification System

In addition to a model, the ICF is also a classification system that allows for the collection of useful information in multiple domains for *all* people, not just those with disabilities. Although the ICF was developed to fill a need, it was not developed to replace the ICD-10 but rather to complement and incorporate the ICD-10. Referring to figure 11.1, the *health condition* component within the model is described using ICD-10 codes.

In WHO's international classifications, health conditions (diseases, disorders, injuries, and so on) are classified primarily in ICD-10, which provides an etiological framework. Functioning and disability associated with health conditions are classified in the ICF. ICD-10 and ICF are therefore complementary and users are encouraged to utilize these two members of the WHO family of international classifications together. ICD-10 provides a "diagnosis" of diseases, disorders, or other health conditions, and this information is enriched by the additional information given by ICF on functioning. Together, information on diagnosis plus functioning provides a broader and more meaningful picture of the health of people or populations, which can then be used for decision-making purposes (WHO 2007, 4).

Coding Scheme

The ICF includes four code components: Body Structures, Body Functions, Activities and Participation, and Environmental Factors. The "health condition" is designated using ICD-10 codes; "personal factors" are not currently coded in the ICF, although they are recognized as an integral component in the ICF model, due to the wide variance across cultures (WHO 2001). Each code set is divided into "chapters" (see figure 11.2). Chapters are referred to as the first-level of classification. Within each chapter there are "branches," referred to as tiered "levels" of classification. Below is an example from Body Structures to illustrate the coding scheme:

Chapter 1: Structures of the nervous system (chapter = first-level classification)

- s120 Spinal cord and related structures (first branch = second-level classification)
  - s1200 Structure of the spinal cord (second branch = third-level classification)
    - s12000 Cervical spinal cord (third branch = fourth-level classification)
    - s12001 Thoracic spinal cord
    - s12002 Lumbosacral spinal cord
    - s12003 Cauda equina
    - s12008 Structure of the spinal cord, other specified
    - s12009 Structure of the spinal cord, unspecified

BODY STRUCTURES

Body structures are defined as anatomy of the body, including organs, limbs, and their components. Within the component of Body Structures (BS), there are eight chapters of codes (see figure 11.2). Every BS code begins with a lowercase s. If a person has a problem with a BS code, it is referred to as an "impairment." To describe the impairment, BS codes have three qualifiers that follow the code (see figure 11.3).

FIGURE 11.2. ICF chapters

Chapter	Part 1: Functioning and Disability		Part 2: Contextual Factors	
	Body Structures	Body Functions	Activities and Participation	Environmental Factors
Chapter 1	Structures of the nervous system	Mental functions	Learning and applying knowledge	Products and technology
Chapter 2	The eye, ear, and related structures	Sensory functions and pain	General tasks and demands	Natural environment and human made changes to environment
Chapter 3	Structures involved in voice and speech	Voice and speech functions	Communication	Support and relationships
Chapter 4	Structures of the cardiovascular, immunological and respiratory systems	Functions of the cardiovascular, haematological, immunological respiratory systems	Mobility	Attitudes
Chapter 5	Structures related to the digestive, metabolic, and endocrine systems	Functions of the digestive, metabolic, and endocrine systems	Self-care	Services, systems, and policies
Chapter 6	Structures related to the genitourinary and reproductive systems	Genitourinary and reproductive functions	Domestic life	—
Chapter 7	Structures related to movement	Neuromusculoskeletal and movement-related functions	Interpersonal interactions and relationships	—
Chapter 8	Skin and related structures	Functions of the skin and related structures	Major life areas	—
Chapter 9	—	—	Community, social, and civic life	—

Source: Adapted from International Classification of Functioning, Disability, and Health (2001) and International Classification of Functioning, Disability, and Health: Child and Youth Version (2007).

Example:

Joe has a complete L4 spinal cord injury. The code for lumbosacral spinal cord is s12002. The appropriately written code would look like this: s12002.4_ _

BS Code	First Qualifier (Extent of Impairment)	Second Qualifier (Nature of Impairment)	Third Qualifier (Location of Impairment)
s12002.	4	—	—

FIGURE 11.3. Body structure qualifiers

First Qualifier Extent of Impairment	Second Qualifier Nature of Impairment	Third Qualifier Location of Impairment
0 NO impairment (none, absent, negligible: 0–4%) 1 MILD impairment (slight, low: 5–24%) 2 MODERATE impairment (medium, fair: 25–49%) 3 SEVERE impairment (high, extreme: 50–95%) 4 COMPLETE impairment (total: 96–100%) 8 not specified 9 not applicable	0 no change in structure 1 total absence 2 partial absence 3 additional part 4 aberrant dimensions 5 discontinuity 6 deviating position 7 qualitative changes in structure, including accumulation of fluid 8 not specified 9 not applicable	0 more than one region 1 right 2 left 3 both sides 4 front 5 back 6 proximal 7 distal 8 not specified 9 not applicable

Source: Adapted from International Classification of Functioning, Disability, and Health (2001) and International Classification of Functioning, Disability, and Health: Child and Youth Version (2007).

FIGURE 11.4. Body function qualifiers

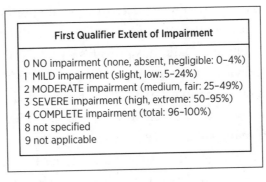

First Qualifier Extent of Impairment
0 NO impairment (none, absent, negligible: 0–4%) 1 MILD impairment (slight, low: 5–24%) 2 MODERATE impairment (medium, fair: 25–49%) 3 SEVERE impairment (high, extreme: 50–95%) 4 COMPLETE impairment (total: 96–100%) 8 not specified 9 not applicable

Source: Adapted from International Classification of Functioning, Disability, and Health (2001) and International Classification of Functioning, Disability, and Health: Child and Youth Version (2007).

BODY FUNCTIONS

Body functions are the physiological and psychological functions of the body. Within the component of Body Functions (BF), there are eight chapters of codes (see figure 11.2). Every BF code begins with a lowercase *b*. If a person has a problem with a BF, it is referred to as an "impairment." To describe the impairment, BF codes have one qualifier that follows the code (see figure 11.4).

Example:

As a result of the spinal cord injury, Joe has no voluntary movement in half of his muscle groups (50 percent = 3 Severe impairment, 50–95 percent). The code for control of voluntary movement functions is b760. The appropriately written code would look like this: b760.3.

BF Code	First Qualifier (Extent of Impairment)
b760.	3

ACTIVITIES AND PARTICIPATION

Activities and participation are the execution of tasks and actions. Within the component of Activities and Participation (A&P), there are nine chapters of codes (see figure 11.2). Every A&P code begins with a lowercase *d*. Although the codes for "Activities" (A) and "Participation" (P) are the same, there is an important distinction. Activities are tasks and actions that are performed in a standardized testing environment, which is the **capacity** qualifier (for example, propelling a wheelchair in the therapy gym). Participation is tasks and actions that are performed in the person's real-life living situation (such as propelling a wheelchair in one's home), which is the performance qualifier. Even though the task or action is the same, the context in which it is performed is different. This distinction recognizes that people perform differently in different settings. The gap between capacity and performance "reflects the difference between the impacts of current and uniform environments, and thus provides a useful guide as to what can be done to the environment of the individual to improve performance" (WHO 2001, 15). If a person has difficulty performing a task or action in a standardized testing environment (Activity, capacity qualifier), it is called an "Activity Limitation." If a person has difficulty performing a task or action in his or her real-life living situation (Participation, performance qualifier), it is called a "Participation Restriction." To describe the level of difficulty, A&P codes have four qualifiers that follow the code and each qualifier uses the same scaling (see figure 11.5). Definitions for each of the qualifiers follow:

FIGURE 11.5. Activity and participation qualifiers

First Qualifier (Performance – With Assistance) Extent of Difficulty	Second Qualifier (Capacity – Without Assistance) Extent of Difficulty	Third Qualifier (Capacity – With Assistance) Extent of Difficulty	Fourth Qualifier (Performance – Without Assistance) Extent of Difficulty
Use for all four qualifiers:			
0 NO difficulty (none, absent, negligible: 0–4%)			
1 MILD difficulty (slight, low: 5–24%)			
2 MODERATE difficulty (medium, fair: 25–49%)			
3 SEVERE difficulty (high, extreme: 50–95%)			
4 COMPLETE difficulty (total: 96–100%)			
8 not specified			
9 not applicable			

Source: Adapted from International Classification of Functioning, Disability, and Health (2001) and International Classification of Functioning, Disability, and Health: Child and Youth Version (2007).

- *Performance* = The person's real-life living situation (for example, home, neighborhood, store, recreation center, residential living facility in which the person resides long term)

  - Performance without assistance = The person's ability to do the task or action in his or her real-life living situation without any assistance from another person.
  - Performance with assistance = The level of difficulty that still remains, despite assistance provided, in ability to do the task or action in his or her real-life living situation.

- *Capacity* = A standardized environment (for example, clinic setting, testing room, therapy gym, doctor's office)

  - Capacity without assistance = The person's ability to do the task or action in a standardized environment without any assistance from another person
  - Capacity with assistance = The level of difficulty that still remains, despite assistance provided, inability to do the task or action in a standardized environment

Example:

A therapist assesses Joe's ability to propel his wheelchair (d465 Moving around using equipment). In the clinic (capacity), he requires 20 percent assistance to propel the wheelchair (1 Mild Difficulty, 5–24 percent). When assistance is provided by the therapist, he has no remaining difficulty (0 No Difficulty, 0–4 percent).

In his neighborhood (performance), Joe requires 50 percent assistance to propel the wheelchair (3 Severe Difficulty, 50–95 percent). When assistance is provided by his spouse, they still have a remaining difficulty of 25 percent (2 Moderate Difficulty, 25–49 percent) because it is difficult for her to help him overcome architectural barriers (such as high curbs). The code for moving around using equipment is d465. The appropriately written code would look like this: d465.2103.

Code	1st Qualifier (Performance – With Assistance)	2nd Qualifier (Capacity – Without Assistance)	3rd Qualifier (Capacity – With Assistance)	4th Qualifier (Performance – Without Assistance)
d465.	2	1	0	3

Special notes:

- When scoring performance with assistance, only consider use of realistic everyday supports (such as spouse). For example, in inpatient rehabilitation the therapist will not be with the person after discharge, so do not consider the therapist as a source of assistance.

- When scoring capacity with assistance or performance with assistance, only score the person's "remaining difficulty." For example, if a person has difficulty with a task, but the assistance of a device or person removes all of the difficulty, the person is said to have "no difficulty."

- Activities in this section consist of blended skills. Don't get caught up in each individual skill, but rather look at the activity as a whole and choose the lowest score.

  - For example, d4554 Swimming is defined as "propelling the whole body through water by means of limb and body movements without taking support from the ground underneath." This requires many skills including: mobility of joints (b710 Mobility of Joint Functions), upper body and lower body strength (b730 Muscle Power Functions), endurance (b740 Muscle Endurance Functions), and control and coordination of voluntary movements (b7601 Control of Complex Voluntary Movements, b7602 Coordination of Voluntary Movement).

ENVIRONMENTAL FACTORS

Environmental factors are the physical, social, and attitudinal environment in which people live and conduct their lives. Within the component of Environmental Factors (EF), there are five

FIGURE 11.6. Environmental factor qualifier

First Qualifier (Extent of Barrier)
e____.0 NO barrier (none, absent, negligible: 0–4%)
e____.1 MILD barrier (slight, low: 5–24%)
e____.2 MODERATE barrier (medium, fair: 25–49%)
e____.3 SEVERE barrier (high, extreme: 50–100%)
e____.4 COMPLETE barrier (total: 96–100%)
e .8 barrier, not specified
e .9 not applicable

First Qualifier (Extent of Facilitator)
e____+0 NO facilitator (none, absent, negligible: 0–4%)
e____+1 MILD facilitator (slight, low: 5–24%)
e____+2 MODERATE facilitator (medium, fair: 25–49%)
e____+3 SUBSTANTIAL facilitator (high, extreme: 50–100%)
e____+4 COMPLETE facilitator (total: 96–100%)
e +8 facilitator, not specified
e .9 not applicable

Source: Adapted from International Classification of Functioning, Disability, and Health (2001) and International Classification of Functioning, Disability, and Health: Child and Youth Version (2007).

chapters of codes (see figure 11.2). Every EF code begins with a lowercase *e*. If an EF hinders a person, then it is called a **barrier**. If an EF helps a person, then it is called a **facilitator**. To describe the extent to which an EF is a barrier or facilitator, one qualifier follows the code (see figure 11.6). If the EF is a barrier, a period is placed after the code. If the EF is a facilitator, a plus sign is placed after the code. EF codes can be listed in a stand-alone format, or they can be paired with the specific A&P code that they affect. Pairing the EF code with the A&P code, however, can be helpful as it allows the reader to clearly understand what particular EF codes are impacting performance in a specific task or action.

Example (Barrier):

Forty percent of the facilities that Joe frequents in his neighborhood are not wheelchair accessible (2 Moderate Barrier, 25–49 percent) resulting in difficulty "moving around using equipment" (d465). The code for design, construction, and building products and technology of buildings for public use is e150. The appropriately written code would look like this: d465.2103, E-Code: e150.2.

Code	Barrier = . Facilitator = +	1st Qualifier (Extent of barrier or facilitator)
e150	.	2

Example (Facilitator):

When in the community, Joe's wife, Mary, assists him with "moving around using equipment" when barriers are present. As noted above, Joe has 50 percent difficulty with this task due to community barriers. Despite Mary assisting Joe, they still have a remaining 25 percent difficulty "moving around using equipment" in the community. Consequently, Mary is a 25 percent facilitator (2 Moderate Facilitator, 25–49 percent). The code for immediate family is e310. The appropriately written code would look like this: d465.2103, E-Code: e310+2.

Code	1st Qualifier (Barrier = . Facilitator = +)	2nd Qualifier (Extent of barrier or facilitator)
e310	+	2

Special Note: Determining the extent of a barrier or facilitator

- Facilitator: Percent of increase from baseline
  - Example: A person has moderate difficulty taking care of plants (40 percent). Assistance from an adaptive gardening device (e1401 Assistive products and technology for culture, recreation, and sport) lessens the person's difficulty to mild difficulty (20 percent). Consequently, the device caused a 20 percent change in a positive direction; therefore, it is a mild facilitator (1, Mild facilitator, 5–24 percent; e1401+1).

- Barrier: Percentage of decrease from baseline
  - Example: A person desires to engage in community sports. The local recreation center does not provide adaptive sports and is against making

adaptations to mainstream sport offerings. Consequently, he only participates in 25 percent of the sports he would like to do. The attitude of the community center staff (e430 Individual attitudes of people in positions of authority) lessens his potential participation by 75 percent; therefore, it is a severe barrier (3 Severe barrier, 50–100 percent; e430.3).

Principles and Guidelines

Once all of the relevant codes for an individual's health situation have been chosen and scored, the scored codes are listed in a **coding string**. To illustrate this, the running code example used in this chapter is provided:

Example:

A gentleman named Joe had a spinal cord injury. Below is a compilation of his codes and scores:

- Complete L4 spinal cord injury: s12002.4_ _.
- Moderate impairment with control of voluntary movement: b760.3.
- Severe difficulty propelling wheelchair in his neighborhood, but with assistance reduces to moderate difficulty. In the clinic, mild difficulty propelling wheelchair, but with assistance reduces to no difficulty: d465.2103.
- Design, construction and building products and technology of buildings for public use is a moderate barrier to moving around with equipment: e150.2.
- Joe's spouse is a moderate facilitator for moving around with equipment in the community: e310+2.

In a database, there is no need for the sentence descriptors shown above. Therefore, Joe's functioning is reduced to only codes (full coding string):

s12002.4_ _
b760.3
d465.2103; E-Codes: e150.2, e310+2

Codes might also be placed into a graph, such as the one below (note: the symbol '---' is being used in the graph to indicate that this is not a possible score at this time):

BODY STRUCTURES		Qualifier	Qualifier Score									
			0	1	2	3	4	5	6	7	8	9
s12002	Lumbrosacral spinal cord	Extent of Impairment					■	---	---	---		
		Nature of the Change										
		Localization										

BODY FUNCTIONS		Qualifier	Qualifier Score									
			0	1	2	3	4	5	6	7	8	9
b760	Voluntary movement	Extent of Impairment				■		---	---	---		

ACTIVITIES & PARTICIPATION		Qualifier	Qualifier Score									
			0	1	2	3	4	5	6	7	8	9
d465	Moving around using equipment	Performance with Assistance			■			---	---	---		
		Capacity without Assistance		■				---	---	---		
		Capacity with Assistance	■					---	---	---		
		Performance without Assistance				■		---	---	---		

ENVIRONMENTAL FACTORS		. Barrier or + Facilitator	Qualifier Score									
			0	1	2	3	4	5	6	7	8	.9*
e150	Design, construction & building products and technology of buildings for public use	.			■			---	---	---		
e310	Immediate family	+			■			---	---	---		

*.9 indicates not applicable, there is no +9

Core Sets

Given the vast array of codes in the ICF and the need to choose codes based upon each person's health experience, identifying and choosing codes can be overwhelming. To provide guidance, **core sets** were developed for specific conditions and populations. There are currently 36 core sets available on various diagnoses and conditions, with several having multiple subsets (see figure 11.7) (ICF Research Branch 2017). More ICF core sets are in development.

The development of a core set goes through a rigorous process consisting of an empirical multicenter study to identify common problems related to the health condition, a systematic literature review on problems associated with the health condition, an expert survey to identify problems considered to be relevant by the experts who treat individuals with the health condition, a qualitative study to identify problems from the point of view of individuals who have the particular health condition, and a structured decision-making and consensus process at an international conference to develop the first version of the core set (Bickenbach et al. 2012). Once a core set is developed and released for use, it continues to be reevaluated and updated as appropriate. Although the core sets can be helpful to the healthcare provider in choosing relevant codes, it should *not* be the sole determinant. As per the first basic coding rule (select an array of codes to form an individual's profile), chosen codes should reflect the *individual's* health experience. Although there are commonalities related to health conditions and situations, no two individuals and their health experience are the same. Consequently, the core sets should be used as a

FIGURE 11.7. ICF core sets

```
┌─────────────────────────────────────────────┐
│  ┌──────────────────────────────────────┐   │
│  │ ICF Core Sets                        │   │
│  │  • Acute Arthritis                   │   │
│  │  • Amputation                        │   │
│  │  • Ankylosing Spondylitis            │   │
│  │  • Autism                            │   │
│  │  • Attention Deficit Hyperactivity Disorder │
│  │  • Bipolar Disorders                 │   │
│  │  • Breast Cancer                     │   │
│  │  • Cardiopulmonary Conditions        │   │
│  │  • Cerebral Palsy                    │   │
│  │  • Chronic Ischemic Heart Disease    │   │
│  │  • Chronic Widespread Pain           │   │
│  │  • Depression                        │   │
│  │  • Diabetes Mellitus                 │   │
│  │  • Geriatric Patients in Post-Acute Care │
│  │  • Hand Conditions                   │   │
│  │  • Head and Neck Cancer              │   │
│  │  • Hearing Loss                      │   │
│  │  • ICF Generic Set                   │   │
│  │  • ICF Rehabilitation Set            │   │
│  │  • Inflammatory Bowel Diseases       │   │
│  │  • Low Back Pain                     │   │
│  │  • Musculoskeletal Conditions        │   │
│  │  • Multiple Sclerosis                │   │
│  │  • Neurological Conditions           │   │
│  │  • Obesity                           │   │
│  │  • Obstructive Pulmonary Disease     │   │
│  │  • Osteoarthritis                    │   │
│  │  • Osteoporosis                      │   │
│  │  • Rheumatoid Arthritis              │   │
│  │  • Schizophrenia                     │   │
│  │  • Sleep Disorders                   │   │
│  │  • Spinal Cord Injury                │   │
│  │  • Stroke                            │   │
│  │  • Traumatic Brain Injury            │   │
│  │  • Vertigo                           │   │
│  │  • Vocational Rehabilitation         │   │
│  └──────────────────────────────────────┘   │
└─────────────────────────────────────────────┘
```

guide for identifying common ICF codes that relate to the person's particular health experience. Healthcare providers must be careful not to limit their scope of evaluation and treatment to only those codes in the core set; otherwise, it defeats the purpose of following an individually tailored biopsychosocial model as advocated in the ICF. (See [Bickenbach et al. 2012] in the resources section at the end of the chapter for information on how to access ICF core sets.)

Basic Coding Rules

WHO recommends that coders follow the rules shown below to increase accuracy of information.

1. Select an array of codes to form an individual's profile: Select the most appropriate codes to describe the person's health experience.

2. Code relevant information: Only choose and score codes that are relevant to the health condition.

3. Code explicit information: Do not make inferences (assumptions) about a person's functioning in other areas. For example, just because a person has difficulty with b1641 Organization and Planning does not mean she or he will have difficulty with d230 Carrying Out Daily Routine.

4. Code specific information: Use the most specific code whenever possible. For example, if a person has an impairment with sustaining attention, score the specific code of b1400 Sustaining Attention rather than the broader code of b140 Attention Functions (WHO 2001).

In addition, qualifiers for a particular code that are not scored should be left blank. For example, if scoring only two qualifiers for a particular A&P code (such as the capacity qualifiers), the remaining performance qualifiers that were not evaluated should be left blank.

Process for Revision and Updates

While there is no specific schedule for updates and revisions, an official update approved annually at the WHO Family of International Classification (WHO-FIC) meeting has been published since 2011 as a simple list of changes. The list identifies the code affected, the original version of the text from the WHO ICF database, and the revisions to the text as approved by the Update and Revision Committee and ratified by the WHO-FIC Council. Proposed revisions are posed to the WHO ICF Update Platform by members of the Functioning and Disability Reference Group. Many of the changes coming forward are related to the plans to merge ICF and ICF for Children and Youth (ICF-CY).

Relationship with Other Terminologies, Classification Systems, and Code Sets

The integration of the ICF into healthcare has been gaining momentum. Functioning Properties have been added to the *International Classification of Diseases 11th Revision* (ICD-11), along with the integration of two WHO ICF-based assessment and survey tools. A new classification being developed called the International Classification of Health Interventions has codes that align with ICF. And, authors are calling for the consideration of the integration of current classification systems, including the ICF, into electronic health records to provide a more comprehensive and robust picture of people's health and functioning. Each of these is further explained next.

ICD-11

A request was made to explore integrating the ICF and the International Classification of Diseases (ICD), which was followed by a special report (Kohler et al. 2012; Selb et al. 2015). The WHO has subsequently added 'Functioning Properties' into the ICD-11 alpha draft (WHO 2011). Functioning Properties include ICF Body Function codes and Activity and Participation codes. The incorporation of Environmental Factor codes is under consideration, along with the development of a Personal Factors classification. Section 3.2 in the ICD-11 Reference Guide states:

> The ICD-11 has been created both to share concepts and be used jointly with the ICF. This partnership may assist with the following tasks: evaluation for general medical practice (e.g., fitness for work), evaluation for social benefits (e.g., disability, pension), payment or reimbursement purposes, needs assessment (e.g., for rehabilitation, occupational assistance, long term care), and outcome evaluation of interventions. Signs and symptoms in the ICD are aligned with body functions in the ICF, and 'factors influencing health status' in the ICD with contextual factors in the ICF. The items of the functioning section of ICD are a subset of the entities contained in ICF. (WHO 2018a)

According to Inside Angle, the ICD-11 will be presented to the World Health Assembly in May 2019 for adoption by member countries, with the earliest implementation January 2022 (Caux-Harry 2018). More information about ICD-11 can be found in chapter 7 of this text and on the WHO website. (See [WHO 2018a] in the resource list at the end of the chapter).

The World Health Organization Disability Assessment Schedule 2.0 (WHODAS 2.0) is a standardized assessment tool that measures health and disability in the adult population in six domains: cognition, mobility, self-care, getting along, life activities, and participation (WHO 2018b). It is used across all diseases and cultures, is applicable in both clinical and general populations, is easy to administer and score (about 5–20 minutes), and directly relates to the ICF (for item correlation with specific ICF codes, see Üstün et al. 2010). The Model Disability Survey (MDS), also developed by the WHO, is a generic population survey for people with and without disabilities that describes how they conduct their lives and the difficulties encountered. The purpose of the survey is to identify barriers, which can be used for a variety of purposes (such as policy development, service development, and monitoring Sustainable Development Goals) (WHO 2018c). Both the WHODAS 2.0 and the MDS have been integrated into the ICD-11 V Supplementary Section for Functional Assessment to allow the user to create individualized functioning profiles and overall functioning scores (WHO 2018d).

International Classification of Health Interventions

International Classification of Health Interventions (ICHI) is being developed by the WHO as a tool to report and analyze health interventions that are utilized across all levels of healthcare by a variety of providers (WHO 2016). The ICHI Beta 2018 is currently open for comments. It has not yet been approved by WHO, it is being updated on a regular basis, and it cannot be used for coding except for field trials. The codes are divided into four sections, of which three (*) align with the ICF: Interventions on Body Systems and Functions (*), Interventions on Activities and Participation Domains (*), Interventions on the Environment (*), and Interventions on Health-Related Behaviors. The codes within each section consist of three axes (or parts): Target (the entity on which the Action is carried out), Action (a deed done by an actor to a Target) and Means (the processes and methods by which the Action is carried out). Individuals can browse and comment on the ICHI Beta 2018. (See [WHO 2018b] in the resource list at the end of the chapter.)

Electronic Health Records

Physiotherapists have called for clinical information system vendors to consider the integration of Logical Observations Identifiers, Names, Codes (LOINC), Systematized Nomenclature of Medicine – Clinical Terms (SNOMED CT), and the ICF into EHRs (Vreeman and Richoz 2015). The authors argue that an EHR that has an ICF-based template could aid in orienting therapists to practice from a biopsychosocial model, increase attention to interventions and environmental modifications, increase awareness and understanding of how interventions targeted at one domain may impact other domains, and further ICF implementation research.

Tools to Access and Use

There are various tools available to assist in the utilization of the ICF, including the ICF browser, ICF checklist, and mobile applications. Each is described next in more detail.

- ICF Browser: The ICF browser provides drop-down lists of the hierarchy of codes within the ICF. A description of each code is provided, along with inclusions and exclusions. The browser also contains a search field to assist in finding specific codes. The browser can be accessed from the WHO ICF website. (See [WHO 2018c] in the resource list at the end of the chapter.)
- ICF Checklist: Providing practical applications by means of computerization and case recording forms, ICF Core Sets and related coding forms have been developed, and continue to be developed, for diagnoses and populations to help clinicians more quickly identify common diagnosis-related codes and document functioning (Bickenbach et al. 2012). Additionally, the WHO developed an ICF Checklist Clinician Form that clinicians can use to elicit and record information. This form can be accessed at the WHO ICF website. (See [WHO 2018c] in the resource list at the end of the chapter.)

- Development of mobile applications: The Dutch-based ICanFunction (mICF) foundation was formed in April 2018. Their project plan overview states, "The International mICF partnership consisting of service users, service providers, specialists in ICF and health informatics are developing a user-friendly mobile application to assist people at point of service delivery to be able to enter what is important to them about their functioning and context so that health services can respond more appropriately. In the background ICF-related data (including patient-reported outcomes) will be amalgamated. This will enable individualized, predictive service provision by utilizing big data models" (mICF 2018). They have a facilitation team that consists of 23 partners from 12 different countries and other individuals are invited to join the International mICF Partnership through application (instructions to join are on their website).

Adoption and Use Cases

Possible future directions for ICF development and application (WHO 2001; WHO 2007; WHO 2018e), along with an update of what is currently being done is described next:

- Use in an electronic environment: A systematic review of the literature from 2001 to 2015 identified 17 publications citing the potential benefits and challenges of incorporating the ICF into EHRs (Maritz et al. 2017). Benefits included the ICF's biopsychosocial perspective of health and interdisciplinary focus. Challenges included the ICF not being structured as a formal terminology and the sheer number of codes (1400+) that could cause potential difficulties in everyday clinical use. As discussed earlier in this chapter, there have been calls to integrate the ICF with other electronic coding systems (Vreeman and Richoz 2015). Such calls appear to have been heard as the process for integrating the ICF into the ICD-11 has begun and we are beginning to see the formation of mobile electronic applications (Caux-Harry 2018; mICF 2018).
- Promoting the use of ICF at country level for the development of national databases: Several countries started the process of streamlining ICF into their health and social information standards and legislation. Development and piloting of ICF-based indicators and reporting systems for use in rehabilitation, home-care, age-care, and disability evaluation are ongoing in Australia, Canada, Italy, India, Japan, and Mexico. ICF-based data sets and questionnaires are also currently used in Australia, Ireland, Mexico, Zimbabwe, and Malawi.
- Education of healthcare professionals: The WHO published education guidelines that call for new approaches to health professionals' education based on the ICF. There is also a related WHO Transformative Education for Health Professionals

website that contains additional resources and case studies. (See [WHO 2013] in the resource list at the end of the chapter for website addresses.)

- Identification of algorithms for eligibility for social benefits and pensions: In 2013, the Social Security Administration in the US put out a call for public opinion about the use of the ICF for disability evaluation related to benefits, although a collection of responses was unable to be found (Social Security Administration 2013). They also released a grant to crosswalk the ICF codes to job requirements of which several projects have been completed (Policy Research, Inc. 2017).

- Development of precise operational definitions of categories for research purposes: The WHO is in the process of developing a standardized manual for healthcare professionals that provides more precise detail about each code (WHO 2013). An exposure draft of the publication is available for comment. Professional organizations representing various disciplines have been involved with the manual's development. At this time, there is no anticipated publication date.

- Development of assessment instruments for identification and measurement: Within various fields of study, work has been done (and continues to be done) to crosswalk current discipline assessment instruments to the ICF (for example, what domain does it relate to, such as BF or A&P; what ICF codes does the assessment measure). The ICF provides a step-by-step process to undertake this endeavor. (See [WHO 2005] in the resource list at the end of the chapter.)

- Research into treatment or intervention matching and establishing links with quality-of-life (QOL) concepts and the measurement of subjective well-being: Much research has been done using the ICF to help identify its relationships with treatment, interventions, QOL, and more. Go to Google Scholar online, enter the key words "International Classification of Functioning, Disability, and Health" and "[a discipline or topic of interest]", and explore what is currently published.

- Development of training and reference centers worldwide: The WHO developed an open-access online ICF eLearning Tool. (See [WHO 2018b] in the resource list at the end of the chapter). It also created an ICF Education Portal "to allow members of the WHO-FIC Network Functioning and Disability Reference Group, WHO-FIC Collaborating Centers, and other collaborators to upload existing tools and documentation that can be freely used by others seeking to improve their understanding and use of ICF" (WHO 2018f).

- Further research on environmental factors: This research is being undertaken to provide the necessary detail for use in describing both the standardized and current living environment, and mapping environmental factors that influence particular situations, such as participating in valued activities post stroke, as well as comparing environmental influences across diagnoses and within different contexts (Jellema et al. 2017; Wong et al. 2017; Thompson et al. 2018).

- Development of codes for the Personal Factors component: There have been calls for further scientific debate about the development of codes for the Personal Factors component (Geyh et al. 2018; Muller and Geyh 2015).
- Study of disability and functioning of family members (such as a study of third-party disability due to the health condition of significant others).

Use Case One: Implementing an ICF Core Set

Scenario-Based Example: A Washington healthcare network operates four outpatient rehabilitation hospitals that specialize in the treatment of individuals with traumatic brain injury (TBI). All four outpatient hospitals track outcome data; however, they do not all track the same data, nor do they track data in the same manner. The Chief Executive Officer (CEO) of the healthcare network decided to implement the utilization of the brief ICF core set for TBI. The CEO formed a committee to evaluate the codes in the core set. Although there were additional codes that could be relevant to treatment (depending upon the unique health situation of the client), they all agreed to begin tracking data on these basic core codes. The committee determined which disciplines would be responsible for scoring each code in the core set. For example, recreational therapy would score d720 Complex interpersonal interactions, d920 Recreation and leisure, and e310 Friends; nursing would score b110 Consciousness functions; social work would score d760 Family relationships; physical therapy would score b760 Control of voluntary movement functions and d450 Walking; and occupational therapy would score d5 Self-care (to name a few). Each discipline utilized their specific assessment methods to arrive at the appropriate ICF code score. Data was tracked at admission and discharge, along with interventions employed. Following six months, data from all four centers were analyzed. The data showed that the clients, on average, progressed in a range of 1.2 to 2.3 ICF levels in all but three codes in the core set. The CEO reached out to another outpatient rehabilitation hospital network in another state (Pennsylvania) that specializes in TBI treatment. The CEO purposefully contacted this network because it was known that the network tracked data using the ICF. The CEO asked about their outcome data related to the three ICF core set codes that were not progressing in her facilities. Through comparing data, it was found that clients being treated in the Pennsylvania network were progressing in the three code areas. Upon further evaluation, it was found that the Pennsylvania network provided intensive community integration training to its clients. This consisted of recreational therapists taking clients out into the community to practice skills and problem-solve in real-life community settings. This was different from the Washington network, which was providing in-clinic only recreational therapy services. As a result, the Washington network decided to implement community integration training for the clients and will reassess the outcomes in another six months.

Use Case Two: Comparing Population Environmental Factors

Scenario-Based Example: Country A and country B collect data on community-dwelling older adults using the ICF. The mortality rate in country A for community-dwelling older adults is much higher than in country B. The two countries compare data in the hope of identifying differences for possible intervention. One of the predominant findings from the comparison was that country A had more Environmental Factor barriers than country B. Country A developed a task force to explore the professional literature related to Environmental Factors and health and found that a positive correlation existed. As a result, country A decided to launch a campaign aimed at changing people's attitudes about older adults and earmarked funds to increase the accessibility of public buildings and neighborhoods.

CHECK YOUR UNDERSTANDING

1. True or false? The ICF is only used for people who have a disability, injury, or disease.

    a. True
    b. False

2. True or false? The ICF coding scheme is comprised of Chapters and Branches.

    a. True
    b. False

3. True or false? Environmental and Personal Factors can positively or negatively impact functioning and health.

    a. True
    b. False

4. True or false? The ICF assumes there is a disablement syndrome.

    a. True
    b. False

5. Match the terms with the appropriate descriptions

    a. Body Structures   ___ Execution of tasks and actions
    b. Body Functions   ___ The physical, social, and attitudinal environment in which people live and conduct their lives
    c. Activities & Participation   ___ The physiological and psychological functions of the body

d. Environmental Factors   ___ Anatomy of the body including organs, limbs, and their components

e. Personal Factors   ___ Internal influences that facilitate or hinder functioning and health

REVIEW

1. Match the terms with the appropriate descriptions

    a. Performance   ___ Difficulty performing a task or action in a standardized testing environment

    b. Capacity   ___ Difficulty performing a task or action in one's real-life living situation

    c. Participation Restriction   ___ A standardized environment

    d. Activity Limitation   ___ The person's real-life living situation

2. Match the letter code with the appropriate ICF component

    a. Body Structures   ___ d

    b. Body Functions   ___ e

    c. Activities & Participation   ___ s

    d. Environmental Factors   ___ b

3. The overall aim of the ICF is to:

    a. Provide a unified and standard language
    b. Provide a framework for the description of health and health-related states
    c. Replace the ICD with a more holistic view of health and health-related states
    d. A and B
    e. None of the above

4. The ICF model reflects which type of model?

    a. Medical Model
    b. Social Model
    c. Biopsychosocial Model
    d. Functional Model

5. The ICF can be used as a:

   a. Statistical tool
   b. Research tool
   c. Clinical tool
   d. Social policy tool
   e. All of the above

6. A client has 75 percent impairment in Orientation Functions. The code for Orientation Functions is b114. Which of the following represents the correct score?

   a. b114.0
   b. b114.1
   c. b114.2
   d. b114.3
   e. b114.4

7. A client is seen in an outpatient treatment facility. In the facility, when assistance is provided by the therapist, the client has no difficulty with dressing. At home, however, when the client does not have assistance, the client has moderate difficulty with dressing. The code for Dressing is d540. Which of the following reflects the appropriately scored code?

   a. d540. 2 0 _ _
   b. d540. _ _ 0 2
   c. d540. _ 2 0 _
   d. d540. _ 0 2 _

8. If an environmental factor is a facilitator, what "mark" is placed after the code?

   a. A star
   b. An equal sign
   c. A period
   d. A plus sign

9. A client has 75 percent difficulty walking. With the use of a walker, the client has 25 percent remaining difficulty. To what extent is the walker a facilitator?

   a. Mild facilitator
   b. Moderate facilitator
   c. Substantial facilitator
   d. Complete facilitator

10. Which of the following is true about core sets?

    a. Codes outside of the core set should not be considered during assessment.

    b. Once a core set is developed, it is not revaluated.

    c. Core sets can be helpful in choosing relevant codes for assessment.

    d. None of the above.

References

Bickenbach, J., A. Cieza, A. Rauch, and G. Stucki. 2012. ICF core sets: *Manual for Clinical Practice*. Boston: Hogrefe Publishing.

Brundtland, G. H. 2002. WHO Conference on Health and Disability. http://www.who.int/ dg/speeches/en/.

Caux-Harry, R. 2018. It is coming: ICD-11 released. https://www.3mhisinsideangle.com/blog-post/ it-is-coming-icd-11-released/?utm_campaign=HIS-1807-US-EDU-NSL-Focus_0717&utm_ medium=email&utm_source=Eloqua&utm_content=HIS-201807-en_US-NSL-Email-Focus-20180717&utm_eloquacontactid=4096851.

Centers for Disease Control and Prevention (CDC). n.d. The ICF: An overview. https://www.cdc.gov/nchs/ data/icd/icfoverview_finalforwho10sept.pdf.

Geyh, S., U. Schwegler, C. Peter, and R. Muller. 2018. Representing and organizing information to describe the lived experience of health from a personal factors perspective in the light of the International Classification of Functioning, Disability and Health (ICF): A discussion paper. *Disability and Rehabilitation*. doi: 10.1080/09638288.2018.1445302.

ICanFunction mHealth Solution (mICF). 2018. Project plan overview. http://icfmobile.org/project-plan-2/ project-plan/.

ICF Research Branch. 2017. ICF core sets projects. https://www.icf-research-branch.org/ icf-core-sets-projects2.

Jellema, S., S. van Hees, J. Zajec, R. van der Sande, M. van der Sanden, and E. Steultjens. 2017. What environmental factors influence resumption of valued activities post stroke: A systematic review of qualitative and quantitative findings. *Clinical Rehabilitation* 31:936–947.

Kohler, F., M. Selb, R. Escorpizo, N. Kostanjsek, G. Stucki, and M. Riberto. 2012. Towards the joint use of ICD and ICF: A call for contribution. *Journal of Rehabilitation Medicine* 44:805–810.

Maritz, R., D. Aronsky, and B. Prodinger. 2017. The International Classification of Functioning Disability and Health (ICF) in electronic health records. A systematic review. *Applied Clinical Informatics* 8:964–980.

Muller, R. and S. Geyh. 2015. Lessons learned from different approaches towards classifying personal factors. *Disability and Rehabilitation* 37: 430–438.

Policy Research, Inc. 2017. Final report on the Social Security Administration's disability determination process small grant program, 2012–2017. https://ddp.policyresearchinc.org/wp-content/uploads/2017/09/ DDP-Final-Report-09182017.pdf.

Selb, M., F. Kohler, M. Nicol, M. Riberto, G. Stucki, C. Kennedy, and B. Üstün. 2015. ICD-11: A comprehensive picture of health, an update on the ICD-ICF joint use initiative. *Journal of Rehabilitation Medicine* 47:2–8.

Social Security Administration. 2013. Notice of solicitation of public and federal agency comments for collaboration on evaluating the World Health Organization International Classification of Functioning, Disability, and Health (ICF) standard for coding functional capability in federal programs. https://www.gpo.gov/fdsys/pkg/FR-2013-01-02/pdf/2012-31593.pdf.

Thompson, C., S. Bolte, T. Falkmer, and S. Girdler. 2018. To be understood: Transition to adult life for people with autism spectrum disorder. *PLoS ONE* 13:e0194758.

Üstün, T., S. Chatterji, N. Kostanjsek, J. Rehm, C. Kennedy, J. Epping-Jordan, S. Saxena et al. 2010. Developing the World Health Organization Disability Assessment Schedule 2.0. *Bulletin of the World Health Organization* 88:815–823.

Vreeman, D. and C. Richoz. 2015. Possibilities and implications of using the ICF and other vocabulary standards in electronic health records. *Physiotherapy Research International* 20:210–219.

Wong, A., S. Ng, J. Dashner, M. Baum, J. Hammel, S. Magasi, J. Lai et al. 2017. Relationships between environmental factors and participation in adults with traumatic brain injury, stroke, and spinal cord injury: A cross-sectional multi-center study. *Quality of Life Research* 26:2633–2645.

World Health Organization (WHO). 2018a. ICD-11 Reference Guide. https://icd.who.int/browse11/content/refguide.ICD11_en/html/index.html#3.2to3.5FunctioningRevisionFeaturesTM|functioning-in-icd-and-joint-use-with-icf|c3-2.

World Health Organization (WHO). 2018b. WHO Disability Assessment Schedule 2.0. http://www.who.int/classifications/icf/more_whodas/en/.

World Health Organization (WHO). 2018c. Model Disability Survey. http://www.who.int/disabilities/data/mds/en/.

World Health Organization (WHO). 2018d. ICD-11 for Mortality and Morbidity Statistics, V Supplementary Section for Functioning Assessment. https://icd.who.int/browse11/l-m/en#/http%3a%2f%2fid.who.int%2ficd%2fentity%2f231358748.

World Health Organization (WHO). 2018e. ICF Application Areas. http://www.who.int/classifications/icf/appareas/en/.

World Health Organization (WHO). 2018f. International Classification of Functioning, Disability and Health (ICF). http://www.who.int/classifications/icf/en/.

World Health Organization (WHO). 2016. International Classification of Health Interventions (ICHI). http://www.who.int/classifications/ichi/en/.

World Health Organization (WHO). 2013. A Practical Manual for Using the International Classification of Functioning, Disability and Health (ICF): Exposure Draft for Comment. http://www.who.int/classifications/drafticfpracticalmanual2.pdf?ua=1.

World Health Organization (WHO). 2011. ICD-11 alpha content model reference guide. http://www.who.int/classifications/icd/revision/Content_Model_Reference_Guide.January_2011.pdf.

World Health Organization (WHO). 2007. *International Classification of Functioning, Disability, and Health: Children and Youth Version.* Switzerland: WHO.

World Health Organization (WHO). 2002. Towards a Common Language for Functioning, Disability, and Health. http://www.who.int/classifications/icf/training/icfbeginnersguide.pdf.

World Health Organization (WHO). 2001. *International Classification of Functioning, Disability, and Health.* Switzerland: WHO.

Resources

Bickenbach, J., A. Cieza, A. Rauch, and G. Stucki. 2012. *ICF Core Sets: Manual for Clinical Practice.* Boston: Hogrefe Publishing.

Hannover Medical School. n.d. Transformative Education for Health Professionals. https://whoeducationguidelines.org/.

ICF Clearinghouse Newsletters (2002–2012). http://www.cdc.gov/nchs/icd/icf.htm.

ICF Research Branch. www.icfresearchbranch.org. Includes links to the ICF Branch Newsletter, ICF core sets, ICF INFO (an international collaborative project which aims to establish the principles to harmonize routinely collected health information based on the ICF), ICF e-learning tool, ICF case studies, ICF-based documentation forms, current ICF-related research programs and projects, ICF-related publications.

World Health Organization (WHO). 2018a. ICD-11. https://icd.who.int/.

World Health Organization (WHO). 2018b. ICHI Beta 2018. https://mitel.dimi.uniud.it/ichi/.

World Health Organization (WHO). 2018c. ICF. www.who.int/classifications/icf/en/. Includes links to the ICF browser, ICF Learning Tool, ICF Checklist, Towards a Common Language for Functioning, Disability and Health (a guide for beginners learning to use), draft of the "How to Use the ICF: A Practice Manual for Using the ICF," ICF core sets, and ICF Education Portal.

World Health Organization (WHO). 2013. Transforming and Scaling Up Health Professionals' Education and Training: WHO Education Guidelines. http://www.who.int/hrh/resources/transf_scaling_hpet/en/.

World Health Organization (WHO). 2005. Cross-walking Assessment Tools to ICF. http://apps.who.int/classifications/apps/icd/meetings/tokyomeeting/P2-20%20Kostanjsek%20cross-walking%20assessment%20tools%20to%20ICF.pdf.

12

Terminologies Used in Nursing Practice

Susan Matney, PhD, RNC-OB, FAAN, FACMI

LEARNING OBJECTIVES

- Explain the historical evolution of terminology and vocabulary systems associated with the nursing profession
- Identify the American Nurses Association (ANA) criteria established for recognizing standardized terminologies
- Differentiate the purpose of nursing terminologies, including:
    - NANDA International (NANDA)
    - Nursing Interventions Classification System (NIC)
    - Nursing Outcomes Classification System (NOC)
    - Clinical Care Classification (CCC)
    - Omaha System
    - PeriOperative Nursing Data Set (PNDS)
    - International Classification for Nursing Practice (ICNP)
- Illustrate how selected nursing terminologies compare with other terminologies and vocabularies used in healthcare systems
- Discuss the use of the Nursing Problem List Subset of SNOMED CT in meeting Meaningful Use criteria
- Compare tools available to access and use
- Identify how nursing terminologies are used in an electronic environment

- American Nurses Association (ANA)
- Clinical Care Classification (CCC)
- Comité Européen de Normalisation (CEN), or European Committee for Standardization
- Domain
- International Classification for Nursing Practice (ICNP)
- International Council of Nurses (ICN)
- International Organization for Standardization (ISO)
- NANDA-I
- Nursing Interventions Classification (NIC)
- Nursing Outcomes Classification (NOC)
- Semantic type
- Taxonomy

Introduction to Nursing Terminologies

Nurses represent the largest group of organized professionals in many countries, including the US. Nurse informaticists play a critical role in terminology and classification systems related to nursing care within the healthcare system worldwide. National and international professional associations collaborate on the development of systems created for a variety of nursing purposes.

For years, nurses have expressed nursing care using different terms to say the same thing. Standardized nursing language is a common language, readily understood by computers and nurses, and used to describe care (Thede and Schwirian 2014). A uniform representation of nursing care supports a complete and unambiguous description for documenting nursing problems, interventions, and outcomes. The use of coded standardized terminology for nurses is vital to bedside nursing and to the nursing profession. The use of standardized nursing terminology will increase the visibility of nursing, enhance data collection used to evaluate and analyze patient-care outcomes, and support greater adherence to standards of care.

This chapter discusses the history of nursing terminology and vocabulary development, describes the elements of the key terminologies currently in use, and includes two use cases illustrating how nursing terminologies are used in practice.

History of Nursing-Related Terminologies

Formalized nursing terminology applications began in the late 1970s with the use of computers to support nursing care. One of the first books to describe computers and their relationship to nursing and healthcare was *Using Computers in Nursing,* by Marion Ball and Kathryn Hannah, published in 1984.

The first terminology systems developed for nursing were called controlled vocabularies. By definition, problems occur in applying a controlled vocabulary for too broad a purpose, so the number of nursing terminologies has increased over time. Controlled means the vocabulary's governance processes ensure that it is structurally sound, accurate, and up to date. Clearly, there is a need in nursing, as in other areas of healthcare, for a mechanism to resolve problems resulting from the use of diverse terminologies. Thus, work continues to further harmonize nursing terminologies or to employ a reference terminology to serve as an interlingua between them (Spackman et al. 1997).

A number of standards organizations, such as the **Comité Européen de Normalisation (CEN), or European Committee for Standardization**, the **International Organization for Standardization (ISO)**, and SNOMED International, work collaboratively to achieve greater harmony between nursing terminologies and other vocabularies used in healthcare applications. This work is expected to culminate in greater synchrony as more electronic health record (EHR) systems are used to document and store patient information.

ANA Recognized Terminologies

In 1991, the **American Nurses Association (ANA)** formed the Committee for Nursing Practice Information Infrastructure (CNPII) to review and recognize nursing languages (Warren and Bakken 2002). This work laid the foundation for the growing knowledge of terminology standards for nursing practice. The CNPII recognized 12 terminologies to be appropriate for clinical practice (Lundberg et al. 2008). The CNPII no longer exists, but the ANA maintains the recognition (ANA 2018a). The ANA has specific criteria terminologies it must meet for approval. The criteria specify that terminologies support all or part of the nursing process. The nursing process steps include assessment, diagnosis, outcome identification (goal), implementation (interventions), and outcome evaluation (ANA 2018b). In addition, the ANA recognition criteria require that (1) the terminologies contain concepts that are unambiguous with a unique identifier; and (2) the terminology developer has an outlined process for maintenance and growth. Table 12.1 lists the ANA-recognized terminologies and lists the ANA-approved terminologies and where they align with the nursing process (ANA 2018a). The Nursing Management Minimum Data Set, Nursing Minimum Data Set, and ABC (see chapter 13) are data and code sets approved by the ANA but not discussed in this chapter.

These current terminologies are used in conjunction with the Nursing Minimum Data Set, the Nursing Management Minimum Data Set, and the natural language found in traditional documentation and information management structures (NMDS 2018; NMMDS 2018).

TABLE 12.1. ANA-recognized terminologies nursing process step alignment

Terminology	Assessment	Diagnosis	Intervention	Goal and Outcome	Other
Alternative Billing Codes					Billing Codes
Clinical Care Classification (CCC)		X	X	X	
International Classification of Nursing Practice (ICNP)	X	X	X	X	
Logical Identifiers Names and Codes (LOINC)	X			X	
North American Nursing Diagnosis International (NANDA-I)		X			
Nursing Intervention Classification (NIC)			X		
Nursing Outcomes Classification (NOC)				X	
Nursing Management Minimum Data Set					Nursing Management Codes
Nursing Minimum Data Set		X	X	X	
Omaha System		X	X	X	
Perioperative Nursing Data Set (PNDS)		X	X	X	
SNOMED CT		X	X	X	

Public Policy and Resources Related to Nursing Terminologies

A number of federal initiatives exist to assist with the adoption of terminologies, including those for the nursing domain. In addition, resources, such as maps, are available to facilitate the exchange of healthcare information.

Interoperability Standards Advisory

The Office of the National Coordinator (ONC) identifies the "best-available" standard vocabularies, code sets, and terminologies, messaging structures, and implementation specifications for the healthcare industry and outlines them in the Interoperability Standards Advisory (ISA) (ONC 2018a). The ISA functions as a road map to interoperability and includes standard

TABLE 12.2. ISA mapping recommendations to SNOMED CT and LOINC

Nursing Process Step	SNOMED Semantic Type	LOINC
Assessment		X
Diagnosis	Clinical Finding	
Intervention	Procedure	
Goal/Outcome	Clinical Finding	X

terminology specifications. The ISA includes recommendations for nursing, endorsing encoding data collected by nurses with LOINC and SNOMED CT for messaging between systems. Table 12.2 illustrates how the nursing terminologies should be mapped to SNOMED CT semantic types (domains) and LOINC based on the steps of the nursing process.

ANA Position Statement

The ISA recommendation motivated the ANA to issue a position statement to reaffirm their support of documentation within EHRs using the ANA-recognized terminologies. They also state that for comparison across health systems and transmission, the ANA-recognized terminologies should be mapped to LOINC and SNOMED CT.

Mapping Resources

SNOMED International purchased SNOMED CT from the College of American Pathologists (CAP). The mappings CAP developed from the nursing terminologies to SNOMED CT were not part of the purchase. Therefore, the only official maps currently available are the ICNP to SNOMED CT equivalency tables (ICNP 2018a). Some of the nursing terminologies have a map set that can be obtained from the terminology developer, but there are no other "official" maps to SNOMED CT.

The Nursing Knowledge Big Data Science Conference first convened in 2013 with an invitation-only think tank (See [UMN 2018] in the resource list at the end of this chapter). One of the objectives that emerged was to facilitate sharable, comparable data by adopting terminologies and standards (Westra et al. 2015). The conference has met annually since and is a working meeting with over 10 workgroups (University of Minnesota College of Nursing 2018). The clinical data analytics workgroup retrieves and validates flowsheet information models across multiple health systems and applies data science methods to create information models (Westra et al. 2018). The resulting information models are handed off to the encoding and modeling group who map to, develop, and disseminate LOINC and SNOMED CT for EHR nursing assessments. They collaborate with the nursing LOINC subcommittee on the development and curation of the LOINC terms. To date, the nursing panels curated and released in LOINC include a wound assessment panel, a pain assessment panel, and a basic nursing physiologic assessment panel (Matney et al. 2017).

The nursing LOINC subcommittee began in 2002. Regenstrief formalized the committee structure in 2017 and required official membership where members can vote on terms developed for nursing. The purpose of the nursing LOINC subcommittee is to "facilitate the development and use of LOINC codes for observations used during key stages of the nursing process, including assessments, goals, and outcomes. Also, to meet the needs for administrative, research, and quality measurement initiatives related to nursing care" (LOINC 2018).

The Clinical Care Classification System (CCC), the Omaha System, and the Nursing Management Minimum Data Set (NMMDS) are integrated into LOINC. LOINC is an open source terminology; therefore, submissions are accepted only from terminologies or instruments that are open source and nonproprietary.

National Library of Medicine UMLS and Nursing Resource

Several of the nursing terminologies discussed in this chapter are listed as source vocabularies in the Unified Medical Language System (UMLS) hosted by the National Library of Medicine (NLM). The most current listing can be found on their website (NLM 2018a). The UMLS maps synonymous concepts from different terminologies to a single identifier. This provides the ability to determine mappings between SNOMED CT and the ANA-recognized nursing specific terminologies.

In 2015, the NLM developed a web resource entitled Nursing Resources for Standards and Interoperability (NLM 2017a; Warren et al. 2015). This resource provides information about why particular standards are pertinent and necessary for use in nursing and nursing documentation. The web page provides a tool to discover synonymous mappings between SNOMED CT, LOINC, and the ANA-recognized terminologies, thus providing a valuable resource for nursing.

Nursing Terminologies

The developers of nursing terminologies are agencies or professional organizations with an interest in the use of terminology or vocabulary in a specific nursing **domain**. Information provided for each terminology will include: 1) the developer or developing body; 2) the terminology purpose and types of nursing content included; 3) development or maintenance processes; 4) relationships or maps to other terminologies; and 5) browsing tools (if they exist).

NANDA International

The **NANDA-I** classification is a set of nursing diagnoses developed by NANDA International. The purpose of the terminology is to provide nursing diagnoses used to describe patients' responses to actual or potential health problems and life processes responses to diseases rather than classifying the conditions of diseases and disorders. The NANDA-I classification was the first to be recognized by ANA. This work enables documentation of nursing practice and facilitates aggregation and analyses to build the body of knowledge related to nursing science. The NANDA-I classification is organized around 13 domains:

- Health promotion
- Nutrition
- Elimination/Exchange
- Activity/Rest
- Perception/Cognition
- Self-perception
- Role relationship
- Sexuality
- Coping/Stress tolerance
- Life principles
- Safety/Protection
- Comfort
- Growth/Development

Within each domain, NANDA-I lists two or more classes. Within the Self-perception domain are the following classes: "Self-Concept, Self-Esteem, and Body Image" (NANDA 2018a). The diagnoses are classified into the classes containing nursing diagnoses. Each nursing diagnosis has a description, a definition, and diagnostic indicator terms. The diagnostics indicator categories include defining characteristics (manifestations, signs, and symptoms), related factors, and two new categories introduced in the 11th edition, associated conditions and at-risk populations. The coding structure is for the nursing diagnoses only, consisting of five digits and carrying no meaning in order to conform to best vocabulary practices.

NANDA-I is committed to increasing the visibility of nursing's contribution to patient care by developing, refining, and classifying phenomena of concern to nurses. NANDA-I's leadership includes a diagnosis development committee that oversees the maintenance and development of nursing diagnoses.

For development of the discipline, the NANDA-I board believes that:

- NANDA-I will be a global force for the development and use of nursing's standardized terminology to ensure patient safety through evidence-based care, thereby improving the healthcare of all people.
- NANDA-I provides the world's leading evidence-based nursing diagnoses for use in practice and to determine interventions and outcomes.
- Nursing diagnoses communicate the professional judgments that nurses make every day to our patients, colleagues, members of other disciplines and the public. Nursing diagnoses define what we know—they are our words (NANDA 2018b).

Organization of the NANDA-I nursing diagnoses has evolved from an alphabetic listing in the mid-1980s to a conceptual system that guides the classification of nursing diagnoses in a multiaxial **taxonomy**. A taxonomy is a hierarchical organization of knowledge. The NANDA-I taxonomy is now available in its entirety in the NANDA International Nursing Diagnoses: Definitions & Classification, 2018–2020 and is on a two-year update cycle. New diagnoses are developed by members and then submitted for review and classification.

Several countries outside the US use the NANDA-I taxonomy and it is translated into a number of languages and widely used in major nursing textbooks. It is the foundation of nursing care planning and is most often used in conjunction with NIC and NOC to provide coverage for the nursing care process and plans. There are no browsing tools for the NANDA-I nursing diagnoses. More information about the NANDA-I taxonomy can be found online (NANDA 2018b).

Nursing Interventions Classification

The **Nursing Interventions Classification (NIC)** is a standardized classification developed by a research team at the University of Iowa. The purpose of NIC is to define interventions that nurses do on behalf of patients in all care domains (NIC 2018). An intervention is defined as "any treatment, based upon clinical judgment and knowledge, a nurse performs to enhance patient/client outcomes" (Butcher et al. 2018, xii).

NIC has many uses, including those related directly to patient care, such as clinical documentation and communication of care across settings and management aspects, including productivity measurement and competency evaluation. Additionally, NIC is referenced in textbooks to discuss nursing treatments and utilized by researchers to study the effectiveness of nursing care. NIC also is implemented in nursing information systems and nursing education programs to structure curricula and to identify competencies of graduating nurses.

NIC is not limited to a specific setting or to only the domain of nursing. This system contains interventions done by other non-physician providers and thus describes their treatments. The system describes interventions for illness treatment, illness prevention, and health promotion for use with individuals, families, and communities. Included with each intervention is a label name, a definition, a unique number (code), a set of activities to carry out the intervention (to define the intervention, not to be coded), and background readings.

The seventh edition of NIC contains 565 interventions organized into 30 classes and 7 domains. The domains are

- Physiological: Basic
- Physiological: Complex
- Behavioral
- Safety
- Family
- Health system
- Community

NIC holds an annual conference where additions are requested. NIC is on a publication update cycle of approximately every four years since 1992. However, an ongoing process for feedback and review is established and modifications to existing interventions or proposals for a new intervention are accepted between editions.

NIC is translated into a number of languages and many countries outside the US use NIC. There are no online browsers for NIC.

Nursing Outcomes Classification

The **Nursing Outcomes Classification (NOC)** is a standardized classification developed by the same research team at the University of Iowa that develops NIC. NOC is a standardized classification of outcomes used to evaluate the outcomes of nursing interventions in all settings and with all patient populations. An outcome is "a measurable individual, family, or community state, behavior, or perception that is measured along a continuum and is responsive to nursing interventions" (NOC 2018).

NOC has many of the same uses as NIC, including clinical documentation, nursing education, and research. Clinical sites use NOC in their evaluations of nursing practice and educational institutions to structure curricula and teach students clinical evaluation. It is possible to apply NOC across the care continuum to follow patient outcomes over an extended time. However, NOC is not limited to the domain of nursing. Other non-physician providers may find NOC outcomes valuable in evaluating their interventions.

The sixth edition of NOC contains 540 outcomes grouped in a coded taxonomy that arranges them within a conceptual framework. The following are included with each outcome:

- A definition
- A list of indicators for evaluating patient status in relation to outcome
- A target outcome rating

- A place to identify the source of data
- A five-point Likert scale to measure patient status
- A short list of references used in developing the outcome

NOC describes outcome levels for individuals, families, and communities grouped into 34 classes and 7 domains. Included with each outcome is a unique code number that facilitates its use in clinical information systems. The domains are

- Functional health
- Physiologic health
- Psychosocial health
- Health knowledge and behavior
- Perceived health
- Family health
- Community health

NOC is developed by a research team at the University of Iowa and has an annual conference where additions are requested. NOC is published every four years. However, regular updates are made for any necessary modifications to existing outcomes or to include new outcomes.

NOC is translated into a number of languages, and many countries outside the US use NOC. There are no online browsers for NOC.

Clinical Care Classification

Clinical Care Classification (CCC) system is a nursing classification designed to document the steps of the nursing process across the care continuum. The CCC system consists of two interrelated taxonomies: the CCC of Nursing Diagnoses and Outcomes and the CCC of Nursing Interventions and Actions. Both taxonomies are classified by care components, or clusters of elements, that represent behavioral, functional, physiological, or psychological care patterns. CCC provides a framework and a unique coding structure for the following purposes (CCC 2017):

- Mapping and linking the two taxonomies to each other and to other health-related classifications
- Assessing, documenting, and classifying patient care in hospitals, home health agencies, ambulatory care clinics, and other healthcare settings

The CCC system came about from the Home Care Project (HCFA No: 17C-98983/3) conducted by Virginia K. Saba and colleagues in 1991 at the Georgetown University School of Nursing. The purpose of the project was to develop a methodology for evaluating and classifying

FIGURE 12.1. Clinical Care Classification System Framework

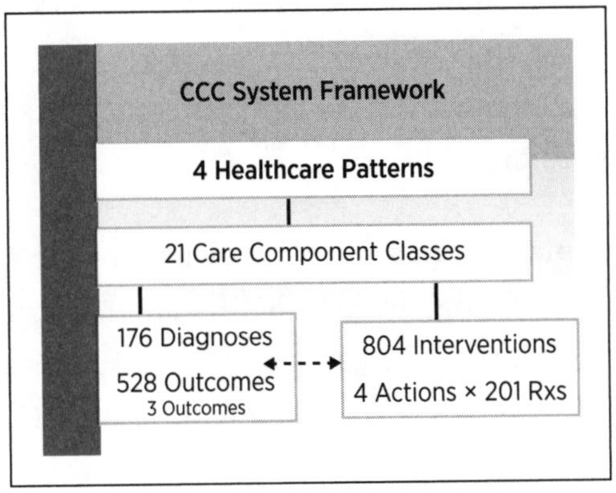

Source: Saba 2012.

patients to determine what resources are required when providing home health services to the Medicare population.

The CCC system consists of a standardized framework that provides a terminology for classifying the steps in the nursing process (see figure 12.1). The framework's top level contains four healthcare patterns 1) physiological, 2) psychological, 3) functional, and 4) health behavioral. Under the healthcare patterns are 21 care components; for example, activity, cardiac, coping, and respiratory. The care components have specific diagnoses, interventions, and outcomes as children.

The CCC system serves as a language for nursing and other health services (physical, occupational, and speech therapy; medical social worker; and home health aide) because data capture is enabled at the point of care. Examples of the uses of this system include:

- Documentation of integrated care processes
- Classification and tracking of clinical care
- Development of evidence-based practice models
- Analysis of patient profiles and populations
- Prediction of care needs and resources

The CCC system is (Saba 2012):

- The basis for the ICNP developed by the **International Council of Nurses (ICN)** and is referenced in the Integration of a Reference Terminology Model for Nurses (ISO 2018).
- Approved by the ISO Technical Committee (TC) 215 Working Group 3 Concept Representation.

- Approved by home health agencies as Medicare Rules Coverage and Conditions of Participation, and also linked to HCFA Forms 485 and 486, and the home health prospective payment system (PPS).
- Available in the public domain, even though it is copyrighted (although its use requires written permission).

There is no specific schedule for updates and revisions of the taxonomies. Content will be revised as clinical requirements change in nursing documentation. The CCC doesn't have an explicit browser but a "code builder" tool was recently released on their website that facilitates building a CCC code following the steps of the nursing process (CCC 2017).

Omaha System

The Omaha System was originally developed by the Omaha Visiting Nurses Association (VNA). Practicing clinicians employed by the VNA of Omaha and seven diverse test sites located throughout the US collected actual patient and family data and submitted them for inclusion in the Omaha System. Numerous other individuals and groups participated in the research as advisory committee members and consultants. From the beginning of the Omaha System's development, the terms, codes, and definitions were not copyrighted; thus, they are equally accessible to practitioners, administrators, students, faculty, and other potential users.

The Omaha System is a comprehensive practice and documentation tool used by nurses, other healthcare providers, and students from the time of client admission to discharge in the home health setting. The system includes 1) a Problem Classification Scheme used during assessment; 2) an Intervention Scheme; and 3) a Problem Rating Scale for Outcomes. These components provide a structure for documenting client needs and strengths, relating clinician interventions, and measuring client outcomes in a simple, yet comprehensive, manner. When the three components are used together, the Omaha System offers a way to link clinical data to demographic, financial, administrative, and staffing data (Omaha System 2017).

Using the Omaha System is comparable to arranging the diverse pieces of a puzzle into a completed picture. When it is implemented accurately and consistently, the data generated describes client needs, related interventions, and client outcomes, as well as interactions among those data. Automated documentation systems based on the Omaha System provide a powerful information management tool for data collection, aggregation, and analysis (Omaha System 2017).

The Omaha System was one of the first vocabularies recognized by the ANA in 1990. Additionally, it is in the Accreditation Standards of the Joint Commission and the Community Health Accreditation Program. It is used internationally. The system's terms, codes, and definitions have been translated into a number of languages including Chinese, Dutch, Estonian, German, Greek, Japanese, Korean, Slovene, Spanish, Swedish, Thai, and Turkish (Omaha System 2017).

The terms, codes, and definitions of the Omaha System are not copyrighted. Individuals who use or write about the Omaha System should reference the source. Software based on the Omaha System also must follow copyright laws in order to use the system.

In 2001, a 12-member Omaha System Advisory Board consisting of representatives from diverse service and educational settings was formed to develop an action plan to review and revise the Omaha System based on comments from survey results of current research and suggestions from users. The goal was to include the revision in the next book about the Omaha System. The most recent edition includes revised terms and definitions, information on how to use the system in diverse settings, and 18 case studies illustrating terms used in the system (Martin 2005). There are nine additional case studies available online (Omaha System 2017). Currently, there is no scheduled process for updates and there are no browsers available.

Perioperative Nursing Data Set

The Association of periOperative Registered Nurses (AORN) developed the Perioperative Nursing Data Set (PNDS) to capture the activities of the operating room nurse (AORN 2018). AORN incorporates this terminology in practice, education, standards, and certification activities to further the documentation, description, and research of this nursing specialty. AORN is the only nursing specialty organization to create their own terminology system and to integrate it in their professional practice artifacts.

PNDS is based on a conceptual framework with the patient and family at the center. There are four domains: safety, physiologic response, behavioral response (patient and family), and the health system. There are nursing diagnoses, nursing interventions, and nurse-sensitive patient outcomes. AORN has updated PNDS's nursing diagnoses to SNOMED CT codes. AORN is responsible for the maintenance and updating of PNDS, which is updated annually. PNDS 4 was recently submitted to the NLM for inclusion in the UMLS.

PNDS is used to document the perioperative patient experience from preadmission through discharge and is incorporated by three major EHR vendors.

The data set has a number of benefits, including consistent clinical documentation, communication between clinicians in various practice settings, benchmarking nursing activities, and evaluating patient outcomes (Lundberg et al. 2008). PNDS is only available within the AORN Syntegrity perioperative nursing documentation system (PNDS 2018). There is not a PNDS browser.

International Classification for Nursing Practice

The **International Classification for Nursing Practice (ICNP)** is a unified nursing language system. It is a compositional terminology for nursing practice that facilitates cross mapping of local terms and existing terminologies. Cross mapping allows comparison of nursing data collected using other recognized nursing vocabularies and classification systems. ICNP can be used to represent nursing diagnoses, interventions, and outcomes.

The International Council of Nurses (ICN) is a federation of 132 national nurses' associations representing millions of nurses worldwide (ICN 2018). ICN has supported the development of ICNP since 1989 and established the ICNP Programme in 2000. ICNP is copyrighted by ICN. Permission to use, translate, publish, and reproduce the terminology is granted on a case-by-case basis. Commercial use requires a licensing fee; other uses are free of charge. The 2005 release of ICNP Version 1.0 was a major change for the terminology. This version was developed using Web Ontology Language (OWL) in the Protégé software environment to support a unified language and compositional approach. A description logics approach allows for explicit definitions, the possibility of multiple classifications, greater granularity, and sensitivity to variation in language and culture. The most recent release of ICNP, with a browser and added content, was made available in May 2017 (ICNP 2018b).

ICNP envisions being an integral part of the global information infrastructure informing healthcare practice and policy to improve patient care worldwide. It can serve as a major force to articulate nursing's contribution to health and healthcare globally and promote harmonization with other widely used classifications and the work of standardization groups in health and nursing (Coenen and Bartz 2010; ICNP 2018c). ICNP represents nursing concepts used in local, regional, national, and international practice, across specialties, languages, and cultures. Using information about nursing practice, ICNP supports decision-making, education, and policy in the areas of patient needs, nursing interventions, health outcomes, and resource utilization. ICNP improves communication in healthcare and encourages nurses to reflect on their own practice and influence improvements in quality of care.

ICNP has a number of representations. The multiaxial representation has seven axes, all of which describe some aspect of nursing practice. The axes are defined as follows (ICNP 2018c):

- *Focus:* The area of attention that is relevant to nursing (for example, pain, homelessness, elimination, life expectancy, knowledge)
- *Judgment:* Clinical opinion or determination related to the focus of nursing practice (for example, decreasing level, risk, enhanced, interrupted, abnormal)
- *Means:* A manner or method of accomplishing an intervention (for example, bandage, bladder-training technique, nutritionist service)
- *Action:* An intentional process applied to or performed by a client (for example, educating, changing, administering, monitoring)
- *Time:* The point, period, instance, interval, or duration of an occurrence (for example, admission, childbirth, chronic)
- *Location:* Anatomical and spatial orientation of a diagnosis or intervention (for example, posterior, abdomen, school, community health center)
- *Client:* Subject to which a diagnosis refers and who is the recipient of an intervention (for example, newborn, caregiver, family, community)

Specific guidelines have been recommended to create nursing diagnosis, intervention, or outcome statements. According to ICN (ICNP 2018c), when using the 7-Axis Model to compose a diagnosis

- A term from the Focus Axis is required.
- A term from the Judgment Axis is required.
- Additional terms from the Focus, Judgment, and other axes are included, as needed.

Table 12.3 provides an example of a combination of concepts from selected axes for the nursing diagnosis of chronic constipation.

A different set of guidelines is used when identifying a nursing intervention. The rules for creating a nursing intervention are as follows (ICNP 2018c):

- A term from the Action Axis is required.
- At least one target term is required. Target terms come from other axes with the exception of the Judgment Axis.
- Additional terms from the Action and other axes are included, as needed.

Figure 12.2 shows the results of a search on "assessing bowel status" found in the catalogue concepts using the ICNP Version 2018 browser.

To provide nursing professionals with a practical way to use ICNP at the point of care, ICN is collaborating with nurses and specialty organizations to develop ICNP Catalogues, or subsets of the terminology. ICNP Catalogues consist of sets of nursing diagnosis, intervention, and outcome statements for certain specialties or settings, or phenomena that are sensitive to nursing interventions, or health conditions (Coenan and Kim 2010; ICNP 2018a). The first catalogue, *Partnering with Individuals and Families to Promote Adherence to Treatment*, was published in 2008 (ICNP 2018a). *Guidelines for ICNP Catalogue Development* were also published in 2008 (ICNP 2018a). The repository has grown to eight ICNP Catalogues, including Community Nursing, Nursing Care of Children with HIV and AIDS, Palliative Care, and others. Figure 12.2 shows the ICNP browser after searching for "assessing bowel status."

TABLE 12.3. Nursing diagnosis

Select AXES	Select CONCEPTS
Focus	Constipation
Judgment	Actual
Time	Chronic
Nursing diagnosis: Chronic constipation	

Source: ICN 2018.

FIGURE 12.2. Search results for "assessing bowel status"

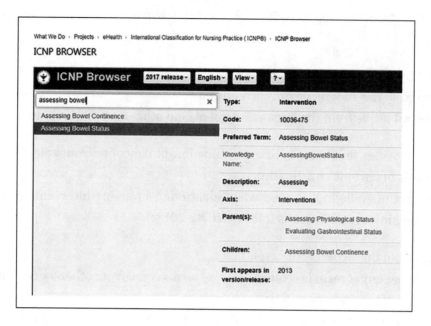

Source: ICNP 2018b.

The International Classification for Nursing Practice Programme is responsible for ensuring that ICNP content reflects the domain of nursing. The ICN staff reviews suggestions from nurses worldwide and forwards them to nursing practice expert reviewers or technical and informatics experts. These individuals utilize specific criteria to recommend acceptance, rejection, or expanded review of the recommendation to add, modify, or inactivate the concept. The ICN staff uses the recommendations to make a final decision and communicates the results to the person submitting the recommendation. ICNP is released every two years.

Recommendations, including new terms and definitions, are accepted through an open process that gives individuals and groups the opportunity to participate in the development of ICNP. There are specific forms on the ICNP website for submitting recommendations.

Adoption and Use Cases

Use Case One: Creating a Nursing Problem List Subset of SNOMED CT

Problem lists have been used to organize the patient record and to provide communication among clinicians caring for a patient. The creation of the idea of a problem list is credited to Lawrence Weed (Weed 1968). The problem list would form the basis of a problem-oriented record that would reflect the critical thinking of the patient care team. This characteristic of a problem list was so compelling that it was adopted in stage one of Meaningful Use (ONC 2018b).

While many think this is a problem list for physicians, the regulations are very clear that it is a patient-focused problem list to which all clinicians caring for a patient contribute. The problem list provides an overview of the patient so that one clinician does not prescribe treatment from a narrow perspective that could interact adversely with treatment prescribed by another clinician such as eye medications, dental prophylaxis, activities of daily living, physical therapy exercises, pain management for surgery, or diabetic regimens.

SNOMED CT is designated as the terminology to populate the problem list. A SNOMED CT subset was created for physician use (NLM 2018b). In 2010, a Nursing Problem List Subset of SNOMED CT was created (NLM 2017b). Members of the International Health Terminology Standards Development Organization's (IHTSDO) Nursing Work Group created this subset (Matney et al. 2012). The problem list was created through a series of queries conducted on NLM's Unified Medical Thesaurus System, which contains SNOMED CT and all ANA-recognized terminologies. The team then validated the list through a methodology explained in the study, including issues of mapping between and among various terminologies (Matney et al. 2012). The problem list is free for download from the NLM.

Additionally, the creation and use of this problem list subset assists in meeting the challenges described in the Institute of Medicine report "The Future of Nursing: Leading Change, Advancing Health." One of the recommendations of this report is that nurses should be able to practice to the full extent of their education and training (IOM 2011). The problem list makes visible the contributions of nursing to patient care and safety.

Use Case Two: Standardizing Nursing Documentation across an Enterprise

Dr. Jane Englebright, Chief Nursing Officer of HCA Healthcare, has been working to simplify and standardize nursing documentation across HCA-affiliated facilities (Englebright et al. 2014). The work began in 2007 with the vision of creating a patient-centric record that guides and informs the provision of safe, effective care by the interdisciplinary team while producing quality data that supports the care of individuals and populations. The goals were to decrease nursing documentation time, respond to nurses' dissatisfaction with documentation burden, and return time to caregiving.

Four different teams were assembled: 1) a steering committee, which provided the vision, guiding principles, and set priorities; 2) a clinical team, which defined evidence-based practice; 3) a technical team, which defined the design and applied informatics science; and 4) subject matter experts, who looked at standards, risk, legal issues, and the like. The first task the teams performed was diagramming workflows through an evidence-based process that included content development, data flow development, and hand-off management.

The teams identified the need for a standard terminology to provide an organizing framework, define domain completeness, enable interoperability, and support research. They chose

FIGURE 12.3. HCA's use of CCC to standardize documentation

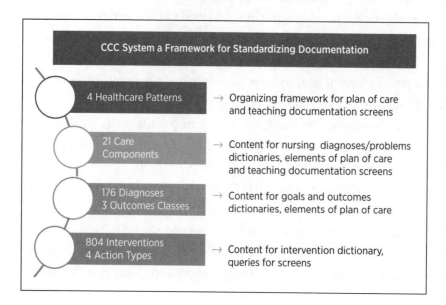

Source: © Jane Englebright 2018.

CCC because it was derived from research nursing documentation, based on the nursing process, and focused on the "essence of care" (Saba 2012). The CCC met their technical requirements of ANA recognition, mapped to SNOMED CT and LOINC, and fit easily into their MEDITECH dictionary framework.

The teams used the CCC domains in various ways as illustrated in figure 12.3. The Healthcare Patterns (described in the CCC section), 21 Care Components, Outcomes Classes, and Intervention and Action types provided the content for the MEDITECH dictionaries used to create the patient-specific, goal-directed care plan.

The use of a consistent framework has had tremendous outcomes. First, standardizing documentation has decreased documentation time by an average of 49 minutes per shift, providing more time at the bedside. Second, routine care across all settings is consistent and standardized. Third, a learning health system has been developed where current evidence has been implemented and future evidence can be derived.

CHECK YOUR UNDERSTANDING

1. Each NIC intervention includes all but one of the following:

    a. Five-point Likert scale

    b. Definition

    c. Unique number

    d. Label name

2. Which of the following statements is consistent with the vision of NANDA International?

   a. Intensity of nursing care must be included in the DRG methodology.
   b. Perioperative nursing care is an important area of future research.
   c. Nursing diagnoses communicate the professional judgments that nurses make every day.
   d. Nursing informatics systems will be subsumed by the acceptance of ICD as a universally recognized reference terminology in the EHR environment.

3. The NIC system includes which of the following?

   a. Interventions for illness prevention
   b. Medication Administration Records (MARs)
   c. Thirty domains with seven classes each
   d. NANDA diagnoses in each NIC

4. The Interoperability Standards Advisory provides recommendations for

   a. Submitting new concepts to SNOMED
   b. Improving nursing terminologies
   c. How to integrate terminologies in an EHR
   d. Standard vocabularies, messaging structures, and implementation specifications for the healthcare industry

5. Which of the following statements is true about NIC?

   a. Interventions in NIC are equivalent to Observables semantic type in SNOMED CT.
   b. NIC fails to meet the uniform guidelines for IS vendors required by the American Nurses Association.
   c. NIC is not limited to only the domain of nursing.
   d. NIC contains two interrelated taxonomies classified by care components.

REVIEW

1. Which two systems have many of the same uses?

   a. NIC and NOC
   b. NOC and NANDA
   c. NIC and NANDA
   d. NANDA and the Omaha System

2. The NANDA Classification is a:

    a. Standardized classification of patient and client outcomes

    b. Set of nursing diagnoses

    c. Standardized classification of interventions

    d. Unified nursing language system into which nursing terminologies can be cross mapped

3. Which of the following statements is false?

    a. NOC is used to classify outcomes.

    b. NOC is recognized by the ANA as one of the standardized languages of nursing.

    c. NOC may be used in all settings and with all patient populations.

    d. NOC is used for reimbursement of nursing care for Medicare patients.

4. The Clinical Care Classification (CCC) system consists of how many interrelated taxonomies?

    a. Three

    b. Two

    c. Four

    d. Five

5. Which system includes the following components: assessment (Problem Classification Scheme), intervention (Intervention Scheme), and outcomes (Problem Rating Scale for Outcomes)?

    a. NIC

    b. Omaha System

    c. NANDA

    d. NOC

6. A term from the _____ is required to create a nursing diagnosis.

    a. Means Axis

    b. Judgment Axis

    c. Location Axis

    d. Client Axis

7. Which of the following is not one of the seven axes of ICNP?

    a. Focus

    b. Means

    c. Beneficiary

    d. Location

8. The first terminology systems developed for nursing were considered:

   a. Taxonomies
   b. Controlled vocabularies
   c. Classification systems
   d. Heuristics

9. The Clinical Care Classification system:

   a. Classifies acute-care hospital episodes into diagnosis-related groups
   b. Was developed entirely from private funding and is a proprietary system
   c. Is not yet part of the Unified Medical Language System (UMLS)
   d. Resulted from work performed for a home care project initiated by the Centers for Medicare and Medicaid Services (formerly the Health Care Financing Administration)

10. The Perioperative Nursing Data Set benefits surgical endeavors because it:

    a. Standardizes a nursing procedure list
    b. Meets compliance requirements
    c. Benchmarks nursing practice
    d. All of the above

References

Association of periOperative Registered Nurses (AORN). 2018. Perioperative Nursing Dataset (PNDS). https://www.aorn.org/syntegrity/products.

American Nurses Association (ANA). 2018a. Inclusion of Recognized Terminologies Supporting Nursing Practice within Electronic Health Records and Other Health Information Technology Solutions. https://www.nursingworld.org/practice-policy/nursing-excellence/official-position-statements/id/Inclusion-of-Recognized-Terminologies-Supporting-Nursing-Practice-within-Electronic-Health-Records/.

American Nurses Association (ANA). 2018b. What is Nursing? https://www.nursingworld.org/practice-policy/workforce/what-is-nursing/.

Butcher, H., G. Bulechek, J. M. Dochterman, and C. Wagner. 2018. *Nursing Interventions Classification (NIC)*, 7th ed. St. Louis, MO: Elsevier.

Clinical Care Classification (CCC). 2017. http://www.sabacare.com.

Coenen, A. and T. Y. Kim. 2010. ICNP: Development of terminology subsets using ICNP®. *International Journal of Medical Informatics* 79(7):530–538.

Coenen, A. and C. Bartz. 2010. ICNP: Nursing Terminology to Improve Healthcare Worldwide. Chapter 11 in *Nursing and Informatics for the 21st Century: An International Look at Practice, Education and EHR Trends*, 2nd ed. Edited by C. A. Weaver, C. Delaney, P. Weber, and R. L. Carr. Chicago, IL: HIMSS.

Englebright, J., K. Aldrich, and C. R. Taylor. 2014. Defining and incorporating basic nursing care actions into the electronic health record. *Journal of Nursing Scholarship* 46(1):50–57.

Institute of Medicine (IOM). 2011. *The Future of Nursing: Leading Change, Advancing Health.* Washington, DC: The National Academies Press.

International Classification for Nursing Practice (ICNP). 2018a. ICNP Catalogues. http://www.old.icn.ch/what-we-do/icnpr-catalogues/.

International Classification for Nursing Practice (ICNP). 2018b. ICNP Browser. http://www.old.icn.ch/what-we-do/ICNP-Browser/.

International Classification for Nursing Practice (ICNP). 2018c. ICNP Information Sheet. http://www.old.icn.ch/images/stories/documents/pillars/Practice/icnp/ICNP_FAQs.pdf.

International Council of Nurses (ICN). 2018. http://www.icn.ch.

International Organization for Standardization (ISO). 2018. http://www.iso.org/iso/home/about.htm.

Logical Observation Identifiers, Names, and Codes (LOINC). 2018. https://loinc.org/committee/nursing/.

Lundberg, C., J. Warren, J. Brokel, G. Bulechek, H. Butcher, J. McCloskey Dochterman, M. Johnson et al. 2008. Selecting a standardized terminology for the electronic health record that reveals the impact of nursing on patient care. *Online Journal of Nursing Informatics* 12(2). http://www.ojni.org/12_2/lundberg.pdf.

Martin, K. S. 2005. *The Omaha System: A Key to Practice, Documentation, and Information Management,* reprinted 2nd ed. Omaha, NE: Health Connections Press.

Matney, S. A., T. Settergren, J. M. Carrington, R. L. Richesson, A. Sheide, and B. L. Westra. 2017. Standardizing physiologic assessment data to enable big data analytics. *Western Journal of Nursing Research* 39:63–77.

Matney, S. A., J. J. Warren, J. L. Evans, T. Y. Kim, A. Coenen, and V. A. Auld. 2012. Development of the nursing problem list subset of SNOMED CT. *Journal of Biomedical Informatics* 45(4):683–688.

NANDA International. 2018a. *NANDA International Nursing Diagnoses: Definitions and Classification* 2018–2020, 11th ed. New York, NY: Thieme Publishers.

NANDA International. 2018b. http://www.nanda.org.

National Library of Medicine (NLM). 2018a. UMLS Source Vocabularies. https://www.nlm.nih.gov/research/umls/sourcereleasedocs/index.html.

National Library of Medicine (NLM). 2018b. Core Problem List Subset of SNOMED CT. https://www.nlm.nih.gov/research/umls/Snomed/core_subset.html.

National Library of Medicine (NLM). 2017a. Nursing Resources for Standards and Interoperability. https://www.nlm.nih.gov/research/umls/Snomed/nursing_terminology_resources.html.

National Library of Medicine (NLM). 2017b. Nursing Problem List Subset of SNOMED CT. http://www.nlm.nih.gov/research/umls/Snomed/nursing_problemlist_subset.html.

Nursing Interventions Classification (NIC). 2018. https://nursing.uiowa.edu/cncce/nursing-interventions-classification-overview.

Nursing Management Minimum Data Sets (NMMDS). 2018. https://www.nursing.umn.edu/centers/center-nursing-informatics/center-projects.

Nursing Minimum Data Sets (NMDS). 2018. https://www.nursing.umn.edu/sites/nursing.umn.edu/files/usa-nmds.pdf.

Nursing Outcomes Classification (NOC). 2018. https://nursing.uiowa.edu/cncce/nursing-outcomes-classification-overview.

Office of the National Coordinator for Health IT (ONC). 2018a. 2018 Interoperability Standards Advisory. https://www.healthit.gov/isa/.

Office of the National Coordinator for Health IT (ONC). 2018b. https://www.healthit.gov/topic/federal-incentive-programs/meaningful-use.

Omaha System. 2017. http://www.omahasystem.org/.

Saba, V. 2012. *Clinical Care Classification (CCC) System Version 2.5*. New York, NY: Springer Publishing.

Spackman, K., K. Campbell, and R. Cote. 1997. SNOMED-RT: A reference terminology for healthcare. *Proceedings of the 1997 AMIA Annual Symposium*. Nashville, TN: American Medical Informatics Association.

Thede, L. Q., and P. M. Schwirian. 2014. Informatics: The standardized nursing terminologies: a national survey of nurses' experience and attitudes--SURVEY II: Participants' Perception of the Helpfulness of Standardized Nursing Terminologies in Clinical Care. *Online Journal of Issues in Nursing* 20(1):9.

University of Minnesota College of Nursing. 2018. https://www.nursing.umn.edu/centers/center-nursing-informatics/news-events/2018-nursing-knowledge-big-data-science-conference-0.

Warren, J. J. and S. Bakken. 2002. Update on standardized nursing data sets and terminologies. *Journal of AHIMA* 73(7):78–83.

Warren, J. J., S. A. Matney, E. D. Foster, V. A. Auld, and S. L. Roy. 2015. Toward interoperability: A new resource to support nursing terminology standards. *CIN: Computers, Informatics, Nursing* 33(12):515–519.

Weed, L. L. 1968. Medical records that guide and teach. *New England Journal of Medicine* 278:652–657.

Westra, B., G. E. Latimer, S. A. Matney, J. I. Park, J. Sensmeier, R. L. Simpson, M. J. Swanson et al. 2015. A national action plan for sharable and comparable nursing data to support practice and translational research for transforming health care. 2015. *Journal of the American Medical Informatics Association* 22(3):600–607.

Westra, B. L., S. G. Johnson, S. Ali, K. M. Bavuso, C. A. Cruz, S. Collins, M. Furukawa et al. 2018. Validation and refinement of a pain information model from EHR flowsheet data. *Applied Clinical Informatics* 9(01):185–198.

Resources

American Nurses Association (ANA). 2014. *Nursing Informatics: Scope and Standards of Practice*. Washington, DC: American Nurses Publishing. https://www.nursingworld.org/nurses-books/nursing-informatics-scope-and-standards-of-practice-2nd-ed/.

European Committee for Standardization. 2018. http://www.cenorm.be/cenorm.htm.

Hardiker, N. and A. Casey. 2000. Standards For nursing terminology. *Journal of the American Medical Informatics Association* 7(6):523–528.

Moorhead, S., M. Johnson, M. Maas, and E. Swanson, eds. 2018. *Nursing Outcomes Classification (NOC)*, 6th ed. St. Louis, MO: Elsevier.

SNOMED International. 2018. "5-Step Briefing." https://www.snomed.org/snomed-ct/five-step-briefing.

University of Minnesota (UMN). 2018. "2013 Nursing Knowledge: Big Data Science Conference." https://www.nursing.umn.edu/centers/center-nursing-informatics/news-events/2013-nursing-knowledge-big-data-science-conference.

13

Other Terminology and Classification Systems

Kathy Giannangelo, RHIA, CCS, CPHIMS, FAHIMA

LEARNING OBJECTIVES

- Identify the World Health Organization family of ICD-derived and -related classifications
- Define the history, use, and purpose of the International Classification of Diseases for Oncology, Third Edition (ICD-O-3)
- Differentiate classifications such as the International Classification of Primary Care (ICPC) from systems such as the International Classification of Diseases (ICD)
- Examine the development of other terminology and classification systems such as the Medical Dictionary for Regulatory Activities (MedDRA) and ABC codes
- Summarize the uses and applications of these systems
- Examine the relationships among the various classifications, terminologies, and code sets
- Compare tools available to access and use these systems
- Differentiate how these systems are used in an electronic environment

KEY TERMS

- ABC codes
- Complementary and alternative medicine (CAM)
- Derived classification
- Differentiation
- Histology
- International Classification of Diseases for Oncology, Third Edition (ICD-O-3)

- International Classification of Primary Care, Second Edition (ICPC-2)
- International Conference on Harmonization (ICH) of Technical Requirements for Registration of Pharmaceuticals for Human Use
- Medical Dictionary for Regulatory Activities (MedDRA)
- Morphology
- Reasons for encounter (RFE)
- Related classification
- Rubrics
- SOAP
- Topography
- WHO Family of International Classifications (WHO-FIC)
- Wonca International Classification Committee (WICC)
- World Organization of Family Doctors (Wonca)

Introduction

Although some terminologies and classifications such as International Classification of Diseases (ICD) have been around for a long time, other terminologies have emerged only in the past 20 or so years because of changes in the healthcare environment. For example, the government found that Current Procedural Terminology (CPT) did not have the detail needed to identify certain services for such things as supplies. Identifying this gap, the Centers for Medicare and Medicaid Services (CMS) developed a code set called HCPCS Level II to meet the operational needs of the Medicare and Medicaid reimbursement programs (see chapter 3). In addition, passage of the Health Insurance Portability and Accountability Act (HIPAA) of 1996 and the identification of standard transaction and code sets have resulted in comments by various organizations noting additional gaps in the current systems. Finally, the movement toward electronic health records (EHRs) also has been an influencing factor in the evolution of, and need for, specific systems.

As discussed in earlier chapters, the World Health Organization (WHO) is a United Nations agency established in 1948 with the objective of working to help people worldwide attain the highest possible level of health. The organization is responsible for the WHO family of international classifications, which includes the International Statistical Classification of Diseases and Related Health Problems, Tenth Revision (ICD-10).

WHO mandates the production of international classifications on health so meaningful and useful frameworks are developed as a common language for use by governments, providers, and consumers. The **WHO Family of International Classifications (WHO-FIC)** is "a suite of integrated classification products that share similar features and can be used individually or jointly to provide information on different aspects of health and on the health care system" (WHO 2016, 4).

There are three reference classifications approved by WHO-FIC:

- *International Classification of Diseases and Related Health Problems* (ICD) (discussed in chapters 1 and 7)
- *International Classification of Functioning, Disability, and Health* (ICF) (discussed in chapter 11)
- *International Classification of Health Interventions* (ICHI)

Additionally, there are derived classifications and related classifications. A **derived classification** is based on one or more reference classifications and may be prepared:

- By adopting the reference classification structure and categories, while providing additional detail beyond that provided by the reference classification
- Through rearrangement or aggregation of items from one or more reference classifications (WHO 2018)

A **related classification** partially refers to a reference classification or is associated with the reference classification at specific levels of structure only and describes important aspects of health or the health system not covered by reference or derived classifications (WHO 2018).

This chapter examines the development, purpose, content, structure, principles and guidelines, and process for revision and updates for the derived classification, **International Classification of Diseases for Oncology, Third Edition (ICD-O-3)**, and the WHO-related classification, **International Classification of Primary Care, Second Edition (ICPC-2)**. In addition, this chapter also includes material on the **Medical Dictionary for Regulatory Activities (MedDRA)**, a system for classifying adverse events associated with medical products, and **ABC codes**, designed for non-physician and alternative medicine health services.

International Classification of Diseases for Oncology, Third Edition

ICD-O is a derived classification of ICD, which is used primarily by tumor or cancer registries to code the **topography** (site) and **morphology** (**histology**) of neoplasms. Over 35 years old, the ICD-O has undergone several revisions. The current version is the third edition, first revision, or ICD-O-3.1. The topography section of the third edition remains the same as in the second edition, but the morphology section was revised. This most recent revision primarily involved new terms, codes, synonyms, related terms, morphology, and behavior code changes on tumors of hematopoietic and lymphoid tissues, the central nervous system, and the digestive system (IARC 2018a).

Developer of ICD-O

WHO published the first edition of ICD-O in 1976. The second edition, a collaboration between WHO and the International Agency for Research on Cancer (IARC), was published in 1990. The second edition was used extensively throughout the world and has been translated into many languages, including Chinese, Czech, French, German, Greek, Italian, Japanese, Portuguese, Russian, Slovak, and Spanish.

Published in 2000, the updated, third edition of ICD-O also was developed by a working party convened by IARC/WHO.

Purpose of ICD-O

The purpose of ICD-O is to provide greater specificity for use by pathologists, clinical oncologists, and cancer registries and others specializing in cancer. The topography code describes the site of origin of the neoplasm and uses the same three- and four-character categories as in the malignant neoplasm section of the second chapter of ICD-10, except those categories that relate to secondary neoplasms and to specified morphological types of tumors. ICD-O also includes a topography for hematopoietic and reticuloendothelial tumors. The morphology code describes the characteristics of the tumor itself, including cell type and biological activity. For example, code M8820/0 is an elastofibroma/benign neoplasm.

Content of ICD-O

ICD-O is based on the structure of ICD-10, but with basic differences. The second chapter of ICD-10, Neoplasms, categorizes the topography and describes the behavior of the neoplasm as follows: malignant, benign, in situ, or uncertain whether malignant or benign. In ICD-10, up to five different categories of codes are needed to describe the neoplasms of a site. Table 13.1 illustrates how five different codes are used in ICD-10 to describe neoplasm of the breast.

In contrast, ICD-O uses one code for topography, and this code remains the same for all neoplasms of a particular site. The code is based on the malignant neoplasm section of ICD-10. Identification of whether the neoplasm is malignant, benign, in situ, or of uncertain or unknown

TABLE 13.1. ICD-10 Alphabetic Index entries for breast neoplasm

	Malignant, Primary	Malignant, Secondary	In situ	Benign	Uncertain and Unknown Behavior
Breast	C50.9	C79.8	D05.9	D24	D48.6

Source: CMS 2018.

behavior is made by the fifth digit in the morphology code. The other digits of the morphology code describe the type of morphology of the neoplasm (for example, adenocarcinoma, carcinoma, squamous cell carcinoma, and so on). Table 13.2 shows how the code stays the same and the morphology code gives the behavior.

Table 13.3 shows how the different sections of the second chapter of ICD-10 correspond to the behavior codes in the morphology codes.

Several abbreviations are used throughout the classification, including:

- M (morphology)
- NOS (not otherwise specified)
- ICD-O (International Classification of Diseases for Oncology)

In ICD-O, NOS appears after topographic and morphologic terms that appear elsewhere in the classification with an additional modifying word or phrase. The NOS is listed first in the Alphabetic Index, followed by the alphabetic listing of modifying words. ICD-O instructs coders to follow a term with NOS when:

- A topographic or morphologic term is not modified,
- A topographic or morphologic term has an adjective that does not appear elsewhere,
- A term is used in a general sense (Fritz et al. 2012).

TABLE 13.2. ICD-O coding of some breast neoplasms

Neoplasm	Code
Malignant neoplasm of the breast (primary, carcinoma)	C50.9 M-8010/3
In situ neoplasm of breast (carcinoma, intraductal, noninfiltrating)	C50.9 M-8500/2
Benign neoplasm of breast (adenoma, apocrine)	C50.9 M-8401/0

TABLE 13.3. ICD-O behavior codes and corresponding sections of chapter II, ICD-10

Behavior Code	Category	Term
/ 0	D10–D36	Benign neoplasms
/ 1	D37–D48	Neoplasms of uncertain and unknown behavior
/ 2	D00–D09	In situ neoplasms
/ 3	C00–C76, C80–C97	Malignant neoplasms, stated or presumed to be primary
/ 6	C77–C79	Malignant neoplasms, stated or presumed to be secondary

Source: Fritz et al. 2012.

357

Structure and Format of ICD-O

ICD-O consists of the following main sections:

I.   Instructions for Use
II. Topography: Numerical List
III. Morphology: Numerical List
IV. Alphabetic Index
V.   Differences in Morphology Codes between Second and Third Editions

Instructions for Use

The Instructions for Use section contains an introduction with historical background, differences between ICD-O and ICD-10, the structure and format of ICD-O-3, and coding guidelines for topography and morphology. This section must be read and followed carefully because it contains the guidelines needed to assign codes correctly.

Topography: Numerical List

The topography section is based on the malignant neoplasm chapter in ICD-10. The codes span from C00.0 to C80.9, and a decimal point separates the subdivisions of three-character categories. ICD-10 categories C43, C45, C46, C81–97, and D00–D48 are not included in the ICD-O-3 nomenclature for topography (IARC 2018b). Figure 13.1 shows the structure of the topography codes and table 13.4 shows an example of the topography—numerical section.

Morphology: Numerical List

Codes in the morphology section have five digits and range from M-8000/0 to M-9989/3. The first four digits of the code give the histology, and the fifth digit, after the slash (/), is the behavior

FIGURE 13.1. Structure of topography code

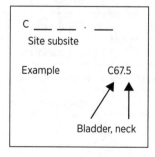

TABLE 13.4. Example from the topography—numerical section

C18		COLON
C18.0		Cecum
		Ileocecal valve
		Ileocecal junction
C18.1		Appendix
C18.2		Ascending colon
		Right colon
C18.3		Hepatic flexure of colon
C18.4		Transverse colon
C18.5		Splenic flexure of colon
C18.6		Descending colon
		Left colon
C18.7		Sigmoid colon
		Sigmoid, NOS
		Sigmoid flexure of colon
		Pelvic colon
C18.8		Overlapping lesion of colon *(see note page 45)*
C18.9		Colon, NOS
		Large intestine *(excludes rectum, NOS C20.9 and rectosigmoid junction C19.9)*
		Large bowel, NOS
	C19	RECTOSIGMOID JUNCTION
C19.9		Rectosigmoid junction
		Rectosigmoid, NOS
		Rectosigmoid colon
		Colon and rectum
		Pelvirectal junction
	C20	RECTUM
C20.9		Rectum, NOS *(excludes skin of anus and perianal skin C44.5)*
		Rectal ampulla

(continued)

TABLE 13.4. Continued

C21	ANUS AND ANAL CANAL
C21.0	Anus, NOS
C21.1	Anal canal
	Anal sphincter
C21.2	Cloacogenic zone
C21.8	Overlapping lesion of rectum, anus, and anal canal *(see note page 45)*
	Anorectal junction
	Anorectum

Source: Fritz et al. 2012.

TABLE 13.5. Example from the morphology—numerical section

880	Soft Tissue Tumors and Sarcomas, NOS
8800/0	Soft tissue tumor, benign
8800/3	Sarcoma, NOS
8800/9	Sarcomatosis, NOS
8801/3	Spindle cell sarcoma
8802/3	Giant cell sarcoma (except of bone 9250/3)
8803/3	Small cell sarcoma
8804/3	Epithelioid sarcoma
8805/3	Undifferentiated sarcoma
8806/3	Desmoplastic small round cell tumor

Source: IARC 2018c.

code. The fifth digit indicates whether the tumor is benign, uncertain whether malignant or benign, in situ, malignant (primary site), malignant (metastatic site), or malignant (uncertain whether primary or metastatic site). Table 13.5 shows an example of the morphology—numerical section.

The behavior refers to the way the tumor acts in the body. A benign tumor can grow in place but does not spread; an in situ behavior indicates the tumor is malignant but still growing in place. Malignant of the primary site indicates the tumor can spread, and metastatic means dissemination from the point of origin and growth at another site. Figure 13.2 illustrates the fifth-digit behavior code for neoplasms.

FIGURE 13.2. Fifth-digit behavior code for neoplasms

Code

/0	Benign
/1	Uncertain whether benign or malignant
	Borderline malignancy
	Low malignant potential
	Uncertain malignant potential
/2	Carcinoma in situ
	Intraepithelial
	Noninfiltrating
	Noninvasive
/3	Malignant, primary site
/6	Malignant, metastatic site
	Malignant, secondary site
/9	Malignant, uncertain whether primary or metastatic site

Source: Fritz et al. 2012.

TABLE 13.6. Histologic grading or differentiation

Code	Grade	Description
1	I	Well differentiated
		Differentiated, NOS
2	II	Moderately differentiated
		Moderately well differentiated
		Intermediate differentiation
3	III	Poorly differentiated
4	IV	Undifferentiated
		Anaplastic
9		Grade or differentiation not determined, not stated, or not applicable

Source: Fritz et al. 2012.

An additional digit is available to identify the histologic grading or **differentiation**. Table 13.6 provides the meanings of this final digit.

The grading codes can be applied to all malignant neoplasms listed in ICD-O when documentation is present that distinguishes the grade or differentiation. For example, to completely code well-differentiated carcinoma, the morphology code would be M-8010/3 1.

There is a separate one-digit code for the cell lineage or immunophenotype for lymphoma or leukemia. This is:

5 T-cell

6 B-cell

   Pre-B

   B-precursor

7 Null cell

   Non T-non B

8 NK cell

   Natural killer cell

9 Cell type not determined, not stated or not applicable

   (Fritz et al. 2012)

Figure 13.3 illustrates the structure of a morphology code.

To completely code with ICD-O, one would use 10 characters. The first four indicate the topographic site, the next four give the morphologic type, followed by one digit for behavior and one digit for grade or differentiation. (The M is not calculated in this number.) Figure 13.4 provides an example of the structure of a complete code.

FIGURE 13.3. Structure of a morphology code

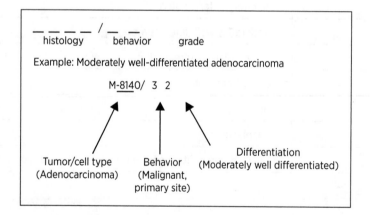

Source: Fritz et al. 2012.

FIGURE 13.4. Structure of a complete code

Diagnostic term:
Well-differentiated squamous cell carcinoma, lower lobe of the lung

C34.3 M-8070/3 1

Alphabetic Index

The Alphabetic Index is available for use in finding both topography (anatomical sites) and morphology (histologic terms). The terms are interspersed in alphabetical order and are listed under both the noun and the adjective. For example, small cell carcinoma is indexed under Carcinoma, small cell, and under Small cell carcinoma.

By knowing the format of the different codes, it is apparent that the topography codes are identified by the letter *C*, the first character of codes in the neoplasms chapter of ICD-10, and the morphology codes begin with the prefix *M-*.

Remember, the first character of ICD-10 codes also may start with the letter *D*, but ICD-O codes are all based on the malignant neoplasm section. The morphology code distinguishes the behavior of the neoplasm in ICD-O.

When topographic (C) and morphologic terms (M) are mixed in the index, they are separated by a space. When three or more terms appear, the term beginning with C or M is in bold type and terms are indented under it. The NOS term is always listed first under the heading in the index rather than in alphabetical order.

The Alphabetic Index also includes some tumor-like lesions and conditions for which no code is provided; instead, a reference is made to *see SNOMED*, which is a reference to the SNOMED CT. The previous versions of ICD-O provided SNOMED CT codes, but ICD-O-3 omitted them. Figure 13.5 shows the format of the Alphabetic Index of ICD-O-3.

Differences in Morphology Codes between Second and Third Editions

The section on differences in morphology codes between second and third editions provides the new ICD-O codes, new morphology terms and synonyms, terms that changed morphology codes, terms that changed from tumor-like lesions to neoplasms, terms deleted from ICD-O-3, and terms that changed behavior codes.

Principles and Guidelines for ICD-O

The coding guidelines for topography and morphology available in the ICD-O-3 consist of Rules A through K. Certain guidelines apply only to topography and some only to morphology, while others apply to both. For example, Rule B. Prefixes states: "If a topographic site is modified by a prefix such as peri-, para-, or the like which is not specifically listed in ICD-O, code to the appropriate ill-defined subcategory C76 (ill-defined site), unless the type of tumor indicates origin from a particular tissue" (Fritz et al. 2012).

Another example of a guideline is Rule C. Tumors involving more than one topographic category or subcategory, which states: "Use subcategory '.8' when a tumor overlaps the boundaries of two or more categories or subcategories and its point of origin cannot be determined" (Fritz et al. 2012).

After the section listing the guidelines, more detail regarding each rule is provided. The rules are listed again, but with more precise guidelines and examples pertaining to each rule.

New case reportability and coding rules for hematopoietic and lymphoid cases were established in 2010 along with new ICD-O histology terms and codes and changes to existing codes. A database and a Hematopoietic and Lymphoid Neoplasm Case Reportability and Coding Manual are the primary resource for abstracting and coding these neoplasms. Several updates have occurred since their initial publication in 2010.

FIGURE 13.5. Alphabetic Index of ICD-O-3

	V	
C52.9		Vagina, NOS
C52.9		Vagina, fornix
M-8077/2	Vaginal intraepithelial neoplasia, grade III (C52._)	
C52.9		Vaginal vault
C72.5		Vagus nerve
M-8077/2	VAIN III (C52._)	
C10.0		Vallecula
C18.0		Valve, ileocecal
C63.1		Vas deferens
	Vascular	
M-8894/0	leiomyoma	
M——	nevus (*see SNOMED*)	
M——	spider (*see SNOMED*)	
C52.9		Vault, vaginal
C49.9		Vein, NOS
C49.5		Vein, iliac
	Vena cava	
C49.4	NOS	
C49.4	abdominal	
C49.4	inferior	
C49.3	superior	
M9122/0	Venous hemangioma	
	Ventral surface of tongue	
C02.2	NOS	
C02.2	anterior	
C02.2	anterior 2/3	

Source: Fritz et al. 2012.

Process for Revision of and Updates to ICD-O

The third edition of ICD-O was developed by a working party convened by IARC/WHO. A special effort was made in this edition of ICD-O to change as few terms as possible. New terms were added at empty spaces. The topography codes remained the same as in the second edition, but morphology codes were thoroughly reviewed and, where necessary, revised to increase their diagnostic precision and prognostic value. As mentioned earlier, most changes reflected the urgent need to code new diagnoses in leukemia and lymphoma.

Since publication of the hard- and soft-cover versions of ICD-O-3 in June 2000, two sets of errata have been created. The first was released May 22, 2001, and the second May 6, 2003. WHO published updates in 2011. The errata included corrections for a number of errors and discrepancies appearing in the hardcover version. Many of the 2011 updates involved new terms and codes, such as 8077/0 squamous intraepithelial neoplasia, low grade, new synonyms, new related terms, new preferred terms, deletions of codes and terms, and behavior code changes.

The tentative publication date of ICD-O-3.2 is 2019.

International Classification of Primary Care

The International Classification of Primary Care (ICPC) has been translated into several languages and is used in a number of countries around the world to classify patient data related to general and family practice and primary care. For example, ICPC is required in electronic prescribing systems in the Netherlands.

In the US, a variation of ICPC, the Reason for Visit Classification, has been used for years to classify the patient's stated reason for the visit or chief complaint in national ambulatory care surveys (CDC 2018). In addition, a project sponsored by the Agency for Healthcare Research and Quality called the Applied Strategies for Improving Patient Safety (ASIPS) used ICPC as its classification system (Pace et al. 2003).

In 2003, WHO recognized the second edition of ICPC as a related classification for the classification of primary care data, and it is considered one of the WHO Family of International Classifications (WHO-FIC). The classification system also has been incorporated into the National Library of Medicine's Unified Medical Language System (UMLS).

Developer of ICPC

The World Organization of National Colleges, Academics, and Academic Associations of General Practitioners/Family Physicians (Wonca), today known as the **World Organization of Family Doctors (Wonca)**, was instrumental in the development of ICPC. Designed by the WONCA Classification Committee (now the **Wonca International Classification Committee [WICC]**), its predecessor, the International Classification of Health Problems in Primary Care (ICHPPC),

TABLE 13.7. Versions of ICPC*

Title	Acronym	Date Published/ Released
International Classification of Primary Care (ICPC)	ICPC-1-v.0.0	1987
International Classification of Primary Care (ICPC), Second Edition	ICPC-2-v.0.0	1998
ICPC-2-E Electronic version, minor revision 1, update version 0	ICPC-2e-v.1.0	2000
ICPC-2-E, minor revision 2, update version 0	ICPC-2e-v.2.0	2002
ICPC-2-E, minor revision 3, update version 0 (corresponds to ICPC Revised Second Edition [ICPC-2-R] book)	ICPC-2e-v.3.0	2005
ICPC-2-E, minor revision 4, update version 0 (corresponds to ICPC-2-R including updates)	ICPC-2e-v.4.0	2008
ICPC-2-E, minor revision 4, update version 1	ICPC-2e-v.4.1	May 2011
ICPC-2-E, minor revision 4, update version 2	ICPC-2e-v.4.2	May 2012
ICPC-2-E, minor revision 4, update version 3	ICPC-2e-v.4.3	September 2013
ICPC-2-E, minor revision 4, update version 4	ICPC-2e-v.4.4	January 2015
ICPC-2-E, minor revision 5, update version 0	ICPC-2e-v.5.0	May 2015
ICPC-2-E, minor revision 6, update version 0	ICPC-2e-v.6.0	April 2017
ICPC-2-E, minor revision 7, update version 0	ICPC-2e-v.7.0	February 2018

*In 2005 WICC decided on a version numbering for the electronic versions that identifies the major version, the minor version, and the update version.

was first published in 1975, followed by a second edition in 1979 and a third (ICHPPC-2-Defined) in 1983. Although deemed an improvement over the International Classification of Diseases (ICD), this system was still considered inadequate for identifying the patient's reason for encounter and problem list.

Further, the system's insufficiencies were recognized at a WHO conference. The National Center for Health Statistics, the WHO North American Collaborating Center, led an effort to address the identified deficiencies with its development of the Classification of **Reasons for Encounter (RFE)** in Primary Care. Under the auspices of WHO, a working party was created, which led to the development of the Reason for Encounter Classification (RFEC). Field trials with members of the WICC were conducted on RFEC, which resulted in the publication of ICPC in 1987. Wonca owns the copyrights to ICPC. Table 13.7 lists the various published versions.

Purpose of ICPC

ICPC enables the labeling of the most prevalent conditions that exist in the community as well as symptoms and complaints. It can classify three important elements of the healthcare encounter:

reasons for encounter (RFE), diagnosis or problems, and process of care. The RFEs are defined as "An agreed statement of the reason(s) why a patient enters the healthcare system, representing the demand for care by that person. The terms written down and later classified by the provider clarify the reason for encounter and consequently the patient's demand for care, without interpreting it in the form of a diagnosis. The reason for encounter should be recognized by the patient as an acceptable description of that person's demand for care" (Bentzen 2003).

Reasons why a patient visits a primary care physician might include symptoms or complaints; known diseases; preventive, diagnostic, or administrative services; and specific treatments. Unlike ICD, which identifies the provider's determination, an RFE classification represents the patient's viewpoint for seeing the provider. This is a key element in the healthcare practitioner's decision regarding the patient's diagnosis and its management.

Content of ICPC

The **SOAP** concept was used in the development of ICPC. SOAP is an acronym for a component of the problem-oriented medical record that refers to how each progress note contains documentation relative to subjective observations. ICPC classifies three of the four elements of the problem-oriented medical record SOAP:

S: Subjective observations by the patient of the problem or the reason for encounter
O: Objective observations not classified with ICPC
A: Assessment or diagnosis of the patient's problem
P: Plans or process of care

ICPC consists of a biaxial configuration, chapters, and components. Whereas ICD has different chapter axes, all 17 ICPC chapters are based on body systems, with additional chapters for general and unspecified issues and social problems. Table 13.8 shows the chapters and their associated alpha characters.

The first character of an ICPC code is the alpha character for the chapter. The next characters in an ICPC code are two digits, referred to as **rubrics**, and represent the second axis components. Each chapter in ICPC is divided into the following seven components (process codes):

- Symptoms and complaints (1–29)
- Diagnostics, screening, and preventive procedures (30–49)
- Medication, treatment, procedures (50–59)
- Test Results (60–61)
- Administration (62)
- Referral and other reasons for encounter (63–69)
- Diseases (70–99)

TABLE 13.8. ICPC chapter titles and associated alpha character

Chapter	Alpha Character
General and unspecified	A
Blood, blood forming organs and immune mechanism	B
Digestive	D
Eye	F
Ear	H
Circulatory	K
Musculoskeletal	L
Neurological	N
Psychological	P
Respiratory	R
Skin	S
Endocrine, metabolic, and nutritional	T
Urological	U
Pregnancy, childbearing, family planning	W
Female genital system (including breast)	X
Male genital system	Y
Social problems	Z

For example, D70, a code for gastrointestinal infection, is found in the chapter D(igestive), disease component 7: D70.

Principles and Guidelines for ICPC

When assigning an ICPC-2 code for the RFE, diagnosis or problems, and process of care, several principles are followed (Soler n.d.). First, the RFE represents the patient's viewpoint for seeing the provider and therefore the ICPC rubric must represent the reason given by the patient. It is incorrect to use the rubrics for recording health problems and diagnoses. Should the individual not be able to describe the problem, then an accompanying person's description can be used. Additionally, when selecting an RFE code, choose the highest level of code specificity and assign multiple codes when more than one RFE is provided. For diagnoses and problems, code the provider's assessment of the patient, which may be a symptom, complaint, or diagnosis. Other options are no disease or health maintenance or preventive measure. When more than one diagnosis or problem is found, each should be coded at the highest level of diagnostic refinement possible. Once a diagnosis has been established, use the inclusions and exclusions, criteria, considerations, and notes to guide appropriate use. For process of care, the codes for the components are uniform throughout all chapters; others are not. The following are guidelines for the components (WICC 2005):

- Component 1 – Symptoms and complaints: Rubrics in this component describe the problem under management (that is, the problem list) when the condition has not been defined.
- Component 2 – Diagnostic, and preventive procedures: Rubrics in this component are used when there is no underlying pathology for the problem being managed and the patient is seeking some type of procedure.
- Component 3 – Medication, treatment, therapeutic procedures: Rubrics in this component are for the naming of processes involved in patient care, such as request for treatment.
- Component 4 – Results: Rubrics in this component describe encounters where the patient is requesting the results of tests done previously.
- Component 5 – Administrative: Rubrics in this component describe encounters for examinations required by a third party, completion of forms, or discussions surrounding the transfer of records.
- Component 6 – Referral and other reasons for encounter. Rubrics in this component describe the reason for the encounter is for a referral to another provider or a provider-initiated reason for the encounter.
- Component 7 – Diagnoses, diseases: Rubrics in this component are used when a practitioner has enough information to determine a diagnosis or disease. Component 7 has five subgroups: infectious diseases, neoplasms, injuries and trauma, congenital anomalies, and other specific diseases. These subgroups are not numerically uniform across chapters.
- Components 1 and 7 function independently in each of the 17 chapters. They are used to classify patient RFEs, presenting symptoms, and diagnoses or problems managed.
- Components 2 and 3 are broadly founded on the ICD-9 Procedures in Medicine and the International Classification of Process in Primary Care.
- Components 2 through 6 are common throughout all the chapters, with each rubric equally valid to any body system.

ICPC's structure results in groups of problems being disseminated among chapters rather than found in their own chapters as in ICD. For example, ICD has a separate chapter for injuries. In ICPC, injuries are found in various chapters depending on the body system to which the injury occurred.

Process for Revision of and Updates to ICPC

WICC is responsible for the maintenance of and updates to ICPC. ICPC-3 work has begun with the formation of the ICPC-3 Consortium. While the Consortium has stated the principles of frequency, evidence-based, simplicity, familiarity, and no excessive subclasses will be retained, a content model will be developed for the classification (PH3C 2018a). Alpha and beta version releases, along with field testing, are expected to occur from December 2019 to September 2020 followed by endorsement by WONCA in May 2021 and publication June 2021 (PH3C 2018b).

Medical Dictionary for Regulatory Activities

The Medical Dictionary for Regulatory Activities (MedDRA) is a terminology designed to facilitate medical product regulation and related electronic data interchange.

Developer of MedDRA

MedDRA was developed under the auspices of the **International Conference on Harmonization (ICH) of Technical Requirements for Registration of Pharmaceuticals for Human Use** to complement ICH's ongoing safety, quality, and efficacy harmonization efforts. MedDRA was based on the U.K. Medicines and Healthcare products Regulatory Agency's medical terminology and is owned by the International Federation of Pharmaceutical Manufacturers and Associations (MedDRA n.d.a.). The FDA has required adverse events and medication errors be coded using MedDRA when submitting reports to the FDA Adverse Event Reporting System (FAERS) database since 2016. The European Union has required MedDRA coding for submissions and safety reporting since January 2003.

Purpose of MedDRA

MedDRA was developed as a tool to be used by drug regulators and pharmaceutical companies to manage clinical information about pharmaceuticals, biologics, vaccines, and drug-device combinations (ICH 2013).

Content of MedDRA

MedDRA has a hierarchical structure in which lowest-level terms (LLTs) are mapped first to preferred terms (PTs), then to a high-level term (HLT), next to a high-level group term (HLGT), and finally to a system organ class (SOC). This dictionary of terms has been translated into several languages including Czech, Dutch, French, German, Japanese, Italian, Portuguese, and Spanish.

TABLE 13.9. MedDRA structural hierarchy

Level	Name	No. of Terms
SOC	System Organ Class	27
HLGT	High-Level Group Term	337
HLT	High-Level Term	1737
PT	Preferred Term	23,389
LLT	Low-Level Term	79,507

Source: ICH 2018a.

FIGURE 13.6. Five-level hierarchy

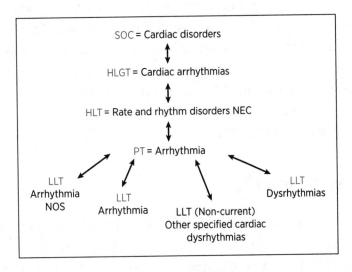

Source: ICH 2018b.

MedDRA is a multiaxial system and includes a five-level hierarchy. Each MedDRA term is assigned an eight-digit code without taxonomic meaning. The levels of structural hierarchy from highest to lowest are depicted in Table 13.9.

Figure 13.6 shows an example of the five-level hierarchy.

Principles and Guidelines for MedDRA

MedDRA terms cover all types of adverse reactions to pharmaceuticals. Although MedDRA is used to report adverse effects of drugs, it does not itself contain codes for drugs. Embedded within MedDRA are many other coding and reporting systems, including:

- The World Health Organization—Adverse Reaction Terminology (WHO-ART©)
- Coding Symbols for a Thesaurus of Adverse Reaction Terms (COSTART)

- International Classification of Diseases, Ninth Revision (ICD-9)
- International Classification of Diseases, Ninth Revision, Clinical Modification (ICD-9-CM)
- Japanese Adverse Reaction Terminology (J-ART)
- Hoechst Adverse Reaction Terminology System (HARTS©)

In addition, the *Diagnostic and Statistical Manual of Mental Disorders*, 5th Edition (DSM-5) was used as the basis for the psychiatry section.

A SOC is the broadest concept in the hierarchy, which is comprised of groupings by etiology, manifestation site, and purpose. One exception to the three groups is SOC Social circumstances, which categorizes factors of a personal nature that could impact on the reported event (ICH 2018c). Related terms in the HLGT and HLT levels are grouped by anatomy, pathology, physiology, etiology, or function. The PT level contains distinct descriptors representing a single medical concept, including symptoms, signs, diseases, diagnoses, therapeutic indication, investigation, surgical or medical procedures, and medical, social, or family characteristics. The LLT level contains synonyms, quasi-synonyms, lexical variants, subconcepts, or identical LLT of the PT to which they are linked. Because LLTs accommodate culturally unique terms, each LLT may not have a translation in all languages. An LLT can be linked to only one PT (ICH 2018c).

Abbreviations Used in MedDRA

The abbreviation NOS stands for "not otherwise specified" and NEC stands for "not elsewhere classified." NOS (for example, in the MedDRA LLT "Pain NOS") indicates that the condition is not included in another LLT (such as "Chest pain" or "Flank pain"). It is often a general term for a condition that has specific instances listed as separate LLTs. The other LLTs may be in multiple SOCs, as the example of different pains indicates.

NEC (for example, in the MedDRA HLGT "Eye disorders NEC") indicates the condition is not classified in any other grouping or within any other SOC under the multiaxial classification schema. Unlike NOS, which is seen exclusively at the LLT level, NEC is seen at the HLT or HLGT level to gather preferred terms that are not easily classified under other HLTs or HLGTs.

Standardized MedDRA Queries

Standardized MedDRA queries (SMQs) are groupings of terms, ordinarily at the PT level, that relate to a defined medical condition or an area of interest (ICH 2018c). They are intended to aid in case identification. SMQs were previously known as special search categories.

The included terms may relate to signs, symptoms, diagnoses, syndromes, physical findings, laboratory and other physiologic test data, and so on related to the medical condition or area of interest (ICH 2018d). LLTs that are not subordinate to an included preferred term are excluded. With the release of MedDRA Version 21.1, there are 103 SMQs. Dehydration was the most recently added.

The following is a simple SMQ providing the terms defined for lactic acidosis (MedDRA n.d.b.):

LACTIC ACIDOSIS, "NARROW" TERMS

Blood lactic acid increased
Hyperlactacidaemia
Lactic acidosis

LACTIC ACIDOSIS, "BROAD" TERMS

Acid base balance abnormal
Acidosis
Anion gap abnormal
Anion gap increased
Blood bicarbonate abnormal
Blood bicarbonate decreased
Blood gases abnormal
Blood lactic acid abnormal
Blood pH abnormal
Blood pH decreased
Coma acidotic
Kussmaul respiration
Metabolic acidosis
PCO2 abnormal
PCO2 decreased
Urine lactic acid increased

Process for Revision of and Updates to MedDRA

The MedDRA Maintenance and Support Services Organization (MSSO), which is the sole licensee and distributor of MedDRA subscriptions, updates MedDRA twice a year on March 1st and September 1st. Commercial, Non-profit/Non-commercial, and Regulator subscriber categories may submit requests for revisions using the WebCR tool. In addition, the MedDRA MSSO staff continually assesses MedDRA for adequacy and makes changes as appropriate. Every change request must include justification for the request. This is a statement of why the change request is necessary, such as an explanation that the concept is required because it is being reported in a clinical trial (ICH 2018e).

Change requests in MedDRA may be both simple and complex. Simple change requests, which are processed with each release, are any changes at the PT level and below in the terminology structure. A simple change request will fall under any of the following categories:

- Add a new PT
- Move a PT
- Rename a PT
- Demote a PT
- Swap a PT with an LLT
- Link a PT to HLT
- Unlink a PT
- Add a new LLT
- Move an LLT
- Rename an LLT
- Promote an LLT
- Change the status of an LLT
- Reassign the primary SOC of a PT
- Add a new term
  (ICH 2018e)

Complex change requests, which are any changes involving HLTs, HLGTs, or SOCs, are processed once a year because they will affect all underlying terms. A complex change request can fall under any of the following categories:

- Add a new SOC, HLGT, HLT
- Rename an SOC, HLGT, HLT
- Merge an HLT
- Merge an HLGT
- Link an HLT to an HLGT
- Link an HLGT to an SOC
- Move an HLT to an HLGT
- Unlink an HLT from an HLGT
- Unlink an HGFT from an SOC
  (ICH 2018e)

All complex changes to the terminology are made once a year in March.

Subscribers requesting revisions to SMQs must use the WebCR tool. Updates to the SMQs occur twice a year at the same time as the MedDRA releases.

The MedDRA MSSO accepts change requests from the organization's subscription point of contact (POC) or those individuals the POC authorizes as requesters. These individuals use the current valid MedDRA ID and Change Request ID assigned to the organization to access the WebCR application on the MSSO website.

ABC Codes

ABC codes fill information gaps in mandated code sets by identifying procedures, treatments, and services performed by integrative health professionals. These codes are a registered vocabulary of HL7 and were incorporated into the NLM's Unified Medical Language System (UMLS) in 1998.

Developer of ABC Codes

ABC Coding Solutions, formally Alternative Link, started the development process of the ABC codes in 1996 via interviews, informal surveys, and case studies. This process was followed by systematic research using formal data collection tools and input from individuals such as those from practitioner associations and experts in the field. The final groups involved were subject matter experts from various backgrounds (for example, coding, claims management, and credentialing). The outcome was five-character alphabetic codes that describe a wide assortment of integrative healthcare practices, two-character bone area treatment identifiers, relative value units (RVUs), and legal practice guidelines.

Purpose of ABC Codes

ABC codes were created to describe the procedures, treatments, and services provided during an encounter with a **complementary and alternative medicine (CAM)**, nursing, or other integrative healthcare provider. This area of healthcare is not identified specifically in other code sets in use today. Figure 13.7 shows the gaps in the national Health Insurance Portability and Accountability Act (HIPAA) code sets addressed by ABC codes.

Molina (2004) states: "Fully deployed and used in conjunction with CPT, HCPCS II, and CDT codes, ABC codes will capture data on an estimated 1.4 billion annual visits to unconventional and nonphysician caregivers and allow for comparisons of the outcomes of these visits to the estimated 1.1 billion visits made to doctors' offices."

FIGURE 13.7. Gaps in the national HIPAA code sets addressed by ABC codes

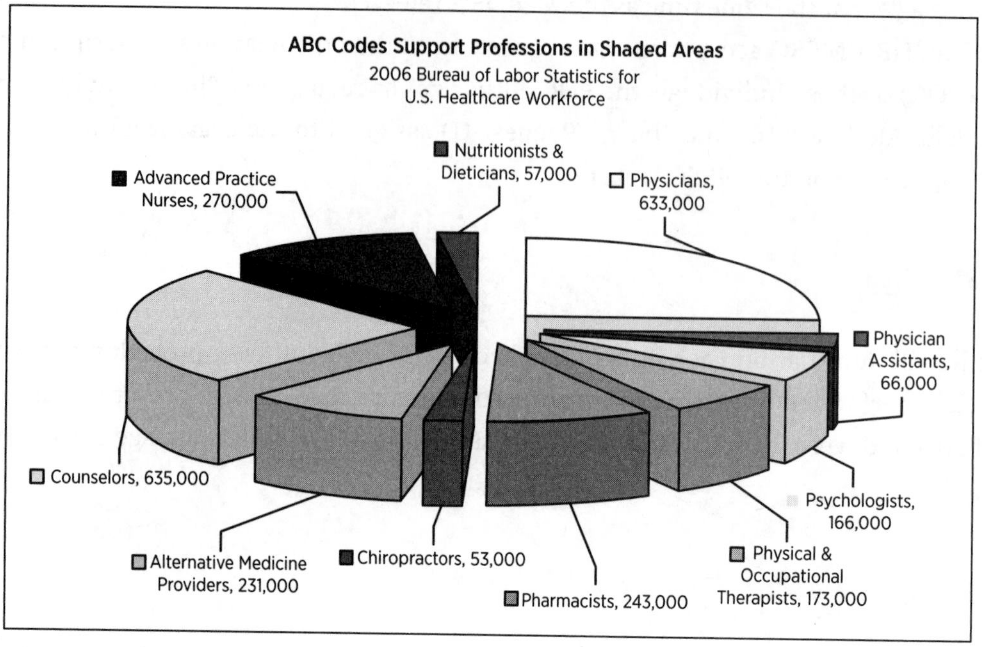

ABC Codes Support Professions in Shaded Areas
2006 Bureau of Labor Statistics for
U.S. Healthcare Workforce

- Nutritionists & Dieticians, 57,000
- Physicians, 633,000
- Advanced Practice Nurses, 270,000
- Physician Assistants, 66,000
- Counselors, 635,000
- Psychologists, 166,000
- Alternative Medicine Providers, 231,000
- Chiropractors, 53,000
- Physical & Occupational Therapists, 173,000
- Pharmacists, 243,000

Note: Shaded-areas indicate gaps in coding targeted by ABC codes.

Source: Alternative Link 2016.

Content of ABC Codes

The five-character alphabetic ABC codes describe a wide assortment of integrative healthcare practices, including what is said, done, ordered, prescribed, or distributed by providers of alternative medicine. Figure 13.8 illustrates the coding hierarchy of an ABC code.

In addition, two-character alphanumeric modifiers are available for osteopaths to identify the area of manipulative treatment (see table 13.10). Modifiers follow the five-character alphabetic ABC code. The two are combined into a seven-character code.

FIGURE 13.8. Coding hierarchy of ABC code

> The coding hierarchy of ABC code is section, subsection, heading, and intervention.
> Using code CBGAA, Acupressure each 15 minutes, as an example,
> C = Practice Specialties section
> B = Somatic education and Massage subsection
> G = Oriental massage heading
> A = Specific intervention, which is acupressure

Source: Alternative Link 2016.

TABLE 13.10. Modifiers to delineate bone area being manipulated

Modifier	Bone
1A	Occipital bone
1B	1st cervical bone (C1)
1C	2nd cervical bone (C2)
1D	3–6 cervical bones (C3–C6)
1E	7th cervical bone (C7)
1F	1st thoracic bone (T1)
1G	2nd thoracic bone (T2)
1H	3rd–6th thoracic bones (T3–T6)
1I (i)	7th through 11th thoracic bones (T7–T11)
1J	12th thoracic bone (T12)
1K	1st–2nd ribs
1L	3rd–6th ribs
1M	7th–10th ribs
1N	11th–12th ribs
1O (o)	1st lumbar bone
1P	2nd–4th lumbar bones (L2–L4)
1Q	5th lumbar bone (L5)
1R	Sacrum
1S	Ilium
1T	Femur or femoral bone
1U	Tibia
1V	Fibula
1W	Talus bone
1X	Calcaneus
1Y	Cuboid bone
1Z	Navicular bone
2A	Cuneiform bones
2B	Metatarsal bones
2C	Foot phalanges
2D	Clavicle

(continued)

TABLE 13.10. Continued

Modifier	Bone
2E S	Scapula
2F	Humerus
2G	Radius
2H	Ulna
2I (i)	Carpal bones
2J	Metacarpal bones
2K	Finger phalanges
2L	Mandible
2M	Hyoid bone
2N	Coccyx
2O (o)	Patella
2P	Maxilla or maxillary bone(s)
2Q	Frontal bone
2R	Parietal bone
2S	Temporal bone
2T	Sphenoid bone
2U	Ethmoid bone
2V	Lacrimal bone
2W	Nasal bone
2X	Vomer bone
2Y	Palatine bone
2Z	Zygomatic bone
3A	Sternum
3B	Tarsal bones

Source: Alternative Link 2016.

ABC Coding Solutions also offers RVUs through a license agreement with Relative Value Studies, Inc. (RVSI) that indicates the financial worth of the procedure, treatment, or service. RVUs are established by RVSI by gathering information from the integrative healthcare practitioners (Alternative Link 2016).

Principles and Guidelines for ABC Codes

ABC codes are used in the same insurance forms (837 Health Care Claim Professional/CMS-1500 and 837 Health Care Claim Institutional/CMS-1450), data fields, software applications, databases, information systems, and business processes as other HIPAA code sets. Figure 13.9 shows a sample superbill for use by a practitioner to identify an encounter.

ABC codes are not intended to replace any of the named HIPAA medical code set standards but, rather, to be used alongside them. According to information on ABC Coding Solutions' website, "ABC codes were designed for computerized documentation and measurement of non-physician and alternative medicine health services provided by over 2 million health professionals. ABC codes are also used to supplement conventional medical codes when filing health insurance claims and can automate reimbursement and comparative effectiveness research" (ABC Coding Solutions 2018).

Process for Revision of and Updates to ABC Codes

ABC Coding Solutions-Alternative Link has the primary responsibility for updating ABC codes. Updating is accomplished through an open and impartial process. New codes or terminology can be added, obsolete codes retired, and codes and terminology modified. Anyone can suggest changes to the ABC codes by submitting an ABC Terminology and Code Request Form to ABC Coding Solutions-Alternative Link.

According to the ABC Coding Solutions' website, requests for updates are checked by an ABC Coding Solutions expert. Once the information is verified, subject matter experts review the proposals and recommendations are made. This process helps to ensure that the ABC codes remain complete and accurate as changes in healthcare practices occur.

Tools to Access and Use

The IARC offers ICD-O-3 and ICD-O-3.1 online as fully searchable electronic resources. A list of ICPC-2 codes is available as a PDF downloadable document and the various ICPC-2e versions may be downloaded from the Norwegian Directorate of Health—Department of Standardization web page. MSSO has a number of tools including a MedDRA Web-Based Browser (WBB) and Desktop Browser (MDB), the WebCR for submitting change requests online, a MedDRA Version Analysis Tool (MVAT), and a number of videocasts for learning MedDRA. ABC Coding Solutions offers an ASCII data file to be used to load the codes into electronic products. A digital ABC Coding Manual is also an option. Find-A-Code provides an ABC code browser.

FIGURE 13.9. Superbill

Superbills for Super-Efficiency

Create a personalized list of coded services on your own form to save and simplify coding.
Call us at 1-877-621-5465 for a price quote.

Sample Group Practice for Oriental Medicine, Reflexology and Massage Therapy
860 Main Street
Anytown, USA 93420

(505) 875-0001 Office
(505) 875-0002 Fax
mail@ABCcodes.com

Tax ID # 99- 999999
State License # 00000

Last Name: _____ First Name: _____
SS#: _____ Referred by: _____
Address: _____ City: _____ State: _____ Zip Code: _____
Home Phone: _____ Work Phone: _____ Cell Phone: _____
E-mail: _____ Miscellaneous: _____
Diagnosis / Complaint: _____

ABC/CPT Code	DESCRIPTION	# / $	ABC/CPT Code	DESCRIPTION	# / $	ABC/CPT Code	DESCRIPTION	# / $
New Wellness Visit w/o ICD Diagnosis			**Multiple Specialties**			**Herbs and Natural Substances**		
ABAAB 99402	Wellness 30 minutes		BAAAF 97039	Cold friction each 20 minutes		GAGAG	Ginseng / ren shen / xi yan she	
ABAAC 99403	Wellness 45 minutes		BABAE 97039	Magnet therapy each 15 minutes		GBAAR	Arctostaphylos uva ursi / uva ursi leaf	
Existing client in-office with ICD diagnosis			BAEAC 97039	Cold laser therapy each treatment		GBHAJ	Hydrastis canadensis / goldenseal	
ACAAG 99203	30 minutes in-office Oriental medicine intake		BBAAH 97110	Postural exercise individual each 15 minutes		GCACQ	Five flower formula / rescue remedy	
ACAAH 99499	10 minutes in-office reflexology intake		BBABY 97139	PNF individual each 15 minutes		GCCBQ	Eucalyptus globulus	
ACAAJ 99215	20 minutes in-office massage therapy intake		BCAAS 97110	Range-of-motion therapeutic exercise individual each 15 min.		GCCCA	Jasminum officinalis	
Existing Client Visit w/o Diagnosis			BDCAD 95999	Electronic muscle testing one region each test		GCCCF	Lavendula officinalis	
ACBAF 99212	20 minutes in-office Oriental medicine intake		BDDAB 95831	Extremity or trunk manual testing each 15 minutes		**Substance Administration**		
ACBAI 99499	20 minutes in-office reflexology intake		**Oriental Medicine Services**			DDADV 97139	Essential oil inhalation each 15 minutes	
ACBAD 99212	10 minutes in-office massage therapy intake		CABAB 97810	Auricular acupuncture each 15 minutes		DDADW 97139	Essential oil compress each 15 minutes	
General Services			CABAE 97810	Acupuncture initial each 15 minutes		**Common Interventions**		
ADBAA 99050	After-hours care until 10 p.m. narrative required		CABAG 97810	Trigger point acupuncture each 15 minutes		ADYAB	Laboratory procedure order no charge	
ADYAL	Specialist referral		CACAB 17999	Cupping each 15 minutes		NAAHI 99199	Body pressure management	
ADYAN	Practitioner referral		CACAC	Ear seeds or pellets each 15 minutes		NAANG 97799	Mobility therapy	
ADZAM	Compounding Oriental herbs each 5 minutes		CACAE 97810	Moxibustion each 15 minutes		CBAAA 99199	Core energetics each 15 minutes	
ADZAX	Therapeutic grade essential oil dispensing		CACAI 97810	Auricular therapy each 15 minutes		CBBBM 97140	Reflexology hand each 15 minutes	
Practice Specialties								
CBBAY 97124	Touch for health™ each 15 minutes		CBCAF 99199	Reiki each 15 minutes		CBECB 97124	Swedish massage each 15 minutes	
CBBBC 97124	Zero balancing™ each 30 minutes		CBEAB 97124	Craniosacral therapy each 15 minutes		CBEBH 97124	Trigger-point therapy each 15 minutes	
CBBBN 97140	Reflexology foot each 15 minutes		CBEAG 97124	Infant massage each 15 minutes		CBEBW 97039	Hot stone therapy each 15 minutes	
CBBBQ 97112	Neuromuscular therapy each 15 minutes		CBEAT 97124	Prenatal massage each 15 minutes		CBGAB 97139	Anma therapy each 15 minutes	
CBCAC 99199	Polarity therapy each 15 minutes		CBEBB 97124	Sports massage each 15 minutes		CBGAK 97139	Tuina each 15 minutes	

Client Self-Care Notes:
_____
_____

 # / $ Represents Number of Units or Fee Charged

Nutritional Items		Supply Items		Charges	
				Services	
				Nutritional/Supply Items	
				Adjustments	
				TOTAL CHARGES	
				AMOUNT PAID	

Practitioner Signature: _____ Date: _____

Patient Signature: _____ Date: _____

CPT® is a registered trademark of the American Medical Association

The sample Superbill above is based on three separate licenses for one practitioner.
To avoid fraudulent billing, be advised not to copy information from this sample.

Source: Alternative Link 2016.

Adoption and Use Cases

ICD-O-3 has been used for over 35 years as the standard tool for coding neoplasms in tumor and cancer registries and in pathology laboratories. In the US, a variation of ICPC, the Reason for Visit Classification, classifies the patient's stated reason for the visit or chief complaint in national ambulatory care surveys. MedDRA is employed in several Food and Drug Administration Centers including the Center for Drug Evaluation and Research, Center for Biologics and Research, and Center for Food Safety and Applied Nutrition. Although ABC codes have not been officially adopted, they have been found to correctly identify procedures, treatments, and services performed by integrative health professionals.

Use Case One: Analyzing Cancer Cases

A cancer registrar evaluated the patient's medical record in order to code and abstract data and then enter this information into the hospital's computer system. In analyzing the case, the registrar noted the pathology report of a biopsy of the right and left tonsils showed diffuse large B cell lymphoma. Upon further review, the record indicated scans were negative for lymphadenopathy and the bone marrow biopsy as benign. Stage was noted by the radiation oncologist as localized bilateral tonsil primary lymphoma. The registrar checked the coding rules to determine if the patient's diagnosis should be coded in ICD-O-3 as multiple primary or one primary neoplasm. Based on Multiple primary rules M2, the register coded this case as a single primary.

Use Case Two: Reporting Adverse Events with MedDRA

The FDA's Adverse Event Reporting System (FAERS) database contains information on adverse event and medical error reports. When electronically submitting postmarketing individual case safety reports (ICSRs), the Specifications for Preparing and Submitting Electronic ICSRs and ICSR Attachments document stipulates the use of MedDRA to code the medical terms for the B2 Data Element Reactions or Events (FDA 2018). The FDA also recommends the use of MedDRA for other data elements such as reported cause of death.

CHECK YOUR UNDERSTANDING

1. Which section remained unchanged in the ICD-O-3 version?

2. The agreed statement of the reason(s) why a patient enters the healthcare system, representing the demand for care by that person, is the definition for which of the following:

   a. Primary diagnosis

   b. Problem list

   c. Process of care

   d. Reasons for encounter

3. Which of the following insurance claim forms may be used to submit ABC codes?

   a. 2711

   b. 2787

   c. 1500

   d. 2700

4. In the MedDRA hierarchy, preferred terms map to:

   a. Lowest-level terms

   b. High-level terms

   c. A system organ class term

   d. A high-level group term

5. What does the fifth digit in the morphology code indicate?

   a. Histology

   b. Grading

   c. Behavior

   d. None of the above

   e. All of the above

REVIEW

1. In ICD-O-3, how many different categories of codes are used to describe the site?

   a. One

   b. Two

   c. Four

   d. Five

2. ICPC consists of a biaxial configuration, chapters, and:

   a. Sections

   b. Components

   c. Subchapters

   d. Titles

3. Which component is addressed by the ICPC-2 code F82, Detached retina?

   a. Component 1
   b. Component 6
   c. Component 7
   d. Component 3

4. True or false? WICC is responsible for maintenance of and updates to ICPC.

   a. True
   b. False

5. True or false? The FDA requires the use of MedDRA to report adverse effects of pharmaceuticals.

   a. True
   b. False

6. Which of the following is not a simple change request in MedDRA?

   a. Add a preferred term
   b. Add a lowest-level term
   c. Add a new term
   d. Add a high-level group term

7. The ABC codes' two-character alphanumeric modifier identifies the:

   a. Area of osteopathic manipulative treatment
   b. Area of acupuncture intervention
   c. Area of heat therapy
   d. Area of massage treatment

8. What does the morphology code in ICD-O-3 identify?

9. True or false? ABC codes are an integral part of HCPCS and follow the same principles and guidelines.

   a. True
   b. False

10. Assign the final two digits for the following statement: Poorly differentiated carcinoma. M-8010/_ _

References

Alternative Link. 2016. *ABC Coding Manual for Integrative Healthcare*. Carlsbad: ABC Coding Solutions.

ABC Coding Solutions. 2018. Why ABC Codes. https://abccodes.com/why-abc-codes/.

Bentzen, N., ed. 2003. *Wonca Dictionary of General/Family Practice*. Copenhagen: Wonca International Classification Committee.

Centers for Disease Control and Prevention (CDC). 2018. Ambulatory Health Care Data. https://www.cdc.gov/nchs/ahcd/index.htm.

Fritz, A. et al., eds. 2012. *International Classification of Diseases for Oncology*, 3rd ed. Geneva: WHO.

International Agency for Research on Cancer (IARC). 2018a. About ICD-O. http://codes.iarc.fr/abouticdo.php.

International Agency for Research on Cancer (IARC). 2018b. Using ICD-O-3 Online. http://codes.iarc.fr/usingicdo.php.

International Agency for Research on Cancer (IARC). 2018c. Morphological Codes. http://codes.iarc.fr/codegroup/2.

International Conference on Harmonisation of Technical Requirements for Registration of Pharmaceuticals for Human Use (ICH). 2018a. What's New MedDRA Version 21.1. https://www.meddra.org/sites/default/files/guidance/file/whatsnew_21_1_english.pdf.

International Conference on Harmonisation of Technical Requirements for Registration of Pharmaceuticals for Human Use (ICH). 2018b. MedDRA Coding Basics. https://www.meddra.org/sites/default/files/page/documents_insert/000140_meddra_coding_basics_webinar.pdf.

International Conference on Harmonisation of Technical Requirements for Registration of Pharmaceuticals for Human Use (ICH). 2018c. Introductory Guide MedDRA Version 21.1. https://www.meddra.org/sites/default/files/guidance/file/intguide_21_1_english.pdf.

International Conference on Harmonisation of Technical Requirements for Registration of Pharmaceuticals for Human Use (ICH). 2018d. Introductory Guide for Standardised MedDRA Queries (SMQs) Version 21.1. https://www.meddra.org/sites/default/files/guidance/file/smq_intguide_21_1_english.pdf.

International Conference on Harmonisation of Technical Requirements for Registration of Pharmaceuticals for Human Use (ICH). 2018e. Medical Dictionary for Regulatory Activities (MedDRA) Change Request Information. https://www.meddra.org/sites/default/files/page/documents/000188_changereq_info.pdf.

International Conference on Harmonisation of Technical Requirements for Registration of Pharmaceuticals for Human Use (ICH). 2013. Understanding MedDRA. http://www.meddra.org/sites/default/files/page/documents/meddra2013.pdf.

Medical Dictionary for Regulatory Activities (MedDRA). n.d.a. About MedDRA. http://www.meddra.org/about-meddra/history.

Medical Dictionary for Regulatory Activities (MedDRA). n.d.b. Standardised MedDRA Queries (SMQs). http://www.meddra.org/how-to-use/tools/smqs.

Molina, S. 2004. ABC codes: An essential tool for health benefit cost management and consumer-driven health plans. *Compensation & Benefits Review* 36(5):71–77.

Pace, W. D., E. W. Staton, G. S. Higgins, D. S. Main, D. R. West, and D. M. Harris. 2003. Database Design to Ensure Anonymous Study of Medical Errors: A Report from the ASIPS Collaborative. http://www.ncbi.nlm.nih.gov/pmc/articles/PMC264430/.

Primary Health Care Classification Consortium (PH3C). (2018a). ICPC-3 Consortium, a 3 Years International Project. http://www.ph3c.org/4daction/w3_CatVisu/en/icpc.html?wCatIDAdmin=1106.

Primary Health Care Classification Consortium (PH3C). (2018b). ICPC-3 Roadmap Milestones. http://www.ph3c.org/4daction/w3_CatVisu/en/doc-about--icpc3.html?wCatIDAdmin=4&wDocID=209&wDocTable=62.

Soler, J. K. n.d. International Classification of Primary Care – Version 2 (ICPC-2): A Brief Overview. http://www.ph3c.org/4daction/w3_CatVisu/en/download-slides.html?wCatIDAdmin=1131.

US Department of Health and Human Services, Food and Drug Administration (FDA). 2018 (February). Specifications for Preparing and Submitting Electronic ICSRs and ICSR Attachments. https://www.fda.gov/downloads/Drugs/GuidanceComplianceRegulatoryInformation/Surveillance/AdverseDrugEffects/UCM601820.pdf.

Wonca International Classification Committee (WICC). 2005. ICPC-2. http://www.ph3c.org/ph3c/docs/27/000098/0000054.pdf.

World Health Organization (WHO). 2018. Derived and Related Classifications in the WHO-FIC. http://www.who.int/classifications/related/en/.

World Health Organization (WHO). 2016. *International Statistical Classification of Diseases and Related Health Problems 10th Revision, Volume 2*, 5th ed. Geneva: WHO.

Part III

HIT Data Standards and Interoperability

Healthcare Data Governance and Data Set Standards

Mary H. Stanfill, MBI, RHIA, CCS, CCS-P, FAHIMA

LEARNING OBJECTIVES

- Explain the importance of data governance
- Explain the functions and characteristics of data quality management
- Distinguish between data dictionary, data element, data element domain, and data set
- Explain the general purpose of healthcare data sets
- Describe how healthcare data sets support the functions and characteristics of data quality
- Examine the relationship between healthcare data sets and code sets, clinical terminologies, and classification systems
- Compare data set standards for interoperability including the Patient Summary Standards Set, the US Core Data for Interoperability, the Uniform Hospital Discharge Data Set, and the Minimum Data Set for Long-term Care
- Compare data set standards for performance and quality measurement including the Outcomes and Assessment Information Set, the Healthcare Effectiveness Data and Information Set, Core Measures for ORYX, and CMS electronic clinical quality measures

KEY TERMS

- Accountability measure
- Artefact
- Candidate class
- Data class

- Data dictionary
- Data element
- Data element domain
- Data governance
- Data quality management (DQM)
- Data set
- Electronic clinical quality measure (eCQM)
- Emerging data class
- FAIR data principles
- Healthcare Effectiveness Data and Information Set (HEDIS)
- Minimum Data Set (MDS)
- Outcomes and Assessment Information Set (OASIS)
- Patient Summary Standards Set (PSSS)
- Provenance
- Resident assessment instrument (RAI)
- Standards set
- Uniform Hospital Discharge Data Set (UHDDS)
- US Core Data for Interoperability (USCDI)

Introduction

The healthcare industry needs **data governance** programs to help manage the growing amount of electronic data. Data governance includes data modeling, data mapping, data audit, data quality controls, data quality management, data architecture, and data dictionaries (Downing 2018). Healthcare data is a fundamental resource that must be consistent, valid, accurate, and used appropriately. This data represents the facts or measurements that, when put into context, become healthcare information. Without data, there is no information. In healthcare settings, data are stored in the individual's health record whether that record is in paper or electronic format. As use of health information technology becomes widespread, however, data are shared and repurposed in new and innovative ways, making data quality more important than ever.

This chapter defines data quality management, data sets, and data dictionaries and illustrates how data set standards, enabled by code sets, clinical terminologies, and classification systems, support the functions and characteristics of quality data outlined in the AHIMA data quality management model. An overview of the FAIR guiding principles for scientific data management is presented as an ideal to aspire to. This is followed by a review of specific examples of data sets commonly used today for health information exchange and interoperability as well as examples of data sets for performance and quality measurement. Part of the data dictionary for the Uniform Hospital Discharge Data Set (UHDDS) is included to illustrate the relationship between a data dictionary and a data set specification.

Developer

Data sets and data dictionaries may be created internally by healthcare providers or produced externally by standards organizations such as the Health Level Seven International (HL7), government agencies such as the Centers for Medicare and Medicaid Services (CMS), or software vendors. The owner of the data dictionary and data set determines the process for revisions and updates.

Purpose and Content

Data quality management (DQM), a key data governance initiative, is defined as the business processes that ensure the integrity of an organization's data (Davoudi et al. 2015). Governance functions ensure that the use and management of data and information is compliant with jurisdictional law, regulations, standards, and organizational policies. The main outcome of DQM is knowledge regarding the quality of healthcare data and its fitness for applicable use in all of its intended purposes. Because of the vast amounts of data available, there needs to be some way to standardize and organize them so they can be managed. Code sets, clinical terminologies, and classification systems enable the numerous portions of data contained in the health record to be standardized. Creating a data set is a method to capture and organize certain data elements in order to turn data into information. Data set standards therefore support data quality management and, as a result, data governance. Figure 14.1 illustrates how data management, data classifications, and data standards and definitions are all functions of data governance.

FIGURE 14.1. Data governance functions

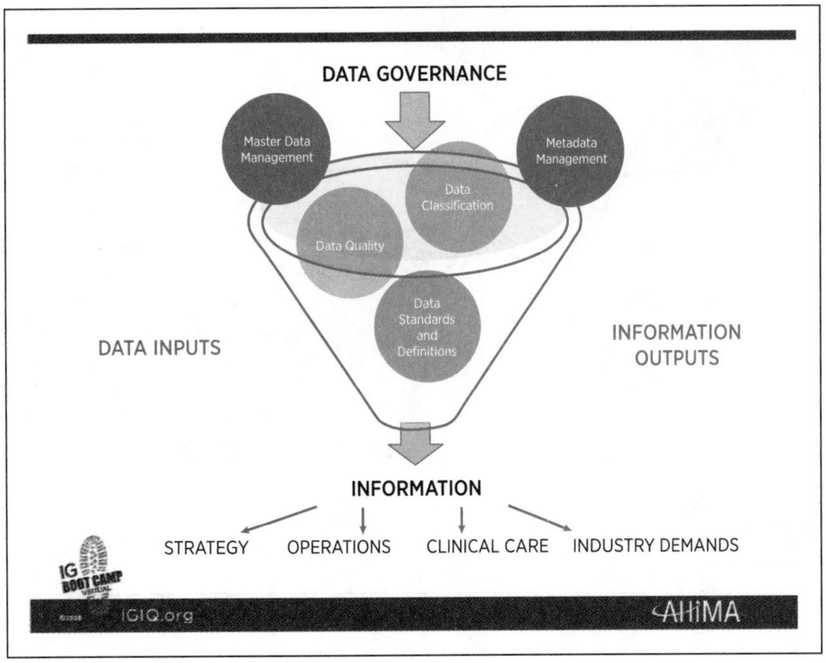

Data Quality Management Model

The AHIMA DQM model (Davoudi et al. 2015) was originally developed to illustrate the different data quality challenges that healthcare professionals face. Figure 14.2 presents a graphic of the DQM domains as they relate to the characteristics of data integrity. Table 14.1 presents the four data quality management functions defined in the AHIMA DQM model and describes how data sets incorporate each function. It also includes examples, using the data sets described later in this chapter, to illustrate these functions. Table 14.2 presents the 10 characteristics of data quality defined in the AHIMA DQM model and describes how data sets exemplify each characteristic.

FAIR Data Principles

Before leaving the subject of data quality management, a brief discussion of the **FAIR data principles** is warranted. The FAIR data principles are a set of guidelines to ensure that data are Findable, Accessible, Interoperable, and Reusable. These principles are not specific to the

FIGURE 14.2. Data quality functions and characteristics

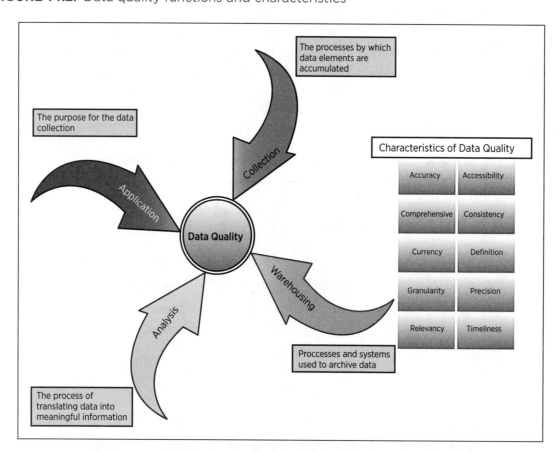

Source: Davoudi et al. 2015.

TABLE 14.1. DQM functions

DQM Function	Data Set Examples
Application (The purpose for the data collection)	Data sets clearly present the purpose, or aim, of collecting the specified data and provide a standard to enable complete data collection with defined values for consistency across applications and systems. Data set standards ensure the data included in the set are valuable and appropriate for the intended purpose of the data set. Examples: UHDDS facilitates collecting comparable health information from hospitals, MDS facilitates data collection from nursing homes, and OASIS gathers data on patients receiving services from a home health agency.
Collection (The processes by which data elements are accumulated)	Data sets standardize data collections by defining the specific standard to be use for a data element and specifying data definitions. They also document the versions of a named data standard, providing a mechanism to communicate updates and changes. Some data sets provide a validated data collection instrument. Examples: The UHDDS data dictionary defines common, uniform data elements and requires diagnoses to be represented with the current version of ICD-10-CM. The RAI is a standard assessment used to collect data on residents in nursing homes.
Warehousing and Interoperability (Processes and systems used to share and archive data)	Data sets define data collectors and data end users for a particular use case. Data sets can reduce redundant data collection and support interoperability. Examples: UHDDS includes guidelines for use of the specified data elements. The PSSS identifies appropriate standards for the defined use case. The USCDI specifies a common set of data classes and identifies transparent processes for data exchange and reuse.
Analysis (The process of translating data into meaningful information)	Data sets provide a context for analyzing (interpreting, using) the data. Data sets allow for appropriate data comparisons at an appropriate (consistent) level of detail. Examples: MDS assessment data is used by CMS for long-term quality monitoring and surveyors find the MDS helpful in identifying potential problem areas to address in the survey process. OASIS includes process items that support measurement of evidence-based practices. HEDIS is designed to provide information to compare the performance of managed healthcare plans.

healthcare industry but are applicable across all scientific domains. The FAIR guiding principles for scientific data management and stewardship, created and endorsed by a diverse group of stakeholders, were first published in 2016. The FAIR principles put specific emphasis on enhancing the ability of machines to automatically find and use data, in addition to supporting its reuse by individuals. These foundational, concise principles emphasize that all research "objects" should be Findable, Accessible, Interoperable, and Reusable for machines and people (Wilkinson et al. 2016). Table 14.3 includes the 15 concise FAIR principles that are applicable to data (or any digital object), metadata (information about that digital object), and infrastructure.

TABLE 14.2. DQM characteristics

DQM Characteristic	Data Set Examples
Data Accessibility (Level of ease to legally obtain protected data)	Data sets provide a mechanism to obtain a group of data. Some data set standards include a specific instrument and process to access data.
Data Accuracy (Extent to which data are free of identifiable errors)	Data sets define the aim for collecting the data and often define acceptable values to aid in data accuracy. Ensuring data accuracy also involves education and training. Many data set owners disseminate training for appropriate use and implementation.
Data Comprehensiveness (Extent to which all required data are collected, documenting exclusions)	Data sets define what to include and how it will be used. The data is comprehensive if all data included in the set are collected. Data sets often define data elements in terms of what is included and what is specifically excluded.
Data Consistency (Extent to which data are reliable, identical, reproducible)	Data sets typically define the data source, types, codes, and calculations to ensure data consistency.
Data Currency (Extent to which data are up to date at a specific point in time)	Data sets document the version of data applicable to specific datum included in the data set. This provides a mechanism to communicate data currency to end users.
Data Definition (The specific meaning of a data element)	Data sets include data definitions to facilitate accurate data collection and document specific attributes of the datum included in the set.
Data Granularity (Level of detail for data quality is defined)	Data sets define the specific terminology (vocabulary) to be used for certain data elements in order to capture data at the appropriate level of detail (granularity).
Data Precision (Degree to which data supports its purpose)	Data sets are designed for specific purposes and define acceptable standards to support the purpose of the data set.
Data Relevancy (Extent to which data are useful for the stated purpose)	Data sets are designed for a specific use, which ensures that data will be relevant for the stated purpose. In addition, the rationale for collecting defined data elements is typically defined.
Data Timeliness (Availability of up-to-date data within a time frame)	Data sets may include time frames for specific data elements. For example, a data set may specify the applicable version for a required code set, clinical terminology, or classification system.

For example, principle F1 defines that both metadata and data are assigned a globally unique and persistent identifier.

The FAIR principles have received worldwide recognition as a useful framework for thinking about sharing data in a way that will enable maximum use and reuse (ANDS 2019). The principles are particularly useful in healthcare because they:

TABLE 14.3. FAIR principles

Findable: The first step in (re)using data is to find them. Metadata and data should be easy to find for both humans and computers. Machine-readable metadata are essential for automatic discovery of datasets and services.	
F1.	(Meta)data are assigned a globally unique and persistent identifier
F2.	Data are described with rich metadata
F3.	Metadata clearly and explicitly include the identifier of the data they describe
F4.	(Meta)data are registered or indexed in a searchable resource
Accessible: Once the user finds the required data, she/he needs to know how they can be accessed, possibly including authentication and authorization.	
A1.	(Meta)data are retrievable by their identifier using a standardized communications protocol
A1.1	The protocol is open, free, and universally implementable
A1.2	The protocol allows for an authentication and authorization procedure, where necessary
A2.	Metadata are accessible, even when the data are no longer available
Interoperable: The data usually need to be integrated with other data. In addition, the data need to interoperate with applications or workflows for analysis, storage, and processing.	
I1.	(Meta)data use a formal, accessible, shared, and broadly applicable language for knowledge representation
I2.	(Meta)data use vocabularies that follow FAIR principles
I3.	(Meta)data include qualified references to other (meta)data
Reusable: The ultimate goal of FAIR is to optimize the reuse of data. To achieve this, metadata and data should be well described so that they can be replicated and/or combined in different settings.	
R1.	(Meta)data are richly described with a plurality of accurate and relevant attributes
R1.1	(Meta)data are released with a clear and accessible data usage license
R1.2	(Meta)data are associated with detailed provenance
R1.3	(Meta)data meet domain-relevant community standards

Source: GoFAIR 2019.

- Support knowledge discovery and innovation
- Support data and knowledge integration
- Promote sharing and reuse of data
- Are discipline independent and allow for differences in disciplines

- Improve the reproducibility and reliability of research
- Allow an organization to stay aligned with international standards
- Enable new research questions to be answered

Various organizations have undertaken the "FAIRification" process, including those in healthcare (Imming 2018), and metrics have been developed to evaluate "FAIRness" (GO FAIR Metrics Group 2019). These early efforts have demonstrated that FAIRness is not easy to achieve but is worthwhile. Though healthcare has a long way to go to meet the ideal set forth in the FAIR principles, data sets that include vocabulary standards with unique and persistent identifiers are consistent with FAIR principles F1 and I2. Likewise, the descriptions and attributes of data elements defined in health data dictionaries are a step in the right direction towards principles F2, F3, and R1.

Data Dictionaries

Data set standards are fundamental to data governance programs and data quality management. Data sets are made up of **data elements**. The International Organization for Standardization (ISO) defines a data element as a unit of data for which the definition, identification, representation, and permissible values are specified by means of a set of attributes (ISO 2013).

The terms *data dictionary* and *data set* have been defined as follows (AHIMA 2017, 70, 72):

- A **data dictionary** is a descriptive list of names (also called representations or displays), definitions, and attributes of data elements to be collected in an information system or database.
- A **data set** is a list of recommended data elements with uniform definitions.

Standardized data sets encourage healthcare providers to collect and report data in a standardized manner (Amatayakul 2017, 300). Identifying the data elements that should be collected and having uniform definitions for common terms ensures that data collected from a variety of healthcare settings will share a standard definition. Standardizing data elements and definitions makes it possible to compare the data collected at different facilities. For example, when data are standardized, the term *admission* means the same thing at City Hospital and at University Hospital. Because both hospitals define *admission* in the same way, they can be compared with each other on such things as number of admissions and percentage of occupancy. When possible, data elements should be represented with a standard code set, clinical terminology, or classification system in order for shared meaning to occur.

The data elements listed in a data dictionary serve as a source for creating a data set. In addition, a data dictionary provides definitions for data elements that comprise a data set and includes each data element's principles and guidelines for use. According to Shakir (1999), the data dictionary includes other information such as **data element domain** that is key to data set creation. Shakir defines data element domain as "a specification of the allowable values for each data element."

Data attributes such as length also are a part of a data dictionary. For example, the UHDDS, which is considered a core data set for hospital reporting, contains a data dictionary where the principal diagnosis, a data element, is defined along with its allowable value, an ICD-10-CM code.

The contents of data sets vary by their purpose. The content of a data set defined for health information exchange, such as the UHDDS, is very different from the content of a data set intended to report performance or quality measures, such as the Outcomes and Assessment Information Set (OASIS). However, data sets are not meant to limit the number of data elements that can be collected. Most healthcare organizations collect additional data elements that have meaning for their specific administrative and clinical operations.

As illustrated by the characteristics in table 14.2, having defined data sets ensures data quality. Furthermore, standardized data sets provide information about the effectiveness of interventions and treatments for specific diseases, thereby improving the quality and safety of healthcare, maximizing the effectiveness of health promotions and care, minimizing the burden on those responsible for generating the data, and helping facilitate efficient reuse of data (Giannangelo 2007).

Data Sets

Health information management (HIM) professionals will likely encounter many types of data sets. Some originate from data reporting requirements from federal initiatives, such as promoting interoperability programs, and others from public initiatives related to standardized performance measures. Data sets may be formed for such activities as research, clinical trials, quality and safety improvement, reimbursement, accreditation, and exchanging clinical information (Giannangelo 2007). The MEDPAR Limited Data Set (LDS), for example, allows researchers to track inpatient history and patterns and outcomes of care over time (CMS 2019a). Acute care hospitals use the Agency for Healthcare Research and Quality (AHRQ) Common Formats when reporting patient safety events. Contained within Hospital Version 2.0a are technical specifications, which include a data dictionary. By defining the Common Formats' data elements and their attributes, standardization is possible.

Data Sets for Health Information Exchange and Interoperability

Data sets may be formed for a variety of reasons. Some are created to collect statistical data for reporting to national and state registries while others collect data for clinical decision support and for computation and reporting of clinical quality measures. In the past, the data elements contained in the data set were captured manually. With the implementation of electronic health records (EHR), data capture occurs when clinical data documentation is done at the time of care.

The data sets for health information exchange and interoperability explored in this section include: Patient Summary Standards Set (PSSS), US Core Data for Interoperability (USCDI), Uniform Hospital Discharge Data Set (UHDDS), Resident Assessment Instrument (RAI), and Minimum Data Set (MDS).

Patient Summary Standards Set

The Joint Initiative on SDO Global Health Informatics Standardization (JIC) is a federation of standards and profiling development organizations (SDOs) that was formed to enable common, timely health informatics standards by addressing and resolving issues of gaps, overlaps, and counterproductive standardization efforts. In 2015, the JIC defined a specific strategic goal to "...contribute to better global patient health outcomes by providing strategic leadership in the specification of sets of implementable standards for health information sharing" (JIC 2018, 7). Stakeholders are often confused by the myriad of choices that exist when conceiving, selecting, and deploying standards in healthcare IT solutions. While most agree that a standardized approach is best, it is often challenging to agree on which specifications are actually the best, given a particular need. The JIC is in a unique position to clarify the choices available to stakeholders and to help them with standards use. JIC can provide authoritative commentary and guidelines about the concurrent use of specifications developed by different SDOs to support appropriate standardization of an informatics business requirement. Thus JIC began working to create **standards sets**. The working definition of a standards set is a "coherent collection of standards and standards artefacts that support a specific use case"(JIC 2018, 7). An **artefact** may be a named standard, profile, guide, or implementation specification used to achieve interoperability.

The first standards set the JIC prioritized for development was the Patient Summary. The JIC chose this as the first Use Case for a Standards Set because there are efforts across the globe at all levels to develop Patient Summaries, which is leading to duplication and potential lack of interoperability. The JIC created the Patient Summary working definition as "the minimum set of information needed to assure healthcare coordination and the continuity of care" (JIC 2018, 8). The use case focused on continuity of care for patients suffering from a pre-existing chronic disease, such as COPD. Thus, the specific Use Case for the **Patient Summary Standard Set (PSSS)** was defined as "access patient summary in acute care setting" (JIC 2018, 13).

The PSSS, first released in January 2018, is a guide to a set of health informatics standards and related materials that can be used to support the implementation of a Patient Summary. Its value is for use in electronic information systems to produce a Patient Summary that can be used in many different countries and by different providers. The PSSS does not recommend specific data standards, rather it provides sufficient detail to enable stakeholders to choose the most suitable standards to meet the requirements for a specific use case. The PSSS provides guidance about relevant standards, standards artefacts, and profiles that meet criteria to meet a specific Use Case for creating and sharing patient summaries. The PSSS guidance document includes a broad perspective on the different types of standards and related materials necessary for this purpose, explains how to assess the conformance of products that claim to use them, and highlights current and emerging practice.

The PSSS guidance document is free and is meant to be informative, not normative. It is predominantly geared toward vendors, health organizations, and government and policymakers who are exploring ways of developing and implementing patient summaries. The PSSS informs these stakeholders about existing or developing standards related to patient summaries. The PSSS guidance document includes the following:

- A clearly defined use case clarifying what is in and out of scope
- Currently available standards that meet specific selection criteria for inclusion
- Standards harmonization requirements
- Framework for conformity assessment
- Implementation guidance
- Information sheets on leading practices

The PSSS addresses data standards for demographic and nonclinical data items as well as standards for clinical data items (JIC 2018, 21). The 2018 release includes 28 required demographic and nonclinical data items, data that must be provided if it is available, and 13 optional demographic and nonclinical data items, data that may be provided based on the availability and the decision of the author or owner. Examples of required demographic and nonclinical data items include patient first and last name, patient ID, and responsible healthcare professional or document author. The 2018 release also includes 28 required clinical data items and an additional 25 optional clinical data items. Examples of required clinical data items include allergies, problems, procedures, and medications. Examples of optional clinical data items include medic alert, do not resuscitate alert, and social history. Approximately 39 standards are included in the first release of the PSSS, with an additional 11 standards evaluated as alternates. Standards are organized to address semantic interoperability as well as technical and functional interoperability. They are categorized to ensure comprehensive coverage. Table 14.4 shows the six standards categories in the PSSS and provides examples of some of the standards included in each category.

According to JIC, the PSSS is subject to the changing landscape in health and will be regularly updated based on user feedback to take into account the evolving nature of standards and related products. This first version is based on standards, artefacts, and profiles as of January 2018. Feedback on the initial release will be collected over a year and an updated version is anticipated in early 2019.

US Core Data for Interoperability

The 21st Century Cures Act defines interoperability in the context of health information technology and sets the expectation that all of a patient's health information that is stored

TABLE 14.4. PSSS Standards Categories

Standard Category	Examples
Standards for Semantic Interoperability	
Data-related Standards (content, format, structure)	ISO: 8601:2004 Date and time format HL7: C-CDA CCD R2.1
Semantic Content-related Standards (terminologies, vocabularies, code sets, terminology binding)	ISO: 3166-1 Country Codes SNOMED International: SNOMED CT Regenstrief: LOINC Universal Code System
Standards for Technical Interoperability	
Transport-related Standards (information exchange, technical, identifiers, exchange services)	HL7: Fast Healthcare Interoperability Resources (FHIR)
Security and Safety Related Standards (security, privacy, safety, consent, data use)	ISO: 27799:2016 Information security management in health using ISO/IEC 27002
Standards for Functional Interoperability	
Functional Service Related standards (business, information governance, systems API's and other)	ISO/HL7 10781:2015 HL7 Electronic health records-system functional model release 2 (EHR FM)
Implementation specification related standards (includes guides, profiles, reference implementations, workflow practices)	ISO 22600-3:2014 Health informatics – Privilege management and access control – Part 3: implementations

Source: JIC 2018, 32–41.

electronically will be able to be exchanged (21st Century Cures Act 2016). The **US Core Data for Interoperability (USCDI)** and its proposed expansion process aim to achieve the goals in the Cures Act by specifying a common set of data classes that are required for interoperable exchange and identifying a predictable, transparent, and collaborative process (ONC 2018a).

In 2015, the US Secretary of Health and Human Services (HHS) issued the 2015 Edition Health IT Certification Criteria final rule (ONC 2015). This 2015 Edition built upon previous rulemaking to facilitate greater interoperability and enable health information exchange. The 2015 Edition adopted the 2015 Edition Common Clinical Data Set (CCDS) definition (ONC 2018b). The CCDS evolved from the initial Meaningful Use Common Dataset that the Office of the National Coordinator for Health IT (ONC) adopted in 2012 (ONC 2015). As part of the ONC's continued efforts to expand the availability of a minimum baseline of data classes that must be commonly available for interoperable exchange, the draft USCDI builds off the CCDS definition and includes two additional data classes (Clinical Notes and Provenance). Clinical Notes is composed of structured (pick list or check box) and unstructured (free text) data. **Provenance** describes the metadata, or extra information about data, that can help answer questions such as when and who created the data. The data classes included in USCDI version 1 are presented in table 14.5.

TABLE 14.5. USCDI Version 1 data classes

USCDI v1 Data Classes	Data Elements	Terminology Standards Named
Assessment and plan of treatment		• Logical Observation Identifiers Names and Codes (LOINC) Database version 2.63 • SNOMED International, Systematized Nomenclature of Medicine Clinical Terms (SNOMED CT) U.S. Edition, March 2018 Release
Care team members		N/A
Clinical notes	Consultation note Discharge summary note History & physical Imaging narrative Laboratory report narrative Pathology report narrative Procedure note Progress note	• Logical Observation Identifiers Names and Codes (LOINC) Database version 2.63
Goals	Patient goals	• Logical Observation Identifiers Names and Codes (LOINC) Database version 2.63 • SNOMED International, Systematized Nomenclature of Medicine Clinical Terms (SNOMED CT) U.S. Edition, March 2018 Release
Health concerns		• Logical Observation Identifiers Names and Codes (LOINC) Database version 2.63 • SNOMED International, Systematized Nomenclature of Medicine Clinical Terms (SNOMED CT) U.S. Edition, March 2018 Release
Immunizations		• CDC IIS: Current HL7 Standard Code Set, CVX -- Vaccines Administered, updates through October 27, 2017 • CDC National Drug Code (NDC) Directory – Vaccine NDC Linker, updates through April 6, 2018
Laboratory	Tests Values/results	• Logical Observation Identifiers Names and Codes (LOINC) Database version 2.63 • SNOMED International, Systematized Nomenclature of Medicine Clinical Terms (SNOMED CT) U.S. Edition, March 2018 Release • The Unified Code of Units for Measure, Revision 1.9
Medications	Medications Medication allergies	• RxNorm, June 4, 2018 Full Release Update • The Unified Code of Units for Measure, Revision 1.9

(continued)

TABLE 14.5. Continued

USCDI v1 Data Classes	Data Elements	Terminology Standards Named
Patient Demographics	First name	
	Last name	
	Previous name	
	Middle name (including middle initial)	
	Suffix	
	Birth sex	Birth sex must be coded in accordance with HL7 Version 3 (V3) Standard, Value Sets for AdministrativeGender and NullFlavor (https://www.healthit.gov/sites/default/files/170299_ f_29_ hl7_v3_agender_and_nullflavor.pdf) attributed as follows: 1. Male. M 2. Female. F 3. Unknown. nullFlavor UNK
	Date of birth	
	Race	• The Office of Management and Budget Standards for Maintaining, Collecting, and Presenting Federal Data on Race and Ethnicity, Statistical Policy Directive No. 15, as revised, October 30, 1997 (https://obamawhitehouse.archives.gov/omb/fedreg_1997standards) • CDC Race and Ethnicity Code Set Version 1.0 (March 2000) (https://www.cdc.gov/phin/resources/vocabulary/index.html)
	Ethnicity	• The Office of Management and Budget Standards for Maintaining, Collecting, and Presenting Federal Data on Race and Ethnicity, Statistical Policy Directive No. 15, as revised, October 30, 1997 (https://obamawhitehouse.archives.gov/omb/fedreg_1997standards) • CDC Race and Ethnicity Code Set Version 1.0 (March 2000) (https://www.cdc.gov/phin/resources/vocabulary/index.html)
	Preferred language	• Request for Comment (RFC) 5646, "Tags for Identifying Languages", September 2009 (http://www.rfc-editor.org/info/rfc5646) See https://tools.ietf.org/html/bcp47
	Address	
	Phone number	
Problems		• SNOMED International, Systematized Nomenclature of Medicine Clinical Terms (SNOMED CT) U.S. Edition, March 2018 Release

TABLE 14.5. Continued

USCDI v1 Data Classes	Data Elements	Terminology Standards Named

Procedures		The code set specified in 45 CFR 162.1002(a)(5):
		• Health Care Financing Administration Common Procedure Coding System (HCPCS), as maintained and distributed by HHS.
		• Current Procedural Terminology, Fourth Edition (CPT-4), as maintained and distributed by the American Medical Association, for physician services and other healthcare services.
		• SNOMED International, Systematized Nomenclature of Medicine Clinical Terms (SNOMED CT) U.S. Edition, March 2018 Release
		• Optional:
		  • International Classification of Diseases ICD-10-PCS 2018
		• Optional for technology primarily developed to record dental procedures:
		  • The code set specified in 45 CFR 162.1002(a)(4) SNODENT, as maintained and distributed by the American Dental Association, for dental services.

Provenance	Author Author time stamp Author organization	N/A
Smoking status		• SNOMED International, Systematized Nomenclature of Medicine Clinical Terms (SNOMED CT) U.S. Edition, March 2018 Release
Unique device identifier(s) for a patient's implantable device(s)		• UDI identifier as described by applicable FDA regulation. (found at https://www.fda.gov/MedicalDevices/Device RegulationandGuidance/UniqueDeviceIdentification/)
Vital signs	Diastolic blood pressure Systolic blood pressure Body height Body weight Heart rate Respiratory rate Body temperature Pulse oximetry Inhaled oxygen concentration BMI percentile per age and sex for youth 2-20	• Logical Observation Identifiers Names and Codes (LOINC) Database version 2.63 • The Unified Code of Units for Measure, Revision 1.9

(continued)

TABLE 14.5. Continued

USCDI v1 Data Classes	Data Elements	Terminology Standards Named
	Weights for age per length and sex Occipital-frontal circumference for children >3 years old	

Source: ONC 2019.

A **data class** is "a high level grouping of similar data types. For example 'Demographics.' A data class is made up of data objects"(USCDI 2018). The USCDI data classes are meant to be iterative and to expand strategically over time. To accomplish this expansion, USCDI identifies additional candidate and emerging data classes.

A **candidate class** is a data class that is considered to be next in line for inclusion in the USCDI. To be in this category, a data class has to have a clear definition and proven applicability across a number of use cases. The data also has to be supported by commonly used standards, including the HL7 Consolidated-Clinical Document Architecture (C-CDA) (HL7 n.d.) and the FHIR standards (FHIR 2018).

An **emerging data class** is the next class in terms of priority. Emerging data classes are considered important to nationwide interoperability, but the need for them to be moved up to candidate classes is still being explored. Once a data class has been proposed by the industry, it will follow a gradual process where it will be promoted to emerging status, then candidate status, and ultimately included in the USCDI. The draft USCDI v1 proposed in January 2018 included 19 candidate data classes to be phased in over three years, from 2019 through 2021. It also specified 29 emerging data classes.

The USCDI expansion process is expected to be conducted on an annual basis. Once a data class is officially included in the USCDI, it will be required for nationwide exchange. This USCDI expansion process limits data classes to a predetermined core, making it realistic for stakeholders to accomplish exchange, while providing a mechanism to expand the core over time. Establishing this process allows adequate time for the industry to implement and upgrade its technology to support the data specified. In this manner, USCDI sets semantic standards for data exchange, to ensure data is accurately captured, accessed, exchanged, and used.

Uniform Hospital Discharge Data Set

Created more than 40 years ago, the **Uniform Hospital Discharge Data Set (UHDDS)** is a core set of data elements that are collected by acute-care, short-term stay (usually less than 30 days) hospitals to report inpatient data elements in a standardized manner. It was developed through the National Committee on Vital and Health Statistics (NCVHS) and has been required by HHS policy since January 1, 1975. Revisions have taken place twice since 1975: in 1984, and again in 1986. Although NCVHS recommended and circulated a revision in 1992 with additional recommendations from an Interagency Task Force in 1993, HHS has made no decisions on any of these recommended revisions.

The UHDDS has become a de facto standard in the hospital inpatient area for data collection by federal and state agencies as well as by public and private data-abstracting organizations (Greenberg 1995). The UHDDS also has had an influence on the UB-04 claim form and the 837I institutional healthcare claim for electronic healthcare transactions on which Medicare and Medicaid data sets are based. In fact, the UB-04 and 837I are major vehicles for collecting UHDDS data elements. When diagnosis-related groups (DRGs) were implemented in 1983, UHDDS definitions were incorporated into the inpatient prospective payment system (IPPS) regulations. Other payers also require use of UHDDS.

The purpose of the UHDDS is to list and define a set of common, uniform data elements. The data elements facilitate collection of uniform and comparable health information from hospitals. An integral part of the UHDDS is the data dictionary, where specific definitions of the core data elements collected on acute inpatient hospitalizations are listed along with each data element's guidelines for use. When UHDDS definitions or principles are ignored, data may be reported inaccurately.

Table 14.6 presents examples from UHDDS's data dictionary.

Resident Assessment Instrument (RAI) and Minimum Data Set (MDS)

A long-term care minimum data set was part of the uniform minimum health data set work done by NCVHS in the mid-1970s. Reports on a long-term care minimum data set were published in

TABLE 14.6. Portions of the UHDDS data dictionary

Data Element	Definition
Personal identification	The unique number assigned to each patient within the hospital that distinguishes the patient and his or her hospital record from all others in that institution
Discharge date	Month, day, and year of discharge
Principal diagnosis	The condition, after study, to be chiefly responsible for occasioning the admission of the patient to the hospital for care
Other diagnosis	All conditions that coexist at the time of admission or that develop subsequently or that affect the treatment received and/or length of stay. Diagnoses that relate to an earlier episode and have no bearing on the current hospital stay are to be excluded.

1980 and 1987. Then in 1987, the Omnibus Budget Reconciliation Act amended sections of the Social Security Act to include requirements for the Secretary of HHS to specify a minimum data set of core elements for use in conducting comprehensive assessments and to designate one or more **resident assessment instruments (RAIs)** based on the minimum data set (MDS).

The RAI process is a federally mandated standard assessment used to collect demographic and clinical data on residents in Medicare- or Medicaid-certified nursing homes and non-critical access hospitals with swing bed agreements. It consists of three components, the **Minimum Data Set (MDS)** Version 3.0, the Care Area Assessment (CAA) process, and the RAI utilization guidelines (CMS 2018a). To meet federal requirements, long-term care facilities must complete an assessment for every resident at the time of admission and at designated reassessment points throughout the resident's stay. The MDS is a tool for implementing standardized assessment and for facilitating care management in nursing homes (NHs) and non-critical access hospital swing beds (SBs). It is far more extensive and includes more clinical data than the UHDDS.

The data collected by the MDS are used to develop care plans for residents and to document placement at the appropriate level of care. The MDS is also used as a data collection tool to classify Medicare residents into Resource Utilization Groups (RUGs), a system used in the PPS for skilled nursing facilities, hospital swing bed programs, and in many State Medicaid case mix payment systems.

Another use of the MDS assessment data is monitoring the quality of care in nursing homes. Providers use the MDS data to assist in their ongoing quality improvement activities. Surveyors use MDS data to help identify potential problem areas to address during the survey process. Finally, CMS uses MDS data as one of the data sources in the Star rating system on the Nursing Home Compare website. The Nursing Home Compare website allows consumers, providers, states, and researchers to compare quality ratings for nursing homes certified by Medicare and Medicaid. The website includes quality of resident care and staffing information for more than 15,000 nursing homes in the US. (Medicare.gov 2019). Quality of resident care measures are derived from MDS data. Quality measures are defined for short-stay and long-stay residents; examples of each are provided in figure 14.3.

Contained in the MDS are items that reflect the acuity level of the resident, including diagnoses, treatments, and evaluations of functional status. Figure 14.4 presents the required components of the MDS that are reported on the RAI, according to the RAI 3.0 User's Manual for version 1.16, published October 2018. The RAI 3.0 User's Manual is an important resource that provides not only an overview of the content of the RAI for nursing homes and the components of the MDS but also instructions on completing and submitting assessments and an item-by-item guide to the MDS 3.0. The item-by-item guide, for example, provides the sources of information and methods for determining the correct response for coding each MDS item. Furthermore, coding instructions and coding tips provide additional clarification on the proper method of recording individual categories and issues to be considered on specific MDS items. This is a key reference to enhance consistency in the reported data elements. In addition, each state has a designated

FIGURE 14.3. Examples of quality of resident care measures

Short-Stay Resident Quality Measures	Long-Stay Resident Quality Measures
Percentage of short-stay residents who were re-hospitalized after a nursing home admission	Percentage of long-stay residents experiencing one or more falls with major injury
Percentage of short-stay residents who have had an outpatient emergency department visit	Percentage of long-stay residents with a urinary tract infection
Percentage of short-stay residents who got antipsychotic medication for the first time	Percentage of long-stay residents who got an antipsychotic medication
Percentage of short-stay residents with pressure ulcers that are new or worsened	Percentage of long-stay high-risk residents with pressure ulcers
Percentage of short-stay residents who improved in their ability to move around on their own	Percentage of long-stay residents whose ability to move independently worsened

Source: Medicare.gov 2019.

RAI Coordinator, whose contact information is available on the CMS website, and a RAI Panel, comprised of experienced RAI Coordinators, that assists CMS and other State RAI Coordinators with questions or comments regarding the MDS 3.0.

Data Sets for Performance and Quality Measurement

A performance or quality measure is a mechanism to assign a quantitative figure to the performance or quality of care by comparison to a criterion. As noted in the previous section, MDS assessment data is used to monitor the quality of care in the nation's nursing homes through MDS-based quality measures (QMs). Additional data sets, designed primarily for performance and quality measurement, explored in this section include: Outcomes and Assessment Information Set (OASIS), Healthcare Effectiveness Data and Information Set (HEDIS), ORYX Performance Measures, and CMS Electronic Clinical Quality Measures (eCQMs).

Outcomes and Assessment Information Set

The **Outcomes and Assessment Information Set (OASIS)** is a standardized data set that represents items of a comprehensive assessment designed to gather and report data about Medicare beneficiaries who are receiving services from a Medicare-certified home health agency (HHA). The OASIS includes a set of core data items that are collected on all adult home health patients whose care is reimbursed by Medicare and Medicaid with the exception of patients

FIGURE 14.4. Components of the MDS

Section	Title	Intent
A	Identification Information	Obtain key information to uniquely identify each resident, nursing home, type of record, and reasons for assessment.
B	Hearing, Speech, and Vision	Document the resident's ability to hear, understand, and communicate with others and whether the resident experiences visual, hearing, or speech limitations or difficulties.
C	Cognitive Patterns	Determine the resident's attention, orientation, and ability to register and recall information.
D	Mood	Identify signs and symptoms of mood distress.
E	Behavior	Identify behavioral symptoms that may cause distress or are potentially harmful to the resident, or may be distressing or disruptive to facility residents, staff members, or the environment.
F	Preferences for Customary Routine and Activities	Obtain information regarding the resident's preferences for his or her daily routine and activities.
G	Functional Status	Assess the need for assistance with activities of daily living (ADLs), altered gait and balance, and decreased range of motion.
GG	Functional Abilities and Goals	Assess the need for assistance with self-care and mobility activities.
H	Bladder and Bowel	Gather information on the use of bowel and bladder appliances, the use of and response to urinary toileting programs, urinary and bowel continence, bowel training programs, and bowel patterns.
I	Active Disease Diagnosis	Code diseases that have a relationship to the resident's current functional, cognitive, mood or behavior status, medical treatments, nursing monitoring, or risk of death.
J	Health Conditions	Document health conditions that impact the resident's functional status and quality of life.
K	Swallowing/Nutritional Status	Assess conditions that could affect the resident's ability to maintain adequate nutrition and hydration.
L	Oral/Dental Status	Record any oral or dental problems present.
M	Skin Conditions	Document the risk, presence, appearance, and change of pressure ulcers as well as other skin ulcers, wounds, or lesions. Also includes treatment categories related to skin injury or avoiding injury.
N	Medications	Record the number of days that any type of injection, insulin, or select medications was received by the resident.
O	Special Treatment, Procedures and Programs	Identify any special treatments, procedures, and programs that the resident received during the specified time periods.
P	Restraints and Alarms	Record the frequency that the resident was restrained by any of the listed devices at any time during the day or night; record the frequency that any of the listed alarms were used.
Q	Participation in Assessment and Goal Setting	Record the participation of the resident, family, and significant others in the assessment, and to understand the resident's overall goals.
V	Care Area Assessment (CAA) Summary	Document triggered care areas, whether or not a care plan has been developed for each triggered area, and the location of care area assessment documentation.
X	Correction Request	Request to modify or inactivate a record already present in the QIES ASAP database.
Z	Assessment Administration	Provide billing information and signatures of persons completing the assessment.

Source: CMS 2018a, 19.

receiving pre- or postnatal services only. Most data items in the OASIS were derived in the context of a CMS-funded national research program (cofunded by the Robert Wood Johnson Foundation) to develop a system of outcome measures for home healthcare (CMS 2019b). It has been reviewed and refined several times since it was originally developed. The OASIS-D data set must be used for all assessments completed on or after January 1, 2019. The OASIS-D data set revision increased standardization across post-acute care settings to enable calculation of standardized, cross-setting quality measures. It includes versions of the OASIS data set for each of the following data collection time points:

- Start of care
- Resumption of care following inpatient facility stay
- Recertification within the last 5 days of each 60-day recertification period
- Other follow-up during the home health episode of care
- Transfer to an inpatient facility
- Death at home
- Discharge from agency

There are over 100 OASIS-D data items. At any one point in time, only a subset of OASIS items is collected (CMS 2019b).

OASIS-D includes items that support measurement of evidence-based practices across the post-acute care spectrum that have been shown to prevent exacerbation of serious conditions, improve care received by individual patients, and provide guidance to HHAs on how to improve care and avoid adverse events. The OASIS-D items encompass sociodemographic, environmental, support system, health status, health conditions, and functional abilities and goals of adult (nonmaternity) patients. CMS provides an extensive OASIS user's manual that includes data element definitions, principles, and guidelines. Chapter 3 of the manual includes item-by-item tips to assist in the completion of the OASIS-D (see figure 14.5 for an example from the manual). Table 14.7 includes examples of OASIS data items from the CMS OASIS-D Guidance Manual.

Data collected through OASIS-D are used to assess the patient's ability to be discharged or transferred from home care services. The data are also used in measuring patient outcomes in order to assess the quality of home healthcare services. Based on the OASIS-D data, CMS provides HHAs with both outcome and process quality measure reports; for example, potentially avoidable events, patient-related characteristics, and patient tally reports. Process quality measures include indicators of how often the HHA follows best practices to improve patient outcomes. Outcome measures include, for example, end-result functional and physical health improvement or stabilization and healthcare utilization measures.

Under the prospective payment program for home health, implemented in 2000, data from OASIS-D also form the basis of reimbursement for provided services. In addition, these data are used to create patient case mix profile reports and patient outcome reports that are used by state

TABLE 14.7. Examples of OASIS-D data items

Item#	Item Description	Collection Time Points	Item Uses
M0020	Patient ID number	Start of care	Administrative
M0030	Start of care date	Start of care	Payment; quality measure
M0032	Resumption of care date	Resumption of care	Quality measure
M0104	Date of referral	Start of care; Resumption of care	Quality measure
M1021	Primary diagnosis, ICD-10-CM and symptom control rating	Start of care; Resumption of care; Follow-up	Payment; Potential quality measure risk adjustment
M1030	Therapies the patient receives at home	Start of care; Resumption of care; Follow-up	Payment; Potential quality measure risk adjustment
M1046	Influenza vaccine received	Transfer; Discharge	Quality measure
M1242	Frequency of pain interfering with patient's activity or movement	Start of care; Resumption of care; Follow-up; Discharge	Payment; Quality measure; Potential quality measure risk adjustment
M1322	Current number of stage 1 pressure injuries	Start of care; Resumption of care; Follow-up	Payment; Potential quality measure risk adjustment

Source: CMS 2019c.

survey staff in the certification process. HHA quality measures that appear on the CMS Home Health Compare website are also based on OASIS-D data.

Healthcare Effectiveness Data and Information Set

The **Healthcare Effectiveness Data and Information Set (HEDIS)** is sponsored by the National Committee for Quality Assurance (NCQA). HEDIS is a set of standard performance measures designed to provide healthcare purchasers and consumers with the information they need to compare the performance of managed healthcare plans. CMS contracted with NCQA to develop these performance measures specifically for special need plans (SNPs). According to CMS, SNPs can use HEDIS performance data to identify opportunities for improvement, monitor and track quality improvement initiatives, and use measurement standards as a point of comparison with other health plans (CMS 2017).

HEDIS is designed to collect administrative, claims, and health record review data. It collects standardized data about specific health-related conditions or issues so that the success of various treatment plans can be assessed and compared. NCQA collects HEDIS data from health plans, healthcare organizations, and government agencies. Administrative measures use data from healthcare claims, hybrid measures use administrative data and data from patient health

FIGURE 14.5. Excerpt from the OASIS-D Manual

OASIS ITEM

(M1021) Primary Diagnosis & (M1023) Other Diagnoses	
Column 1	Column 2
Diagnoses (Sequencing of diagnoses should reflect the seriousness of each condition and support the disciplines and services provided)	ICD-10-CM and symptom control rating for each condition. Note that the sequencing of these ratings may not match the sequencing of the diagnoses
Description	ICD-10-CM/Symptom Control Rating
(M1021) Primary Diagnosis a.	V, W, X, Y codes NOT allowed a. [ ][ ][ ][ ][ ][ ] □0 □1 □2 □3 □4
(M1023) Other Diagnoses b.	All ICD-10-CM codes allowed b. [ ][ ][ ][ ][ ][ ] □0 □1 □2 □3 □4
c. _____	c. [ ][ ][ ][ ][ ][ ] □0 □1 □2 □3 □4
d. _____	d. [ ][ ][ ][ ][ ][ ] □0 □1 □2 □3 □4
e. _____	e. [ ][ ][ ][ ][ ][ ] □0 □1 □2 □3 □4
f. _____	f. [ ][ ][ ][ ][ ][ ] □0 □1 □2 □3 □4

ITEM INTENT

- M1021: the intent of this item is to accurately report and code the patient's primary home health diagnosis and document the degree of symptom control for that diagnosis. The patient's primary home health diagnosis is defined as the chief reason the patient is receiving home care and the diagnosis most related to the current home health Plan of Care.
- M1023: the intent of this item is to accurately report and code the patient's secondary home health diagnosis and document the degree of symptom control for each diagnosis. Secondary diagnoses are comorbid conditions that exist at the time of the assessment, that are actively addressed in the patient's Plan of Care, or that have the potential to affect the patient's responsiveness to treatment and rehabilitative prognosis.

TIME POINTS ITEM(S) COMPLETED

- Start of care
- Resumption of care
- Follow-up

RESPONSE-SPECIFIC INSTRUCTIONS

- HHA clinicians and coders must comply with the ICD-10-CM Official Guidelines for Coding and Reporting when assigning primary and secondary diagnoses to the OASIS items M1021 and M1023. See Chapter 5 for link.

Source: CMS 2019b.

records, while survey measures use data collected in surveys of health plan members. NCQA collects non-survey data through the Interactive Data Submission System (IDSS) and health plans and PPOs submit HEDIS survey data through the Healthcare Organization Questionnaire (HOQ) (NCQA 2018a). The health record data are combined with enrollment and claims data and analyzed according to HEDIS specifications.

HEDIS data form the basis of performance improvement (PI) efforts for health plans. They also are used to develop physician profiles. The goal of physician profiling is to positively influence physician practice patterns.

HEDIS contains more than 90 measures across the following six domains of care:

- Effectiveness of Care
- Access/Availability of Care
- Experience of Care
- Utilization and Risk Adjusted Utilization
- Health Plan Descriptive Information
- Measures Collected Using Electronic Clinical Data Systems

The measures are related to conditions such as heart disease, cancer, diabetes, asthma, chlamydia infection, osteoporosis, and rheumatoid arthritis. They include data related to patient outcomes and data about the treatment process used by the clinician in treating the patient.

An example of a HEDIS measure is comprehensive diabetes care. Other examples of HEDIS effectiveness of care measures include:

- Immunizations for adolescents
- Adult BMI assessment
- Medical assistance with smoking and tobacco use cessation
- Antidepressant medication management
- Breast cancer screening
- Statin therapy for patients with cardiovascular disease and diabetes
- Follow-up care for children prescribed ADHD medication (NCQA 2018b)

Health plans often release data from HEDIS studies publicly to document substantial positive effects on the health of their clients. Results are compared over time and with data from other sources. From the data, health plans determine opportunities for PI and develop potential interventions. Furthermore, NCQA reports include Health Plan Ratings, Quality Compass, and the State of Health Care Quality Report (NCQA 2018c).

NCQA publishes health insurance ratings annually based partially on health plans' HEDIS data. The health plans are rated on a scale from 0 to 5 and the data is published online in September, so that consumers can consider a health plan's rating when they choose health plans during year-end open enrollment. NCQA's Quality Compass provides performance information on health plans and includes national, regional, and state benchmarks. Quality Compass is an online database that provides up to three years of HEDIS performance trends (NCQA 2018d). Lastly, NCQA's State of Health Care Quality report is also published annually in the fall and looks at health plans' collective improvement over time. NCQA is currently working to incorporate digital quality measures to create more efficient data collection and reporting. They plan to convert to digital between 20 to 25 HEDIS measures each year over the next three years. An initial package of six digital measures will be available in the 2019 HEDIS release (NCQA 2018e).

HEDIS is an example of a population-based data collection tool. It illustrates the need for developing standardized data definitions and uniform collection methods. It also emphasizes the importance of data quality management.

ORYX Performance Measures

The Joint Commission is one of the largest users of healthcare data and information. Its primary function is the accreditation of hospitals and other healthcare organizations. In 1997, the Joint Commission introduced the ORYX initiative to integrate outcomes data and other performance measurement data into its accreditation processes. The goal of the initiative is to promote a comprehensive, continuous, data-driven accreditation process for healthcare facilities (Joint Commission 2018a).

The Joint Commission categorizes its process performance measures into accountability and non-accountability measures. ORYX focuses on accountability measures, measures that meet specific criteria to be used for purposes of accountability (for accreditation, public reporting, or pay for performance, for example).

The ORYX initiative uses nationally standardized performance measures to improve the safety and quality of healthcare. The ORYX initiative integrates outcomes and other performance measures into the accreditation process through data collection about specific core measures (Joint Commission 2018a). The measures include the minimum number of data elements needed to provide an accurate and reliable measure of performance.

Since 2016, ORYX performance measurement has included both chart-abstracted measures and electronic clinical quality measures (eCQMs). Accredited hospitals utilize ORYX chart-based vendors to abstract chart-based data throughout the year and submit the data to the Joint Commission. Accredited hospitals collect eCQM data, which can be electronically submitted via the Joint Commission's Direct Data Submission Platform (DDSP), from the EHR. Beginning with calendar year 2019, all hospitals will submit eCQM data via the DDSP (Joint Commission 2018a).

Since 2003, the Joint Commission and CMS have worked to align performance measures so that common measures are identical. The Joint Commission's move to incorporate electronic measures is part of an initiative to reduce the burden of data collection. The Joint Commission intentionally adopted existing CMS eCQMs, consistent with their commitment to continue to align measures as closely as possible with CMS. The Joint Commission and CMS efforts to align common measures resulted in the creation of one common set of measure specifications document, the Specifications Manual for National Hospital Inpatient Quality Measures (Joint Commission 2018b). This manual is used by both organizations and contains common (identical) data dictionary and measure information forms. The manual's data dictionary includes an alphabetic list of the data elements required to calculate category assignments and measurements for the measures. eCQM specifications are defined in value sets available on the internet (discussed further in the next section, CMS Electronic Quality Measures). Using the defined data elements in the manual and value sets ensures standardized and comparable data across facilities.

CMS Electronic Clinical Quality Measures

In 2015, Congress passed the Medicare Access and CHIP Reauthorization Act (MACRA). This bill instituted Medicare payment reform that is designed to lower healthcare costs and improve the quality of patient care (CMS 2018b). The Merit-based Incentive Payment System (MIPS) is a key component of the MACRA Quality Payment Program (QPP). Under MIPS, the Meaningful Use (MU) Medicare incentive program, Physician Quality Reporting System (PQRS), and Value-Based Modifier (VBM) program were consolidated into one program (Quality Payment Program 2019a). MIPS was implemented in January 2017 for eligible providers who bill Medicare more than $90,000 annually or provide care for more than 200 Medicare patients a year (Quality Payment Program 2019b).

The MIPS program scores eligible providers in four categories:

- Quality Measures Requirements (the previous PQRS program)
- Promoting Interoperability Requirements (the previous Meaningful Use program formerly referred to as "Advancing Care Information")
- Improvement Activities Requirements
- Cost Measures Requirements (the previous value-based modifier program)

Eligible providers who score as top performers can earn bonus money, while eligible providers who do not achieve the score threshold of the MIPS program stand to lose 5 percent of their Medicare fee reimbursement in the upcoming year.

The quality measures requirements performance category "measures healthcare processes, outcomes, and patient care experiences" (Quality Payment Program 2019c). To meet the quality requirements, eligible providers must submit data for a specified number of quality measures. For example, MIPS participants were required to submit data for at least six measures for January 1 through December 31, 2018 (Quality Payment Program 2018). Eligible providers select the quality measures to report that are most relevant to their specialty and patient population.

CMS has defined **electronic clinical quality measures (eCQMs)** for eligible clinicians participating in the QPP. eCQMs use data from electronic health records (EHR) or health information technology systems to measure healthcare quality (eCQI Resource Center 2019). eCQMs are assigned a specific unique CMS eCQM identifier, which is a semantic identifier that includes the version number. For the MIPS program, measures are designated as a specific type, such as process versus outcome, and some of the measures are flagged as "high priority." Eligible providers receive higher scores for reporting on outcomes measures or high priority measures.

Table 14.8 provides examples of eCQM measures defined for eligible providers in the 2019 performance period.

CMS maintains an inventory of all quality measures used by CMS in various quality, reporting, and payment programs. The inventory also includes measures under development and those submitted for consideration in the pre-rulemaking process. The CMS measures inventory tool (CMIT) provides access to this compilation of measures and is updated multiple times per year (CMS 2018c). The CMIT includes each measure listed by program. For example, the CMIT, as of August 2018, included thousands of measures with 687 quality measures specified for use in the MIPS program.

TABLE 14.8. Examples of eCQMs for 2019

Measure Title	eMeasure ID	Measure Description	Measure Type	High Priority
Children Who Have Dental Decay or Cavities	CMS75v7	Percentage of children, age 0–20 years, who have had tooth decay or cavities during the measurement period	Outcome	X
Diabetes: Hemoglobin A1c (HbA1c) Poor Control (>9%)	CMS122v7	Percentage of patients 18–75 years of age with diabetes who had hemoglobin A1c > 9.0% during the measurement period	Intermediate Outcome	X
Colorectal Cancer Screening	CMS130v7	Percentage of adults 50–75 years of age who had appropriate screening for colorectal cancer	Process	
Appropriate Testing for Children with Pharyngitis	CMS146v7	Percentage of children 3–18 years of age who were diagnosed with pharyngitis, ordered an antibiotic and received a group A streptococcus (strep) test for the episode	Process	X
Preventive Care and Screening: Influenza Immunization	CMS147v7	Percentage of patients aged 6 months and older seen for a visit between October 1 and March 31 who received an influenza immunization OR who reported previous receipt of an influenza immunization	Process	
Appropriate Treatment for Children with Upper Respiratory Infection (URI)	CMS154v7	Percentage of children 3 months–18 years of age who were diagnosed with upper respiratory infection (URI) and were not dispensed an antibiotic prescription on or three days after the episode	Process	X

Source: eCQI Resource Center 2018.

eCQM value sets specify coded values that are allowed for the data elements within the eCQM. The value set includes a list of codes acceptable or valid for a specific data element in the measure, descriptors of those codes, the code system from which the codes are derived, and the version of that code system. Value sets are found in the Value Set Authority Center (VSAC). The VSAC is a repository of value sets, published by a variety of measure stewards, that is hosted by the National Library of Medicine (NLM) in collaboration with ONC. It provides downloadable access to all official versions of value sets specified by the CMS eCQMs (NLM 2018).

As an example, the value set for eCQM CMS122v7, included in table 14.8, specifies that this measure is only relevant for patients with a diagnosis of Type 1 or Type 2 diabetes; patients with a diagnosis of secondary diabetes due to another condition should not be included. In addition, the initial patient population is defined as patients 18 to 75 years of age with diabetes with a visit during the measurement period. Furthermore, the value set for this measure specifically identifies 304 ICD-10-CM diabetes codes for use in identifying the patient population for reporting on this measure.

Electronic specifications of data elements for clinical quality measures, organized in a consistent manner according to a standard information model, enable the measures to be collected and reported consistently, reliably, and effectively. Furthermore, this standardized approach enables automation of structured data capture, thus reducing the burden of manual abstraction and reporting.

Adoption and Use Cases

Many data sets have been incorporated into federal law and are thus required for use by affected healthcare organizations. For example, in 1983, when Section 1886(d) of the Social Security Act was enacted, UHDDS definitions were incorporated into the rules and regulations for implementing an inpatient prospective payment system based on diagnosis-related groups (DRGs). These definitions are still required for reporting inpatient data for reimbursement under the Medicare program. Other data sets are tied to quality measurement initiatives, accreditation programs, and federal and state regulations.

Use Case One: Data Elements for Registries

The National Institutes of Health describes a registry as "a collection of information about individuals, usually focused around a specific diagnosis or condition" (NIH 2018). Registries provide an organized mechanism to collect, store, retrieve, analyze, and disseminate information on individuals. Federal and state governments as well as universities, hospitals, and organizations create patient registries for a number of purposes including determining the incidence of disease, conducting research, and examining trends of disease over time.

Data elements are a key piece of a patient registry and provide the ability to collect uniform data. Clinical data standards, which define common core datasets for conditions, are ideal for collecting consistent data elements but are difficult to implement uniformly for effective data exchange. One area where a number of groups have worked on standardizing data is for cancer registries. For example, the North American Association of Central Cancer Registries (NAACCR) developed data standards for use by central registries and hospital-based registries to promote uniform data standards across regional and national databases (NAACCR 2018).

Use Case Two: Reporting a Quality Measure

A cardiology practice would like to earn quality measure bonus points under the MIPS program to meet their overall goal to improve their score. To do that they intend to replace a process quality measure that they have been reporting with an outcome measure that is designated as a high priority under the MIPS program. The practice is currently analyzing their data to determine if they are ready to report eCQM CMS124v7, Controlling high blood pressure. To report this quality measure, they need to determine the percentage of their patients who are 18 to 85 years of age, have a diagnosis of hypertension, and have a blood pressure reading under 140/90 mmHg.

To identify the initial population, for the denominator of the measure, they first selected patients within the defined age range who had one of the essential hypertension ICD-10-CM codes specified in the value set for this measure. Based on denominator exclusions in the measure specifications, they subsequently excluded patients with the following codes specified in the value set:

- ICD-10-CM codes for end-stage renal disease
- CPT/HCPCS/SNOMED CT codes for dialysis
- CPT/HCPCS/SNOMED CT codes for kidney transplant
- ICD-10-CM codes for kidney transplant recipient
- ICD-10-CM/SNOMED CT codes for pregnancy

The practice is currently testing the results of this selection criteria to confirm they have identified the correct initial patient population. When they initially attempted this last year, there was a significant error rate revealing discrepancies in how the providers were identifying transplant patients. That has since been corrected, and they are hopeful the results will be more reliable. They are also working to determine how to effectively exclude patients who receive hospice care during the measurement period.

For the numerator, they will use EHR structured data fields where blood pressure is recorded on each patient visit and extrapolate blood pressure readings for the patients in the defined population. If a patient has multiple blood pressure readings on the same date, they will extract the lowest systolic and the lowest diastolic reading. Extrapolated data includes the systolic and diastolic blood pressure with the date the blood pressure was recorded. Additional data includes the patient identifier (so they can spot check and validate the data), the patient's race, ethnicity, and sex, as well as the payer type. A formula applied to the extrapolated data flags each record to indicate if the blood pressure is below the desired threshold of 140/90 mmHg.

CHECK YOUR UNDERSTANDING

1. OASIS forms the basis for measuring patient _____.

2. Which of the following is *not* part of a data dictionary?

   a. Allowable values for a data element
   b. Length of a data element
   c. List of standard data to collect
   d. Definition of a data element

3. Which of the following is *not* a characteristic of data quality in the AHIMA DQM model?

   a. Accuracy
   b. Consistency
   c. Interoperability
   d. Precision

4. Which of the following statements is true?

   a. Data dictionaries limit how aggregate data can be viewed.
   b. Data sets and data dictionaries communicate data standards so that data can be collected and used consistently.
   c. Hospitals have been unable to agree on a uniform data set for reporting inpatient data.
   d. PSSS is the mandated data standard for exchanging patient summaries.

5. The principal diagnosis for inpatient acute care hospital inpatients is defined in which of the following data sets?

   a. UHDDS
   b. HEDIS
   c. OASIS
   d. USCDI

REVIEW

1. The purpose of the _____ is to list and define a set of common, uniform data elements that facilitate collection of comparable health information for hospital inpatients.

2. Which of the following is not one of the data quality management functions defined in the AHIMA DQM model?

   a. Collection
   b. Warehousing
   c. Application
   d. Ownership

3. True or false? The FAIR principles are intended to improve computer automated search and use of data.

   a. True
   b. False

4. The Resident Assessment Instrument is triggered by the data collected by the:

   a. OASIS
   b. PSSS
   c. MDS
   d. HEDIS

5. Which of the following data sets defines the payment diagnosis for home care patients?

   a. MDS
   b. UHDDS
   c. USCDI
   d. OASIS

6. Which of the following best describes the USCDI data set?

   a. An assessment instrument for long-term care data
   b. Specifies a common set of data classes for interoperability
   c. Uses data for inpatient analysis
   d. Collects patient summary information for continuity of care

7. HEDIS data is collected from:

   a. UB claims
   b. 1500 claims
   c. Health record review
   d. All of the above

8. Which of the following is a set of performance measures used in the accreditation process for healthcare facilities?

   a. eCQMs
   b. HEDIS
   c. ORYX
   d. UHDDS

9. Which one of the following statements is false?

   a. eCQMs measure healthcare processes and outcomes.
   b. eCQMs' semantic identifiers specify values that are allowed for the data elements.
   c. eCQMs use data from electronic health records.
   d. eCQMs resolve the problem of manual record review.

10. Which of the following is not one of the data classes in the USCDI?

    a. Problems
    b. Medications
    c. Medication allergies
    d. Functional status

References

Amatayakul, M. K. 2017. *Electronic Health Records: A Practical Guide for Professionals and Organizations,* 5th ed. 2013 Update. Chicago, IL: AHIMA.

American Health Information Management Association (AHIMA). 2017. *Pocket Glossary of Health Information Management and Technology*, 5th ed. Chicago: AHIMA.

Australia National Data Services (ANDS). 2019. The FAIR Data Principles. https://www.ands.org.au/working-with-data/fairdata.

Centers for Medicare and Medicaid Services (CMS). 2019a. MEDPAR Limited Data Set (LDS) – Hospital (National). https://www.cms.gov/Research-Statistics-Data-and-Systems/Files-for-Order/LimitedDataSets/MEDPARLDSHospitalNational.html.

Centers for Medicare and Medicaid Services (CMS). 2019b. Outcome and Assessment Information Set OASIS-D Guidance Manual, Effective January 1, 2019. https://www.cms.gov/Medicare/Quality-Initiatives-Patient-Assessment-Instruments/HomeHealthQualityInits/Downloads/draft-OASIS-D-Guidance-Manual-7-2-2018.pdf.

Centers for Medicare and Medicaid Services (CMS). 2019c. Outcome and Assessment Information Set OASIS-D Guidance Manual, Effective January 1, 2019. Appendix C: OASIS-D Items, Time Points and Uses. https://www.cms.gov/Medicare/Quality-Initiatives-Patient-Assessment-Instruments/HomeHealthQualityInits/Downloads/draft-OASIS-D-Guidance-Manual-7-2-2018.pdf.

Centers for Medicare and Medicaid Services (CMS). 2018a. Long-Term Care Facility Resident Assessment Instrument 3.0 User's Manual, Version 1.16. https://downloads.cms.gov/files/1-MDS-30-RAI-Manual-v1-16-October-1-2018.pdf.

Centers for Medicare and Medicaid Services (CMS). 2018b. What's MACRA? https://www.cms.gov/Medicare/Quality-Initiatives-Patient-Assessment-Instruments/Value-Based-Programs/MACRA-MIPS-and-APMs/MACRA-MIPS-and-APMs.html.

Centers for Medicare and Medicaid Services (CMS). 2018c. CMS Measures Inventory. https://www.cms.gov/Medicare/Quality-Initiatives-Patient-Assessment-Instruments/QualityMeasures/CMS-Measures-Inventory.html.

Centers for Medicare and Medicaid Services (CMS). 2017. Healthcare Effectiveness Data and Information Set (HEDIS). https://www.cms.gov/Medicare/Health-Plans/SpecialNeedsPlans/SNP-HEDIS.html.

Davoudi, S., J. A. Dooling, B. Glondys, T. D. Jones, L. Kadlec, S. M. Overgaard, K. Ruben, and A. Wendicke. 2015. Data quality management model (2015). *Journal of AHIMA* 86(10): expanded web version. http://bok.ahima.org/doc?oid=107773#.XDPMPlxKhaQ.

Downing, K. 2018. Data Governance Defined. https://www.ehidc.org/sites/default/files/resources/files/AHIMA%20presentation.pdf.

eCQI Resource Center. 2018. 2019 Performance Period Eligible Professional/Eligible Clinician eCQMs. https://ecqi.healthit.gov/eligible-professional-eligible-clinician-ecqms/2019-performance-period-epec-ecqms.

eCQI Resource Center. 2019. eCQMs. https://ecqi.healthit.gov/ecqms.

Fast Healthcare Interoperability Resources (FHIR). 2018. Standards Overview. https://www.hl7.org/fhir/overview.html.

Giannangelo, K. 2007. Unraveling the data set, an e-HIM essential. *Journal of AHIMA* 78(2):60–61.GO FAIR. 2019. FAIR Principles. https://www.go-fair.org/fair-principles/.

GO FAIR Metrics Group. 2019. FAIR Metrics. http://fairmetrics.org/.

Greenberg, M. 1995. History of health care core data set development. Attachment 1 to Common Core Health Data Sets, 1/31/95 (unpublished).

Health Level Seven International (HL7). n.d. CDA Release 2. http://www.hl7.org/implement/standards/product_brief.cfm?product_id=7.

Imming, M. 2018. FAIR Data Advanced Use Cases: From Principles to Practice in the Netherlands. https://www.surf.nl/en/fair-data-advanced-use-cases-from-principles-to-practice.

ISO/IEC 11179. 2013. Information technology — Metadata registries (MDR) -Part 3: Registry metamodel and basic attributes. Geneva, Switzerland: International Organization for Standardization.

Joint Commission. 2018a. (October 12). Facts About ORYX for Hospitals (National Hospital Quality Measures). https://www.jointcommission.org/accreditation/performance_measurementoryx.aspx.

Joint Commission. 2018b. Specifications Manual for National Hospital Inpatient Quality Measures. https://www.jointcommission.org/specifications_manual_for_national_hospital_inpatient_quality_measures.aspx

Joint Initiative Council (JIC). 2019. Joint Initiative on SDO Global Health Informatics Standardization. http://www.jointinitiativecouncil.org/.

Joint Initiative Council (JIC). 2018. Patient Summary Standards Set Guidance Document, January 2018 v1.0. http://www.jointinitiativecouncil.org/registry/Patient_Summary_Standards_JIC_Jan_2018.pdf.

Medicare.gov. 2019. Nursing Home Compare. https://www.medicare.gov/nursinghomecompare/.

National Committee for Quality Assurance (NCQA). 2018a. HEDIS Data Submission. https://www.ncqa.org/hedis/data-submission/.

National Committee for Quality Assurance (NCQA). 2018b. HEDIS Measures and Technical Resources. https://www.ncqa.org/hedis/measures/.

National Committee for Quality Assurance (NCQA). 2018c. Reports and Research. https://www.ncqa.org/hedis/reports-and-research/.

National Committee for Quality Assurance (NCQA). 2018d. Quality Compass: Benchmark and Compare Quality Data. https://www.ncqa.org/programs/data-and-information-technology/data-purchase-and-licensing/quality-compass/.

National Committee for Quality Assurance (NCQA). 2018e. The Future of HEDIS. https://www.ncqa.org/hedis/the-future-of-hedis/.

National Institutes of Health (NIH). 2018. List of Registries. https://www.nih.gov/health-information/nih-clinical-research-trials-you/list-registries.

National Library of Medicine (NLM). 2018. Value Set Authority Center. https://vsac.nlm.nih.gov/welcome.

North American Association of Central Cancer Registries (NAACCR). 2018 (October). Data Standards and Data Dictionary, Volume II. https://www.naaccr.org/data-standards-data-dictionary/.

Office of the National Coordinator for Health Information Technology (ONC). 2019. US Core Data for Interoperability (USCDI) Version 1. https://www.healthit.gov/isa/us-core-data-interoperability-uscdi.

Office of the National Coordinator for Health Information Technology (ONC). 2018a. Draft US Core Data for Interoperability (USCDI) and Proposed Expansion Process. https://www.healthit.gov/sites/default/files/draft-uscdi.pdf.

Office of the National Coordinator for Health Information Technology (ONC). 2018b. 2015 Edition Common Clinical Data Set (CCDS) Reference Document Version 1.3. https://www.healthit.gov/sites/default/files/ccds_reference_document_v1_1.pdf.

Office of the National Coordinator for Health Information Technology (ONC). 2015. 2015 Edition Health Information Technology (Health IT) Certification Criteria, 2015 Edition Base Electronic Health Record (EHR) Definition, and ONC Health IT Certification Program Modifications. https://www.federalregister.gov/documents/2015/10/16/2015-25597/2015-edition-health-information-technology-health-it-certification-criteria-2015-edition-base.

Quality Payment Program. 2019a. MIPS Overview. https://qpp.cms.gov/mips/overview.

Quality Payment Program. 2019b. About MIPS Participation. https://qpp.cms.gov/participation-lookup/about.

Quality Payment Program. 2019c. Quality Measures Requirements. https://qpp.cms.gov/mips/quality-measures.

Quality Payment Program. 2018. Quality Measures Requirements, PY 2018. https://qpp.cms.gov/mips/quality-measures?py=2018.

Shakir, A.M. 1999. Tools for defining data. *Journal of AHIMA* 70(8):48–53.

21st Century Cures Act. Public Law No: 114-255. 2016. https://www.congress.gov/bill/114th-congress/house-bill/6.

US Core Data for Interoperability (USCDI) Task Force. 2018. USCDI Task Force Draft Recommendations. https://www.healthit.gov/sites/default/files/facas/2018-04-18_USCDI_TF_DraftRecommendations-508.pdf

Wilkinson, M. D., M. Dumontier, I. J. Aalbersberg, G. Appleton, M. Axton, A. Baak, N. Blomberg, et al. 2016. The FAIR guiding principles for scientific data management and stewardship. Scientific Data 3:160018. doi: 10.1038/sdata.216.18.

15

Data Interchange Standards

Jay Lyle, PhD

LEARNING OBJECTIVES

- Explain the general purpose of healthcare data interchange standards
- Categorize standards development organizations and stakeholders
- Examine the relationship between healthcare data interchange standards and vocabularies, terminologies, and classification systems
- Compare the purposes of the major healthcare data interchange standards

KEY TERMS

- Accredited Standards Committee (ASC) X12
- American National Standards Institute (ANSI)
- Behavioral standards
- Clinical Data Interchange Standards Consortium (CDISC)
- Clinical Document Architecture (CDA)
- Consolidated CDA (C-CDA)
- Content standards
- Designated Standards Maintenance Organization (DSMO)
- Digital Imaging and Communications in Medicine (DICOM)
- Electronic data interchange (EDI)
- Fast Healthcare Information Resources (FHIR)
- Foundational interoperability
- Harmonization
- Health Information Technology for Economic and Clinical Health (HITECH) Act
- Implementation guide (IG)

- Institute of Electrical and Electronics Engineers Standards Association (IEEE-SA)
- Integrating the Healthcare Enterprise (IHE)
- Interoperability Standards Advisory (ISA)
- Meaningful Use (MU)
- National Council for Prescription Drug Programs (NCPDP)
- National Technology Transfer and Advancement Act (NTTAA)
- Normative standard
- Office of the National Coordinator for Health Information Technology (ONC)
- Profile
- Promoting Interoperability (PI)
- Quality Reporting Document Architecture (QRDA)
- Reference Model
- SCRIPT
- Semantic interoperability
- Specifications
- Standards development organization (SDO)
- Structural interoperability
- Transport standards
- Workgroup for Electronic Data Interchange (WEDI)

Introduction

To manage healthcare data and information resources, health information management professionals must be knowledgeable not only in the various types of vocabulary, terminology, classification systems, and data sets, but also in the standards used in the exchange of data. There are many varieties of healthcare data interchange standards. Some are suitable for a paper-based environment; others are created expressly for use in an electronic world.

Data standards are the conventions we use to communicate clearly. They are not limited to the electronic exchange of data; the International Classification of Diseases (ICD) was used to agree on common boundaries for morbidity definitions many decades before the first computer network communication. But the electronic exchange of information requires a much more thorough standardization effort to allow machines to use the information as intended, without the assistance of human interpreters to put the data in proper context.

In this chapter, we will use a set of use cases to illustrate the standards development process and the effects their respective constraints have on the outcomes. All three of these examples, and most of the standards that may be encountered in healthcare data management, will be from the second, structural layer, with more or less support for certain semantic features.

Use Case One: Prescription. A clinician in private practice writes a prescription for a patient and submits it to a pharmacy. Primary example: National Council for Prescription Drug Programs (NCPDP) SCRIPT.

Use Case Two: Patient summary. A provider has a new patient and wishes to view existing documents about the patient (content layer). Primary example: Health Level Seven (HL7) Consolidated Clinical Data Architecture (C-CDA) Continuity of Care Document (CCD).

Use Case Three: Document access. A provider has a new patient and wishes to view existing documents about the patient (transport layer). Primary example: Integrating the Health Enterprise (IHE) Cross-Enterprise Document Sharing (XDS).

Levels of Interoperability

A key factor in understanding the variety of data exchange standards in the marketplace today is the level of interoperability they promise to support. The most commonly cited definitions for levels of interoperability come from the Healthcare Information and Management Systems Society (HIMSS 2018):

- **Foundational interoperability** "allows data exchange from one information technology system to be received by another and does not require the ability for the receiving information technology system to interpret the data."

    - This first level includes transport tools like fax machines, email, and the World Wide Web. They are a necessary technical platform for electronic data exchange, but they are not specific to the healthcare domain, and are not addressed in this chapter.

- **Structural interoperability** is "an intermediate level that defines the structure or format of data exchange (i.e., the message format standards) where there is uniform movement of healthcare data from one system to another such that the clinical or operational purpose and meaning of the data is preserved and unaltered. Structural interoperability defines the syntax of the data exchange. It ensures that data exchanges between information technology systems can be interpreted at the data field level."

    - Most of the data standards discussed in this chapter work primarily at the second, structural, level: they specify fields, boundaries, and organization. A receiving system will understand where to look in an incoming message for the patient name field, or the discharge diagnosis; but it doesn't necessarily understand what that code means. This definition could be taken as a general definition of what health data interchange standards do.

- **Semantic interoperability** "provides interoperability at the highest level, which is the ability of two or more systems or elements to exchange information and to use the information that has been exchanged. Semantic interoperability takes advantage of both the structuring of the data exchange and the codification of the data including vocabulary so that the receiving information technology systems can interpret the data. This level of interoperability supports the electronic exchange of patient summary information among caregivers and other authorized parties via potentially disparate electronic health record (EHR) systems and other systems to improve quality, safety, efficiency, and efficacy of healthcare delivery."

  - Data standards at this third level include clinical decision support standards such as Arden Syntax and the Clinical Quality Language (CQL). Structural standards also tend to support a limited level of semantic engineering; for instance, the system will know whether the value in the patient gender field is actually a gender code. Receiving systems may also be able to infer appropriate actions from these codes—for example, understanding how to use drug code values in automated clinical decision support, such as a drug interaction check. However, reliable semantic processing of unanticipated content—"semantic interoperability"— is a feature that continues to elude system designers and standards designers alike: no current standard can be realistically characterized as fully supporting semantic interoperability.

Level two standards, structural interoperability standards, are primarily about putting things in their place. They will also, to a greater or lesser extent, specify what is permitted in those places. An NCPDP SCRIPT prescription, for instance, will typically use a standard code to identify a drug, so that both sender and recipient will understand what the request is about. The most widely used specification for these codes is the FDA's National Drug Codes (NDC), though the National Library of Medicine's RxNorm is also used. This is a case where the structural specification, SCRIPT, and the terminology specification, NDC, are distinct and independent, and are in fact specified by different organizations. Other fields in the SCRIPT message are stipulated by the SCRIPT specification itself—primarily values that are more tightly related to the structure of the specification or the interaction process, such as the fill status or message receipt acknowledgement.

So, level two structural standards may depend on ancillary standards to specify terminology. Many structural standards include some level of internal terminology specification, but most also refer to existing terminologies for key elements that the specification authors recognize as better served by those terminologies. Examples of terminologies include, in addition to the NDC codes used in prescriptions, Logical Observation Identifiers Names and Codes (LOINC)

FIGURE 15.1. Classification into structure and terminology standards

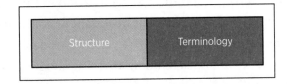

values for observation kinds, International Classification Tenth Revision Clinical Modification (ICD-10-CM) for morbidities, ICD-10 Procedure Coding System (ICD-10-PCS) and Current Procedural Terminology (CPT) for procedures, SNOMED CT for a variety of clinical domains, and RxNorm and Med-RT (replacement and successor to NDF-RT) for drugs. Figure 15.1 divides standards into structure and terminology standards. Terminology standards tend to focus on terminology, structural standards often address both structure and terminology.

Within the category of structural standards, another key factor in standardizing data exchange is the level of specificity that can be achieved. Standards that are specific to healthcare operate at a semantically more detailed layer than just a level one (foundational interoperability) standard, which includes platforms and tools such as fax machines. Healthcare standards identify questions and permissible answers and a syntactical field structure in which to place these answers, as well as workflow assumptions to govern acknowledgement of receipt and technical channels, such as a fax machine, over which to transport the data.

Degrees of Specificity

Within the interoperability levels defined by HIMSS, degrees of specificity the standard achieves can be distinguished. Some standards are designed to be very abstract: they are designed to support more specific derived standards that have implicit relationships to one another. These general-level standards are called **Reference Models**. Examples include the HL7 Reference Information Model (RIM) and ISO's Electronic Health Record Communication standard EN 13606. These standards are not designed to be implemented directly, but rather to provide a common framework for the design of more concrete specifications. The HL7 RIM, for instance, defines an "Act" class that, in downstream specifications, shows up as interventions coded as ICD-10-PCS values, as immunizations coded as Centers for Disease Control (CDC) CVX codes, as laboratory observations coded as LOINC tests, and as assertions of problems coded as ICD-10 CM or SNOMED CT values. Not all specifications are based on reference models, but the HL7 C-CDA is.

The second degree of specificity consists of the standard **specifications** themselves, for example, NCPDP SCRIPT or the Continuity of Care Document (CCD). The specifications serve named purposes, and they often provide sufficient detail to implement without further guidance. However, they sometimes leave some things underspecified for implementers, and a third level may be necessary.

The third degree of specificity is the **profile**. The profile finishes the specification by constraining any ambiguities and options left in a specification so that implementers in a particular community can communicate clearly, without irrelevant or confusing extra decisions. It will often be published in an **implementation guide (IG)**, an artifact designed to be handed to a software developer who, ideally, does not need to know anything about the subject matter; the guide should contain all the information necessary to build the message. Any terminology requirements that the specification leaves open, for instance, must be precisely specified or, if that's not possible, designed to support free text (with the processing requirements appropriate to text, instead). Other fields may be further constrained with business rules specific to interfaces in a certain community of participants; the number of times an element may repeat may be reduced, or an onset date may be required to be later than a birth date.

This is a general framework that cannot neatly classify every standard. Note that there are specifications that are detailed enough to require no additional profiling (for example, NCPDP SCRIPT), and there are profiles that require further refinement to support implementation.

The specificity that can be achieved varies. Some standards are very specific, supporting, for instance, immunization reporting, or public health lab results. These standards are specified in minute detail, and they are as a result very robust. For example, immunization systems routinely exchange data with minimal exceptions, errors, or oversight, and that data can be used by the recipient organization in the provision of care. Other standards attempt to represent broader domains, up to and including everything in a patient record that might be of interest to a consulting clinician, or to a care team taking over for a transferred patient. Due to the breadth and volume of content that might be included in these transfers, these standards have not achieved the level of specificity or robustness seen in immunization messages, even when they are thoroughly profiled.

Any or all three of these degrees of specificity may involve some level of terminology assignment, and the result can sometimes be an overlapping set of artifacts as shown in figure 15.2.

FIGURE 15.2. Classification of standards by specificity

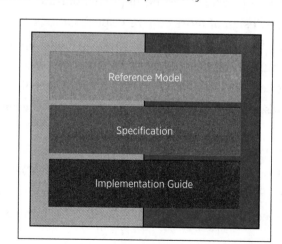

The HL7 RIM specifies some terminology bindings for structural properties, but it leaves terms for clinical properties unspecified. The CDA specification specifies some clinical terminology bindings, and it leaves others for specific implementation guides to specify.

Additional Considerations for Interchange Standards

These interoperability layers and degrees of specificity give a comprehensive overview of static data specifications, but the data doesn't just sit there; people use it. A third consideration in this classification is the ways people find and use this information: **behavioral standards**, as opposed to **content standards**. Behavioral health data interchange standards are those that describe messaging protocols, workflows, and algorithms to be executed by the communicating systems. They can be divided into push and pull standards. Does someone need to ask for it, or does it flow based on some underlying process? A lab report is requested when the order is placed, so when the report is ready, it is pushed to that provider without further request: access to the lab report is defined by the order, prior to the existence of the report. A CCD, on the other hand, is typically not the result of an order; it is a digest of existing information, and a provider who wants it must search for it and request it. Access in this case depends on a discovery process; both access and discovery processes can be standardized.

In addition to the discovery and access standards, a discussion of processes includes security: How are participants in these exchanges authorized to find and view this sensitive information? Security constraints are also an integral part of any exchange standard, as figure 15.3 reflects.

In this diagram, an instance of patient data (a CCD, a SCRIPT prescription, or some other standardized package of information) can be discovered and retrieved by a provider, but both discovery and access are controlled by standardized security policies. Among the security regulations constraining health data exchange in the US, the Health Insurance Portability and Accountability Act (HIPAA) is the most comprehensive, but there are many other constraints. They are realized in specifications such as the IHE's Cross-Enterprise Document Sharing (XDS)

FIGURE 15.3. Classification of behavioral standards

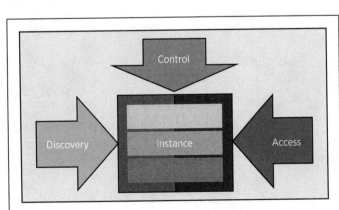

and Audit Trail and Node Authentication (ATNA). These standards tend to function at the foundational level of interoperability, but there are cases where they are controlled by data at the structural or semantic layers, such as when access to a patient record is restricted because the patient has a condition listed in a regulation.

The last dimension to consider is the stakeholders who influence the designs of these standards (see figure 15.4). The standards don't implement themselves, stakeholders define and adopt them to meet business objectives. Some of those objectives may be tightly constrained; for example, HIPAA regulations define non-negotiable requirements on implementers. Others may be a matter of priority, such as facilities that rely on revenue from Medicare and Medicaid claims must comply with policies from the Centers for Medicaid and Medicare (CMS) to enable certain payments; those that don't may choose not to comply with these policies.

Also note that the primary stakeholders, the patients, don't typically have time, expertise, or resources to participate in this process. They may be represented by their caregivers such as large healthcare systems, by government agencies such as the CDC or the Veterans Administration, by legislators who pass laws such as HIPAA or the Affordable Care Act, or by other patient advocacy groups.

The most motivated stakeholders are those with the most resources at stake: the software vendors who may have to comply with standards. Also well represented are the insurers and payers who need to understand the standards in order to transact business and provider organizations large enough to have standards development budgets.

If the three use cases introduced on page 457 are classified, then SCRIPT and the Continuity of Care Document in use cases one and two are content standards, specifying structure and some terminology at different levels of specificity, as in figure 15.5.

The Cross-Enterprise Document Sharing standard in use case three describes how these assets may be identified and retrieved, and it fits in the behavioral standards view shown in figure 15.6.

FIGURE 15.4. The standards development environment

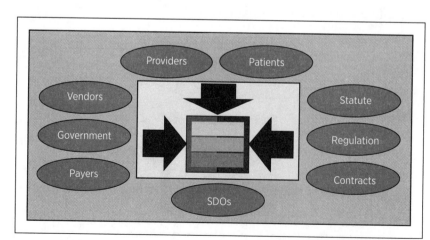

FIGURE 15.5. Classification of SCRIPT and CCD standards

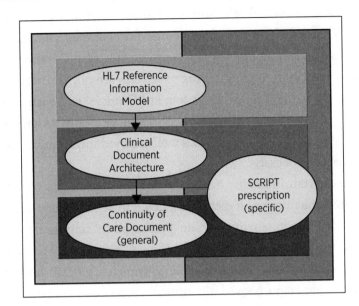

FIGURE 15.6. Classification of XDS standard

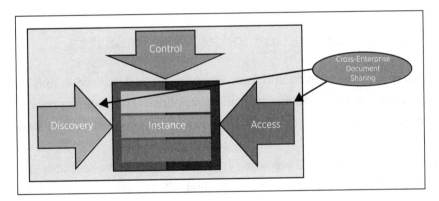

Those interested in identifying standards used for specific purposes in the US may consult the **Interoperability Standards Advisory (ISA)**, a guide published by the **Office of the National Coordinator for Health Information Technology (ONC)** to help clarify the current state of standards regulation (ONC 2018a). The primary source of truth for the content of the ISA is the *Federal Register* but navigating the cross-references and updates to that asset is extremely difficult, and the ISA provides an authoritative summary of the current landscape. It is updated annually.

Standards Drivers

Standards are expensive, so they aren't created without compelling business reasons. In many industries, these reasons are sufficiently clear that stakeholders have come together without encouragement. Healthcare is different, for two primary reasons. First, the information is complex. Financial instruments and telecommunications equipment can be complex, but they encompass services that are defined by human beings; for example, a bank deposit is completely described by its entry in a ledger. Human health is the surface manifestation of the most complex system known, in which most of the underlying processes are not well understood. Second, the ramifications of a mistake in an accounting system are financial and easily remedied. A mistake in a clinical setting could harm a patient, possibly critically or fatally. As a result, the industry has been slow to commit its business processes to a well-defined information architecture that can be managed by automated processes.

Within healthcare, certain domains have been well standardized based on their business requirements. Functions that can be efficiently managed in separate organizations tend to repay effort spent on standardization, so medication prescription standards and lab reports have been well-established for years. Functions with minimal variability can also be easily standardized, so registration functions like "admit-discharge-transfer" (ADT) have been standardized. Additionally, functions that require special technical resources may benefit from aggregation, so imaging services have been standardized. More general clinical processes, however, have not been standardized, until recently.

Health Data Standardization in the United States

For domains that are more complex and interdependent, standardization may not evolve from market priorities. In these cases, if standardization happens, it happens as a result of government action. There have been three primary regulatory events driving health data standardization in the US.

The first event, the **National Technology Transfer and Advancement Act (NTTAA)** of 1995, gave the US Office of Management and Budget (OMB) authority to direct federal agencies to use "voluntary consensus standards" unless inconsistent with law or impractical. OMB Circular A119 describes a voluntary consensus **Standards Development Organization (SDO)** as an organization possessing the attributes of balance of interest, due process, an appeals process, and consensus. Consensus is defined as agreement, but not necessarily unanimity, and compliant bodies include processes to resolve all objections by interested parties. In addition to voluntary consensus standards, the circular identifies "government-unique standards" that are developed for use by the federal government (such as the Federal Information Processing Standards, or FIPS). It does not mention de facto standards—standards adopted by an industry purely due to their prevalence and irrespective of any procedural or organizational authority. Any of these forms of standards can be mandated by law (OMB 1998).

The second event was the passage of the Health Insurance Portability and Accountability Act (HIPAA). This act was originally motivated by public perceptions of the difficulty of switching insurance companies, and the portability features were expected to have an impact on portability across care settings as well. Much of the act, however, dealt with privacy concerns, and while financial transactions were standardized (primarily through Accredited Standards Committee (ASC) transactions), the ability to transfer data among providers was actually impeded.

In addition to mandating specific transaction standards, the HIPAA provisions established a regulatory category of organization—**Designated Standards Maintenance Organization (DSMO)**—to maintain the standards adopted and criteria for the process to be used in such maintenance. Many, but not all, DSMOs are SDOs accredited by the **American National Standards Institute (ANSI)**, such as ASC X12, Health Level Seven (HL7), and **National Council for Prescription Drug Programs (NCPDP)**. Others include the National Uniform Billing Committee (NUBC) and the National Uniform Claim Committee (NUCC). Under the HIPAA regulations, the Secretary of Health and Human Services (HHS) is required to consult with the DSMOs before adopting any standard for electronic healthcare transactions.

The third event was **Meaningful Use (MU)**, the result of the staggering cost of healthcare in the US and the belief that data standardization could help control costs. In addition, increasing recognition that medical errors are a serious problem, and that many errors can be avoided by better compliance with clinical guidelines, has convinced many that more standardized representation of patient data will support better quality care. Despite these perceptions, many clinicians resist data standardization because standardized quality processes have difficulty dealing with the variety of situations that they encounter and because capturing data in standardized forms inevitably imposes costs on the care process, degrades quality, or both.

Whatever the merits of standardization, this stalemate was broken by the financial crash of 2007. The American Recovery and Reinvestment Act of 2009 (ARRA) was an economic stimulus package designed to pull the economy out of recession, and it included the **Health Information Technology for Economic and Clinical Health (HITECH) Act**. HITECH was designed to modernize healthcare by promoting and expanding the adoption of health information technology. A key provision of HITECH was the Meaningful Use, an initiative to encourage adoption of electronic health records by specifying what it meant for such a system to "meaningfully" use data from other systems, and by tying Medicaid and Medicare payments to proof that such a system was in use. In 2018, CMS rebranded MU to **Promoting Interoperability (PI)** to indicate the focus on increasing health information exchange and patient data access.

Within that legislation and subsequent regulation are requirements for certain functional capabilities and use of certain standards within those systems, and a requirement that those systems be tested and certified by a federally recognized certification body.

The PI standards regulations, found in 42 CFR 170 (2015), identify standards to be used in the following operations and transactions:

- Storage of patient data, including demographics, problems, medications, and the like
- Interactions with clinical decision support
- Query, transmission, display, and incorporation of summary records

- Electronic prescribing
- Clinical information reconciliation
- Capture and export of clinical quality measures
- Security and transport-layer specifications

Standards specifications are grouped under several headings:

- Transport standards: §202 (for example, Direct, XDR)
- Content standards: §205 (for example, CCD, C-CDA, NCPDP SCRIPT, HL7 V2.5)
- Terminology standards: §207 (for example, SNOMED CT, LOINC, RxNorm)
- 2014 EHR certification criteria: §314
- 2015 EHR certification criteria: §315

The standards specified by PI already existed, in more or less mature forms, but this policy change meant that stakeholders were much more motivated to make them work. Lab, pharmacy, and imaging standards have not changed under PI, but the management of care coordination depends on more complex interactions, and the standards available in 2007 have been greatly expanded.

In the use cases in this chapter, SCRIPT was standardized before PI. The CCD existed, but has achieved much greater traction since PI, and its profile has been refined and its implementations more effectively integrated. XSD also existed before PI but has been more aggressively adopted since then.

Note that the content domains for standardization are subject to change. The initial PI lists 15 "common clinical data elements" that EHRs are expected to be able to exchange; the more recent efforts, now termed US Core Data for Interoperability (USCDI) adds 7 more, with a prospective calendar for increasing scope gradually over time (ONC 2018b).

All agencies are directed to use standards where appropriate under NTTAA; HHS has authority to require conformance to specific standards under HIPAA, and it has authority to promote specific standards by making payment for certain services dependent on adoption under PI.

The Standards Development Process

At a high level, a standard progresses through three phases:

1. Design
2. Profiling
3. Implementation

The design phase begins when a need is recognized by stakeholders with resources to begin work. This need may be in response to a market opportunity, as with the DICOM imaging standards or NCPDP's universal claim form, to regulatory constraint, as with HIPAA transactions, or to a combination of circumstances like Meaningful Use, which uses government incentives rather than regulation to encourage compliance.

The process of defining the standards is constrained by rules that ensure all stakeholders have a chance to influence the design, and that no single stakeholder has undue influence. These rules are set in the US by ANSI, and they are informed by rules defined by the International Organization for Standards (ISO), to which ANSI is the official US representative. ANSI publishes its process requirements in *ANSI Essential Requirements: Due process requirements for American National Standards*, where key items include openness, lack of dominance, balance, and written procedures for coordinating conflicting perspectives.

During the process of standards development, interested parties will implement draft versions of the standards in their systems to confirm that they support requirements and that they are technically feasible. This trial implementation activity is a significant part of the cost of the standardization process.

If a standard supports communities with divergent needs, it will be left in a somewhat ambiguous state, the ambiguities to be resolved by profiling. Profiling has two meanings. The first is constraint profiling, the activity of specifying standards constraints that may not be universally appropriate. For instance, CDA document headers have no patient race property because different countries have different concepts of race and ethnicity (Morning 2008). In the US, however, race is a required field to support auditing for equity purposes. As a result, US profiles specify that CDA documents include the Office of Management and Budget (OMB) classifications for race and ethnicity. Implementers who are interested in ensuring that the standards support requirements and are technically feasible will continue to test their ability to implement at the profiling stage.

Profiling also refers to the activity of creating implementation guides that specify not only additional constraints, but how to integrate multiple standards. The 360 Exchange Closed Loop Referral (360X) from Integrating the Healthcare Enterprise (IHE), for instance, describes how to use both CDA documents and HL7 V2 messages in referral transactions.

Many SDOs create their own profiles or create standards that may be specific enough to not require profiling. However, even when a standard is technically specific enough to support implementation, a profile may be useful to guide implementers in making shared assumptions about context and integration with other technologies.

The principal healthcare IT standards-profiling organization is Integrating the Healthcare Enterprise (IHE), which selects healthcare IT and cross-industry standards to develop implementation guides based on market requirements. These have been used to define system integration and conformance specifications. IHE operates at the international level, and its profiles are available at no cost.

Many other organizations contribute to profiling, most notably including efforts chartered by the ONC. The names of the ONC efforts change over time and have included Health Information

Technology Standards Panel (HITSP), the Standards and Interoperability Framework (S&I Framework), the Health IT Standards Committee (HITSC) and Health IT Policy Committee (HITPC), and now the Health Information Technology Advisory Committee (HITAC).

Both base standards and profiles may be balloted as **normative standards** – standards that carry the legitimacy and enforceability of the completed SDO process. The process of agreeing that a standard should become normative is the subject of the ANSI process definition, which specifies that an SDO support the ability for stakeholders to comment and to negotiate mutually satisfactory resolutions to comments before the final standard is published.

At a high level, the process looks like what is shown in figure 15.7.

In figure 15.7, the specification of the standards, including the committee meetings, document draft activities, balloting and negotiation, all happen within the green ovals. While this specification work is in process, stakeholders are examining the proposals to ensure they meet requirements and are feasible. The requirements analysis can be done by any stakeholder, but feasibility is the special domain of the implementer. Implementers will be committed to use the standards, so they have significant interest in ensuring that they work, which they confirm by implementing them.

The blue ovals show implementation activity, much of which occurs during the standards design process. If an implementer discovers a problem with some assumption in the design, he or she will be able to influence the design before it becomes a commitment.

The red ovals illustrate third-party testing activities. Implementers may believe that they have succeeded in implementing a standard, but the only way to be sure is through an independent testing process. The two primary channels for this are industry conformance testing and regulatory certification testing. Conformance testing includes events such as IHE Connectathons,

FIGURE 15.7. Standards development process

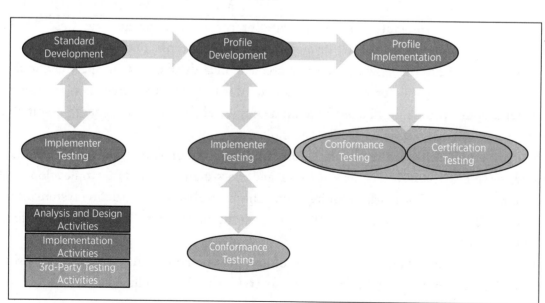

where vendors meet and test their exchanges with one another. These events don't test the standard; they are designed to ensure the implementer meets the standard and to allow vendors to list their products in a product registry that identifies the IHE profiles and roles that have been proven.

Authorized Certification and Testing Bodies (ATCBs) accredited by ANSI conduct certification testing. ATCBs inspect healthcare IT systems for conformance with standards-based criteria for clinical application functions, security, and interoperability specified in the PI regulations. Use of ATCB-tested and certified systems enables healthcare providers to qualify for meaningful use incentives and other regulatory and policy-based benefits.

The length of the standards development process is measured in years. Specific changes, such as an update to a mature standard, may make it through ballot in as little as one year. The FHIR family of standards, famed for its rapid uptake, began in 2012 and will publish its first normative artifacts in 2019.

A final consideration in the standards development process is the number of organizations with similar goals doing this work. The volume of work in progress means that it is not possible for every stakeholder to be fully aware of all of the other related efforts under way, and it is fairly common to discover that a specification is partially or even completely redundant. When two specifications overlap, the question of which is redundant is a matter of perspective, and the ensuing work to bring them into alignment is called **harmonization**. In some organizations, such as HL7, harmonization is a formal part of the development process, designed to minimize the chance of redundant specifications making it into publication. In the cross-organization case, there is no overarching governance to enforce harmonization, so it tends to occur when business drivers cause it.

Stakeholders

The standards development process is supported by a wide variety of participants. These include standards advocates, standards developers, software vendors, clinical institutions, payers, and the research community.

Standards Advocates

Advocates push for the establishment of standards for policy reasons. These may include goals such as improving care quality, reducing costs, or even, as in the case of HITECH, stimulating the economy.

Advocacy organizations influence and facilitate the standards process at every step. National governments are prominent standardization advocates, often sponsoring, funding, and staffing standards activities. Private-sector stakeholders include advocacy organizations such as health

IT and finance advocates and software vendors, implementers, and users. Consumers also have a stake in standards, although they are underrepresented in standards advocacy.

Advocacy organizations can serve a convening and coordinating role, identifying the need for a standard for a particular use case, and coordinating the development and implementation of it across multiple stakeholders. Vendor associations and medical professional societies can serve a similar role.

Many US government agencies are influential stakeholders, including

- ONC, lead agency charged with formulating the federal government's health information technology strategy and coordinating federal health IT policies, standards, and investments
- The National Institute for Standards and Technology (NIST), charged by HITECH with supporting conformance and certification activities
- CMS, which leverages payment to encourage participation in standards and quality programs including Medicare Access and CHIP Reauthorization Act of 2015 (MACRA), the Quality Payment Program, and Ambulatory Payment Classifications (APCs) prospective payment systems, as well as overseeing standards for HIPAA, maintaining the Medicare Severity Diagnosis Related Groups (MS-DRGs), and publishing ICD-10-PCS
- The Agency for Healthcare Research and Quality (AHRQ), which promotes uniform, accurate, and automated healthcare data
- The National Library of Medicine (NLM), which is responsible for the Unified Medical Language System that develops and distributes electronic "knowledge sources" and lexical programs, such as RxNorm
- The Departments of Veterans Affairs (VA) and Defense (DOD), which both contain very large healthcare provider organizations with strong participation in standards value-chain organizations
- CDC, which is responsible for population health at the national level. CDC actively participates in numerous standards development efforts, including the National Center for Health Statistics (NCHS), which is responsible for ICD-10-CM.

In addition, there are many nongovernmental advocacy organizations. Some have broad agendas, such as promoting healthcare IT interoperability standards, and others have a narrower focus, such as promoting patient privacy. They influence the healthcare standards value chain through their publications, educational forums, orchestrated public comment on standards, lobbying, and similar channels.

Advocacy organizations can be placed in several categories:

- Healthcare provider advocates, which represent licensed healthcare professionals and care-providing enterprises. Examples include the American College of

Physicians (ACP), the American Hospital Association (AHA), the American Nurses Association (ANA), the College of American Pathologists (CAP), and the Radiological Society of North America (RSNA). Some of them develop and publish standards, such as CPT and the Diagnostic and Statistical Manual of Mental Disorders (DSM).

- Healthcare financial advocates, including both providers and benefit plans that pay for care. Examples include the Healthcare Financial Management Association, the Council for Affordable Quality Healthcare (CAQH), the Leapfrog Group, and the **Workgroup for Electronic Data Interchange (WEDI)**.

- Healthcare IT advocates, which promote healthcare IT standardization. Examples include AHIMA, the American Medical Informatics Association (AMIA), the Center for Health Transformation, the Healthcare Information and Management Systems Society (HIMSS), the EHR Association (EHRA), the National Quality Forum (NQF), and the Medical Imaging and Technology Alliance (MITA).

- The academic community for cross-industry technologies and clinical informatics, which provides intellectual capital from research, sponsors standardization activities, influences government actions, conducts educational forums, and consults with value-chain organizations. For example, HL7 was fostered at Duke University, and the LOINC code set was developed and is maintained by the Regenstrief Institute in collaboration with Indiana University.

- Healthcare consumers, although they are underrepresented in healthcare IT standardization advocacy. Organizations with relevant agendas include AARP, Medic Alert, Patient Privacy Rights, and consumer-oriented activities within AHIMA and HIMSS.

Market Stakeholders

Software vendors, implementers, and users are economic stakeholders. They influence standards development and implementation through participation and funding. Their balance of interest is both strategic and tactical. Health Information Exchange (HIE) organizations are especially dependent upon standards, those being the underpinnings of the organization.

Developers of Standards

Many consensus-based SDOs are accredited by ANSI, while others have a liaison relationship with the International Organization for Standardization (ISO), and some, like the Internet Engineering Task Force (IETF) and the World Wide Web Consortium (W3C), stand on their own. Professional societies and trade associations may also develop standards. Consensus-based SDOs are the primary developers of data exchange standards. ANSI accredits the developers of voluntary consensus standards in the US to increase global competitiveness in a variety of industries, including healthcare.

Accredited Standards Committee (ASC) X12

In 1979, ANSI chartered the **Accredited Standards Committee (ASC) X12** to develop standards for **electronic data interchange (EDI)**, the most common technical channel for industry interfaces prior to the internet. In 2014, ASC X12 became ANSI accredited as an SDO (ASC X12 2018).

Two boards support the Steering committee: The Procedures Review Board (PRB) ensures that standards development at ASC X12 follows due process, and Policies And Procedures (P&P) has a more general charter to support the Steering Committee in overseeing policies and procedures.

Four subcommittees are responsible for industry-specific standards: Finance (X12F), Transportation (X12I), Supply Chain (X12M), and Insurance (X12N). Three subcommittees support these industry groups. Communications & Controls (X12C) is responsible for "Standards, Guidelines, and Reference Models that govern technical components of the X12 EDI Standard and for other work products that apply across the industry specific subcommittees" (ASC 2017a). Technical Assessment (X12J) is responsible for "the technical integrity of Accredited Standards Committee (ASC) work products developed by the subcommittees" (ASC 2017b). External Code Lists Oversight (X12-02) oversees maintenance of X12 external code lists.

There are also caucuses to promote industry involvement. The Dental Caucus promotes the interest of dental providers, and the Provider Caucus promotes the interest of all providers. Clearinghouse Caucus and Connectivity Caucus have very similar missions, which are "to develop and promote the improvement of EDI Network interconnectivity and peer-to-peer connection between two networking organizations" (ASC X12 2018). Figure 15.8 illustrates an example of the specification for an X12 element.

Use of Implementation Guides

X12 standards are commonly used within the healthcare industry for administrative data that supports reimbursement and insurance-related messaging. HIPAA stipulates the use of many X12 specifications. Healthcare organizations that use HIPAA-defined transactions must use the ANSI ASC X12N standard formats.

The X12N implementation guides explain the proper use of a standard for a specific business purpose. For example, an implementation guide provides details on how each transaction is to be implemented, including field sizes, data definitions, and conditions (whether specific fields are mandatory or situational). Implementation guides also are the primary reference documents used by businesses implementing the associated transactions.

ASC X12N specifications are incorporated into the HIPAA regulations by reference.

FIGURE 15.8. X12 data element

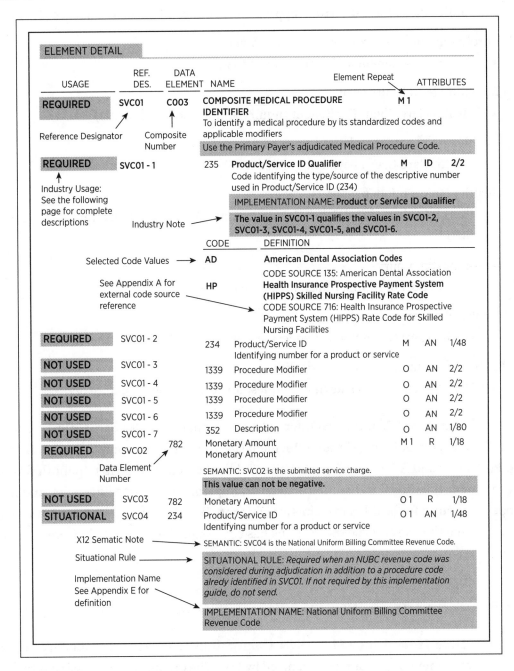

Source: ASC 2010, 9.

The following is a list of the HIPAA-specified transactions and their corresponding X12 specification numbers:

(A) Health claims or equivalent encounter information
- Health Care Claim and Coordination and Benefits (837)

(B) Health claims attachments
  - Additional Information to Support a Health Care Claim or Encounter (275)

(C) Enrollment and disenrollment in a health plan
  - Benefit Enrollment and Maintenance (834)

(D) Eligibility for a health plan
  - Health Care Eligibility Benefit Inquiry and Response (270/271)

(E) Health care payment and remittance advice
  - Health Care Claim Payment/Advice (835)

(F) Health plan premium payments
  - Payroll Deducted and Other Group Premium Payment for Insurance Products (820)

(G) First report of injury
  - First Report of Injury, Illness or Incident (148)

(H) Health claim status
  - Health Care Claim Status Request and Response (276/277)

(I) Referral certification and authorization
  - Health Care Services Review: Request for Review and Response (278)

Note that items B and G, Additional Information to Support a Health Care Claim or Encounter (275) and First Report of Injury, Illness or Incident (148), are not yet required. Section 1104 of the Patient Protection and Affordable Care Act directed the Secretary of HHS to publish final regulations to establish national transaction standards, implementation specifications, and a single set of operating rules for healthcare claims attachments (PPACA 2010). As of late 2018, no regulation stipulating the use of these transactions has been published, though they are listed in the ONC's ISA.

Clinical Data Interchange Standards Consortium

The **Clinical Data Interchange Standards Consortium (CDISC)** is a voluntary consensus standards development organization recognized by ISO. The organization's mission is to develop and support interoperable data standards for medical research and related areas of healthcare (CDISC 2018).

CDISC coordinates with other international standards development efforts, including IHE and HL7. CDISC and HL7 have a memorandum of understanding under which the two organizations have jointly developed standards, including the Biomedical Research Integrated Domain Group (BRIDG) Model, which is a domain analysis model that harmonizes the CDISC standards among each other. BRIDG has been mapped to the HL7 RIM, and it is also published as an OWL graph to support logical and semantic web operations (BRIDG 2018). CDISC also participates in activities in the Quality, Research, and Public Health domains of IHE (see below), promoting use of its standards in IHE profiles that support medical research activities. CDISC has developed standards to support research globally and has coordinating committees in Europe, Japan, and China.

CDISC has created a suite of standards that supports clinical research from the protocol through data collection, analysis, and reporting, including several that were developed for use in electronic submissions to regulatory agencies like the Food and Drug Administration. Foundational standards lay the groundwork to support data exchange. The Study Data Tabulation Model (SDTM) is a reference model for regulatory submission of case report form data tabulations from clinical research studies, and is a base standard used with other CDISC specifications. The Operational Data Model (ODM) is an XML-based content and format standard for the acquisition, exchange, reporting or submission, and archival of Case Report Form (CRF)-based clinical research data and adheres to regulatory requirements for audit trail information. The Clinical Data Acquisition Standards Harmonization (CDASH) specification is a CDISC content standard for basic data collection fields in case report forms. CDISC is aligned with SDTM such that data collection in CDASH format minimizes the resources needed to produce SDTM downstream, thus streamlining the clinical research process. BRIDG is another foundational effort of CDISC.

Data Exchange standards include specifications that may or may not be based on the foundational standards. Clinical Trial Registry (CTR)-XML, Dataset-XML, and Define-XML are XML

FIGURE 15.9. Selected CDISC standards in the classification of standards by specificity

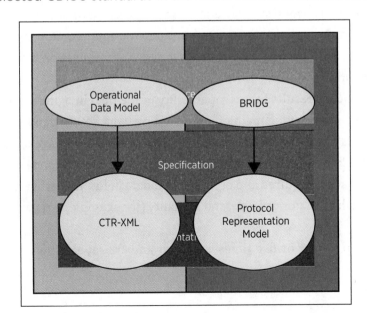

languages for transmission of trial submissions and datasets based on ODM and SDTM foundational standards (see figure 15.9).

CDISC works with stakeholders in autoimmune, cardiovascular, neurology, and other specialty domains to guide study tool standard development. Their coordination with the National Cancer Institute Enterprise Vocabulary Services (NCI-EVS) has resulted in significant terminology development work (see chapter 16).

Digital Imaging and Communications in Medicine

The first (1985) and second (1988) versions of a standard for transferring images and associated information between imaging devices and systems were developed by the American College of Radiology (ACR) and the National Electrical Manufacturers Association (NEMA). These organizations created a joint committee and developed the **Digital Imaging and Communications in Medicine (DICOM)** standard. First available in 1993, DICOM is a standard for the interchange of computerized biomedical images and image-related information within and between healthcare providers.

The DICOM standard contains specifications addressing many of the domains of standard design, including domain information design, terminology, message exchange protocols, network support, storage requirements for media files, and security, though many of the lower-level protocols are not necessary when the content standards are carried as payloads in other standards, such as CDA (NEMA 2018). The DICOM standard has been incorporated into the product designs of many diagnostic medical imaging vendors. Its application is rapidly spreading to every medical profession that uses images, including cardiology, dentistry, endoscopy, mammography, ophthalmology, pathology, radiation therapy, radiology, surgery, and so on. Originally designed to support picture archiving and communication systems (PACS), DICOM images are now integrated into more generally useful standards such as HL7 CDA templates and IHE profiles. Using DICOM can result in the transfer of medical images in a multivendor environment, ease the development and expansion of picture archiving and communication systems, and interface with clinical information systems.

The DICOM standard results in interoperability of medical imaging equipment by defining services for storing and retrieving media files, including workflow around storage commitment and off-line retrieval. The file formats provide flexible options for images, from simple two-dimensional grayscale images to four-dimensional nuclear magnetic resonance images, and they are tagged with a library of required and optional metadata fields indicating the patient, provider, and image details such as anatomy, angle, and modality (for example, x-ray vs. PET scan) (NEMA 2018).

Updates occur up to four or five times each year and are republished on the website under Prior Editions.

Health Level Seven International

Health Level Seven International (HL7), founded in 1987, is a voluntary consensus standards development organization recognized by ISO and accredited by ANSI. The organization's mission is to provide standards for interoperability that improve care delivery, optimize workflow, reduce ambiguity and enhance knowledge transfer among healthcare providers, government agencies, the vendor community, fellow SDOs, patients, and other stakeholders. The number "7" in the name of the organization refers to the application level (the highest level) in the seven-layer communication model known as the Open Systems Interconnection (OSI) model. Thus, HL7 works at the healthcare domain level and does not specify lower-level supporting technologies.

Most HL7 member countries have official "affiliate" organizations, but because HL7 was formed in the US and draws most of its members and funding from the US, it has been well-aligned with US interests, and no US affiliate has been established. There is a US realm steering committee, which assumes some of the duties normally undertaken by an affiliate, but it has limited authority. The lack of a specified US stakeholder complicates the difficulty of coordinating a coherent US position on standards design issues.

The organization is governed by a board, and structured into four steering divisions, guided by a Technical Steering Committee (TSC) and Architecture Review Board (ARB). The Clinical steering division defines "the requirements and solutions to support the needs for communicating information related to the creation, management, execution and quality of messages, services, resources and documents." The Administrative steering division "focuses on the creation of basic patterns and common messages, including knowledge representation and access, that are used to convey domain specific content." The Infrastructure steering division "focuses on providing the fundamental tools and building blocks that other Work Groups should use to build the standards." And the Organizational Support steering division "develops projects and products providing direct support to the work groups" (HL7 2018).

Within each division, work groups develop and maintain the standards. Work groups are semi-permanent structures in the organization, usually lasting for several years or even decades. Standards are created by work groups and approved by the membership of the organization by vote.

Key standards created by HL7 include

- Version 2 Messaging Standard
- Version 3 Product Suite
- Clinical Document Architecture (CDA)
- Fast Health Information Resources (FHIR)

Other standards include the Clinical Context Object Workgroup specification (CCOW) and a set of standards to support quality reporting.

Version 2 Messaging Standard

The Version 2 Messaging standard (V2) is one of the most widely implemented standards used for exchange of clinical data in the world. For intrafacility communication, such as ADT and lab reports, Version 2 is by far the dominant standard. V2 was built in the age of EDI, and its syntax uses defined characters—usually pipes (|)—to indicate field boundaries. The most current version of V2 is 2.8, with version 2.9 under discussion. Most implementations follow the American Recovery and Reinvestment Act of 2009, which specifies version 2.5. This is an example of what many would consider inappropriate specificity in statute, as it impedes adoption of further refined versions of the standard, though the versions tend to be largely backward compatible.

Responsibility for the chapters in the Version 2 standard is distributed throughout various HL7 Workgroups. For example, Control (chapter 2) and Query (chapter 5) are the responsibility of the Infrastructure and Messaging Workgroup.

Implementers of V2 noticed that its specification is not quite as precise as it could be, and the implementation guides that were developed tended to result in incompatible implementations. A key component of this incompatibility was the use of "Z-segments," additional parts of the standard that are fully defined in the implementation guide, and therefore inaccessible to anyone outside of the community responsible for the guide. For implementers of individual interfaces this posed no problem, but for stakeholders who wanted to communicate across these community boundaries—for health information exchanges, patient transfers, or merger-based organizational consolidation—these segments presented a problem. Architects at HL7 developed a solution for this problem: a new specification family based on a reference model that would allow any additional data element to be modeled consistently. This way, an interface developer who needed a field no one else had anticipated could model the element in the reference model, and then other participants could understand what the element was. This insight was the genesis of HL7 Version 3 and its foundational Reference Information Model (RIM).

There are many opinions about why the V3 program did not work, but the general perception was that the investment in architectural overhead did not pay sufficient dividends in either ease of implementation or semantic interoperability. V3 can work with sufficient investment—it has been adopted by the National Health Service in the United Kingdom and by Canada Health Infoway, and adoption was attempted in Japan and the Netherlands—but the required investment level is too high for most communities. In an article posted in 2011, HL7 architect Grahame Grieve argued, among other things, that "the V3 design process is technology and platform agnostic – but that just makes implementation more costly" (Grieve 2011).

If the difficulty of V3 lies in its abstraction, then implementing a more concrete subset of V3 should be easier, and this is what has happened with Clinical Document Architecture (CDA).

Clinical Document Architecture

Clinical Document Architecture (CDA) was developed to be an interchange standard to support electronic documentation of patient encounters and services (for example, lab reports and imaging studies). CDA uses the RIM to specify an XML document header that can be used to index and search for documents. This header may include an attached file, such as a pdf or a scanned image of a document, or it may include an XML body. The body contains section narratives, and those sections may also include detailed structured representations of clinical data following the Clinical Statement pattern of the HL7 RIM. A CDA header with an attachment is referred to as a "level 1" CDA, one with inline XML text sections is "level 2," and one with structured data is "level 3," as shown in figure 15.10.

CDA is the basis for several widely used and internationally adopted implementation guides, including the Continuity of Care Document (CCD), the harmonized collection of 12 CDA document templates called **Consolidated CDA (C-CDA)**, and the **Quality Reporting Document Architecture (QRDA)**. The CCD was originally developed as a US-based implementation guide, but it has been adopted in whole or in part internationally, including by IHE and numerous national programs in Europe and the Asia/Pacific region.

The Joint Initiative Council (JIC), a consortium of SDOs including ISO Technical Committee 215 and others, has embarked on a project to develop an International Patient Summary, building on the work done at ASTM and HL7. The C-CDA is recognized in the Meaningful Use Certification criteria and is the HL7 designated successor to the original CCD specification. The ONC's 2015 requirements cite C-CDA version 2.1, as "Release 2.1 largely provides compatibility with Release 1.1 while maintaining many of the improvements and new templates in Release 2.0" (ONC 2015).

The QRDA draft standard for trial use (DSTU) layers quality-reporting capabilities onto the CDA standard for the exchange of electronic clinical quality measure (eCQM) data. It enables the reporting of measure specific events at the patient level, and aggregating measure scores at the population level. QRDA defines three categories of output: Category I, containing individual

FIGURE 15.10. CDA levels

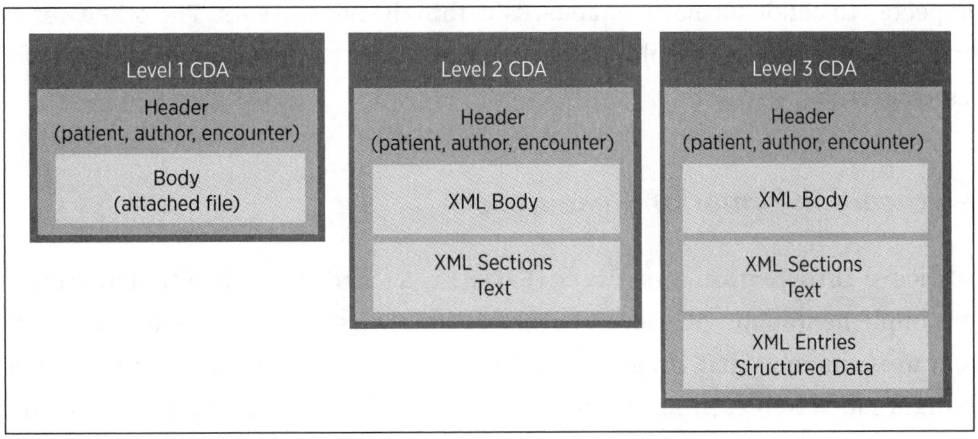

449

patient data; Category II, identifying which patients appear in each cohort associated with a quality measure; and Category III, providing aggregated measure scores. QRDA Category I and Category III formats (DSTU3) are specified in the certification criteria as being the standard format for reporting quality measure data to CMS for the Meaningful Use program (ONC 2015).

The Health Quality Measure Format (HQMF) is a standard specification for defining a quality measure, including those informing QRDA reports. HQMF is also based on the HL7 RIM, but it is not a CDA document. The HQMF and QRDA standards address two different sides of the same issue: how to describe a quality measure, and how to report a quality measurement. They rely on two other standards, the CMS-sponsored Quality Data model (QDM) to lay out how quality data should be structured, and HL7 Clinical Quality Language (CQI) to express logic that is human readable yet structured enough for processing electronically.

Another standard that applies V3 to a constrained domain is the Structured Product Labeling (SPL) specification. This specification defines how to describe regulated products such as pharmaceuticals. These descriptions are used in official transactions with the Food and Drug Administration such as drug trials and adverse event reporting as well as for the management of package insert information. Apart from CDA documents, HQMF, and SPL, V3 is not used in the US.

CDA provides a way to implement HL7 V3 data, but it is not a solution to the interoperability problem. Meaningful Use requires reconciliation of medications, allergies, concerns, and immunizations, but the CDA specification is loose enough that supporting automated management of these tasks has proven extremely difficult. This generality is by design: CDA was built to represent documents, such as progress notes and discharge summaries. Those documents reflect the detailed and nuanced outcome of expert clinical judgment: they tend not to have a lot of predefined structure, and it is unrealistic to expect to be able to impose such structure on this information in a programmatic way. There are specifications that use CDA as a transport device for very specific information, but that is not what the specification is designed to do.

The recognition of the difficulty of V3, and the limits on how well CDA could address that difficulty, led HL7 to take a "fresh look" at its offerings and their usefulness. This effort spawned two programs. One, the Clinical Information Modeling Initiative (CIMI), was an effort to produce more detailed clinical artifacts. That effort continues to wrestle with methodological issues, and it is not expected to ballot normative standards within the next 2 years. The other was driven by a focus on producing implementable specifications, and it is called Fast Healthcare Information Resources, or FHIR.

Fast Healthcare Information Resources

Fast Healthcare Information Resources (FHIR) is a standard for health data exchange that focuses on implementation with several ramifications. First, FHIR does not define technical channels; it uses channels that already exist. The "resources" of the name refer to an architectural paradigm called Representational State Transfer, or REST. REST is the architecture of the

World Wide Web, defined as using web addresses (URLs) to identify information resources and hypertext transfer protocol (http) to exchange them. FHIR does not mandate the use of REST, but it is built in a way that, with REST, leverages the simplicity and robustness of the web architecture (Fielding 2000).

Second, FHIR tries to specify what can be easily and pragmatically agreed on in the core standard, and to leave unusual requirements to local communities. That is, the core specification is extensible, and issues that threaten to derail or delay agreement can be handled by those who find them important in extensions. This approach allows participants in the standards process to secure agreement on common and fundamental decisions in a timely manner, without requiring resolution on difficult or unusual questions.

Note that FHIR is not constrained by any assumptions about the scope of exchange, as CDA was. Users can exchange a Discharge Summary document in FHIR and can also request and receive a single lab test result, or any intermediate structure.

FHIR also tries to leverage recent developments in methodology, notably Agile development practices designed to promote delivery of working products with minimal overhead. These practices help deliver results more quickly, but they must be managed carefully to avoid contravening standards development rules. ANSI conducts audits to ensure that participation in the process is not impeded for any group.

The extensibility of FHIR means that its predictability can be compromised. The tool FHIR provides to address this issue is the profile, a set of constraints and extensions on a set of FHIR resources that is agreed to by a community. FHIR is a lot like V2 in this way: the core is well understood by a broad community, but there may be extensions that are not. The key to interoperability for FHIR, then, is a clear enunciation of the profiles to be used in a particular realm. This is much easier in countries with a single-payer healthcare market. In the US, the government is wary of over-regulating, and it has striven to support interoperability standards without being too directive. An industry coalition known as the Argonauts produced a set of profiles on FHIR DSTU2, and then the body nominally charged with coordinating nationwide standards agreements, the ONC, produced a set of profiles on FHIR DSTU3. The Argonaut and ONC profiles are similar but not completely compatible without some level of transformation—owing partly to the fact that they are built on different releases of FHIR. Release of FHIR V4 occurred in late December 2018; ONC is working on plans to profile it.

Note:

> HL7 standards were labeled "draft standard for trial use" (DSTU) prior to their acceptance as normative standards. However, it was felt that the word "draft" was creating excessive uncertainty, so it has been changed: the term is now "standard for trial use" (STU). Standards already published as DSTU, however, retain that designation.

Integrating the Healthcare Enterprise (IHE)

Integrating the Healthcare Enterprise (IHE) is a consortium of health IT vendors, providers, government and nonprofit organizations, and standards development organizations. The organization promotes the coordinated use of established standards such as DICOM and HL7 to address specific clinical need in support of optimal patient care. Systems developed in accordance with IHE communicate with one another better, are easier to implement, and enable care providers to use information more effectively. The mission of IHE improves healthcare by providing specifications, tools, and services for interoperability by engaging with clinicians, health authorities, industry, and users to develop, test, and implement standards-based solutions to vital health information needs. IHE provides two kinds of guidance: implementation guides ("integration profiles") that make SDO specifications easier to use, and a technical framework providing common understanding on the exchange infrastructure underlying those profiles.

IHE is governed by a board of representatives from sponsoring organizations, domain committees, and national and regional deployment committees of Member Organizations. Sponsoring organizations are members of IHE that sponsor a domain or national or regional deployment committee. These are usually professional societies but can also be government agencies in the case of regional deployment committees. IHE serves several clinical domains associated with different clinical specialties, including Anatomic Pathology, Cardiology, Dental, Laboratory, Patient Care Coordination, Pharmacy, and Radiology, as well as support domains such as IT Infrastructure Quality Research and Public Health. There are also several standing committees. Regional deployment committees have been set up in 18 nations and the European Union, and they are structured into broader organizational units to cover Asia and the Pacific, Europe, and North America.

Domain committees are responsible for the IHE technical frameworks for their respective domains. They are usually structured into a planning and technical work group. A domain has one or more organizational sponsors who provide support to the domain and act as its secretariat. The technical framework is developed as a collection of profiles. A profile can be viewed as an implementation guide addressing a specific use case. For example, one of the IT Infrastructure Profiles is the Sharing Value Set Integration, a profile that provides a means through which healthcare systems can use a centrally managed common nomenclature. Profiles describe the actors (components of systems or applications), their required behaviors, and the transactions that those actors participate in.

Volume I of any IHE Technical Framework describes the profiles, providing an overview and general description of what the participants in the interaction do. Volume II describes the transactions and their content. A profile is developed in an approximately 18-month-long cycle that begins with a profile proposal, develops into a public comment publication, and is followed up by a version designated for trial implementation at Connectathon events. After achieving a specified set of implementation goals, these profiles are incorporated into the technical framework as final text. Until they have been incorporated, they are published as supplements to the technical framework.

The regional deployment committees are responsible for regional activities related to profile development, including regional education, demonstrations at regional events, and testing of newly developed profiles by implementers at Connectathons. IHE Connectathons allow suppliers of healthcare IT products that implement IHE profiles to demonstrate their conformance to the profiles and their ability to interoperate. The event is preceded by an approximately three-month period where vendors are able to unit test their products using assigned testing materials. At the Connectathon, the vendors bring their systems to a single location for a week-long testing session. Vendors who meet the goal of performing successful transactions with at least three other vendors for each transaction type in the target profile may list their products as meeting the profile. The IHE maintains a database of test results that is accessible to the public (IHE 2018).

IHE does not develop content standards. Instead it describes how standards can be used together to solve a problem in a profile. IHE profiles are themselves considered to be standards by national and international bodies. Significant IHE profiles include the following, some of which are represented in figure 15.11:

- Content profiles, such as
    - Nuclear Medicine Image (NMI), a profile on DICOM
    - Immunization Content (IC), a profile on CDA
- Infrastructure, such as
    - Cross-enterprise Document Sharing (XDS), a profile on ebXML
    - Audit Trail and Node Authentication (ATNA), a profile on IETF technologies
- Composite profiles, such as
    - Scheduled workflow (SWF), a profile on HL7 V2 and DICOM

FIGURE 15.11. Select IHE profiles

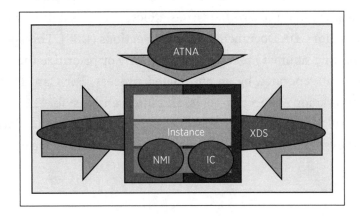

Several IHE specifications have been indirectly referenced in the PIs certification criteria or incorporated into other standards that have been named in that criteria. The Cross-Enterprise Document Sharing (XDS) family of specifications is one of the most widely used international specifications to support health information exchange in regional, national and multinational projects. XDS describes a collection of actors, transactions and metadata that provides a standards-based specification for managing the sharing of documents among healthcare enterprises. Some of those same transactions and metadata have also been used to describe a method of point-to-point exchange and routing between two different communicating systems in the Cross-Enterprise Document Reliable Interchange (XDR) profile, as well as federation in the Cross-Community Access (XCA) profile and file share and manual media transfer in the Cross-Enterprise Document Media Interchange (XDM) profile.

The XDM and XDR profiles are referenced by specifications created by ONC for The Direct Project for secure email of medical documents. The XCA and XDR profiles are also used in the specifications developed by ONC for the eHealth Exchange, formerly called the Nationwide Health Information Network (NwHIN). Authentication of computer systems, encryption of data and audit of transactions are key needs in electronic exchange. These are supported by the IHE Audit Trail and Node Authentication profile. Node authentication is enabled by the exchange of X.509 certificates—a standardized method of authentication defined by the International Telecommunications Union. Encryption is enabled by use of the Transport Layer Security (TLS), an Internet Engineering Task Force (IETF) protocol.

Radiology scheduled workflow (SWF) was one of the first IHE profiles to be developed. Parts of it have been adapted to similarly named profiles in the cardiology and laboratory domains of IHE. It describes the departmental workflow necessary to manage imaging equipment and information systems in imaging settings.

The Sharing of Laboratory Reports (XD-LAB) profile provides an HL7 CDA representation of a laboratory study and has been used by several national and regional health information exchanges to support exchange of labs. Some have viewed XD-LAB as a replacement for the HL7 Version 2 laboratory reporting standard, and it is being adopted in some countries. However, the robustness of the V2 specification, the breadth of its installed base, and its identification in PI regulations suggest that change is not likely in the US without some other business driver.

IHE has also weighed in on one of the issues affecting the usability of CDA documents by drafting a specification for CDA Document Summary Sections (DSS). This specification provides guidance for constructing summary text that might clarify or prioritize the contents of a potentially lengthy document generated by an automated process. For Care Plans, for instance, it identifies relationships among concerns, goals, and interventions; for Encounter summaries, it specifies date-based rules for identifying relevant procedures and medications. DSS is in a trial state, but it is a good example of how SDOs can support and enhance one other's work.

Institute of Electrical and Electronics Engineers Standards Organization

The **Institute of Electrical and Electronics Engineers Standards Association (IEEE-SA)** is a nonprofit standards-setting body that has been in existence for over a century. IEEE-SA is an engineering organization, and their specifications tend to live at a very technical level. One set of standards developed by IEEE-SA is the Point-of-care medical device communication standards, which pertain to communication of patient data from medical devices (patient monitors, ventilators, infusion pumps, and so on). These standards are designed to be technically robust interface specifications for device communication. Their primary driver is predictable and safe communication between machines, and they do not tend to provide a high degree of usability or legibility for human consumers.

With more than 850 standards and more in development, IEEE-SA has an established standards development process that follows five principles: due process, openness, consensus, balance, and right of appeal (IEEE-SA 2019a). Working groups and sponsors are key to the process as is the Project Authorization Request (PAR). A sponsor is responsible for the development and coordination of the standards project, supervising the standards project from inception to completion, and the maintenance of the standards after their approval by the IEEE-SA Standards Board (IEEE-SA 2013).

There are also five committees involved in the standards development process: New Standards Committee (NesCom), Standards Review Committee (RevCom), Procedures Committee (ProCom), Patent Committee (PatCom), and Audit Committee (AduCom) (IEEE-SA 2019a). The IEEE-SA website provides a summary with supporting documents on each of the six stages of the standards development life cycle. Figure 15.12 provides an overview.

FIGURE 15.12. Overview of the standards development life cycle

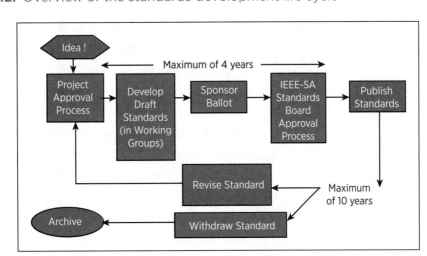

Source: IEEE-SA 2019b.

National Council for Prescription Drug Programs

Many standards result from government attempts to support the general welfare by incenting behavior that the market won't reward by itself. Sometimes, however, an industry recognizes market-driven benefits without government intervention. The National Council for Prescription Drug Programs (NCPDP) participates aggressively in standards development for interactions between providers, pharmacies, and payers. In its overview white paper (NCPDP 2009), the organization characterizes its three main standards in terms of quantified cost savings per interaction. NCPDP standards have been written into broad government regulations, but they came into being to support operational efficiency.

In the early 1970s, NCPDP grew out of efforts to standardize drug codes and pharmacy identifiers, and by 1981 it had developed the Universal Claim Form (UCF), a standard paper form for streamlining the process of submitting drug claims across the nation.

By the late 1980s, the growth of managed care was turning more pharmacy business from cash to receivables, tightening cash flow for pharmacies. NCPDP responded with the NCPDP Telecommunication Standard, supporting automated submission of claims. Version 5.1 of the standard was subsequently written into the Health Insurance Portability and Accountability Act (HIPAA) of 1996.

NCPDP developed and published an electronic prescribing standard, **SCRIPT**, in 1997. This standard extends the automated management of medication data from the pharmacy into the provider domain by automating the transfer of information from a prescribing clinician to a pharmacy. A key driver for this effort was medical errors. Handwritten prescriptions are famously difficult to read, and the Institute of Medicine's seminal report *To Err Is Human* identifies several kinds of errors in prescription-writing that can be solved by standardizing prescriptions (IOM 2000). The study does not provide a rationalized assessment of costs, but it cites studies indicating such cost impacts as "$3.9 billion was spent in 1983 to manage the preventable gastrointestinal adverse effects of nonsteroidal anti-inflammatory drugs" (Bloom 1998). Standardization on SCRIPT prescriptions would support not just accurate transmission from provider to pharmacist, but the ability to check comprehensively for interactions, compliance, and utilization.

NCPDP still publishes a paper Universal Claim Form, but the Telecommunication standard has largely displaced it for pharmacy interactions with payers including eligibility, authorization, and billing claims. Both Telecommunications and SCRIPT leverage external terminologies published by the National Cancer Institute's extensive terminology operation. This touchpoint illustrates the value of cooperation—NCPDP uses selected Drug Enforcement Administration (DEA) terms from the NCI—and its risks—distinct episodes of cooperation have resulted in different value sets for dose units, which require harmonization when both are used.

HIPAA, the Medicare Prescription Drug Improvement and Modernization Act (MMA), the HITECH Act, and PI require the use of NCPDP standards.

Workgroup for Electronic Data Interchange

In addition to SDOs, a supporting organization that assists in the development or production of standards is the Workgroup for Electronic Data Interchange (WEDI). WEDI was formed in 1991 by the Secretary of HHS and named in the HIPAA legislation as an advisor to the Secretary of HHS on administrative simplification standards (WEDI 2018). WEDI supports the various stakeholders using EDI transactions in healthcare, including health plans, providers, vendors, and government agencies. WEDI does not develop EDI standards, but rather uses the collective knowledge of its member stakeholders to inform SDOs and improve EDI standards.

Use Cases

The following use cases illustrate some of the kinds of standards currently in use in the US with reference to the information outlined in this chapter.

Use Case One: Prescription

A clinician in private practice writes a prescription for a patient and submits it to a pharmacy.

By the late 1980s, there was a general recognition of the quality issues surrounding hand-written prescriptions, which combined the variability of habit and convention across organizations with the idiosyncrasies of medical penmanship. Vendors began supporting "e-prescribing," but their interfaces were not standard, so providers were slow to adopt them. Unlike the claims case, the cost savings were not obvious, and those that existed (primarily around error avoidance) were not clearly aligned with the interests of those who would be investing in the technology. NCPDP saw an opportunity and engaged pharmacies and providers to design a new standard, NCPCP SCRIPT.

The SCRIPT standard supports transactions such as New Prescription, Change, Refill, and Cancel from the provider side, supported by Response messages from the pharmacy. Responses might indicate, in addition to confirmation, changes to prescriptions, and reasons for making those changes. Note that, however compelling the general case for this function may have been, its adoption was slower than that for NCPDP Telecommunication. This may be because the provider-to-pharmacy transaction can be supported by point-to-point software, whereas the clearinghouse functions the pharmacies transact with each other and with providers require a common language. If the efficiency requirement can be met by nonstandard software, there is less demand for the standard—at least until it is written into regulation, as it was in the 2015 Meaningful Use certification criteria.

SCRIPT also demonstrates the interdependence of standards. SCRIPT specifies a drug identifier, but the version currently specified in the federal ISA does not require it to be encoded in a standard terminology. Most implementations do provide such an identifier, and most use the

FDA's National Drug Code (NDC). This code system was developed to support pharmacovigilance, primarily of products in development, and it supports very detailed specification not only of drug but manufacturer, packaging, and lot. Resolving that level of detail is not necessary for prescribing, and it is expensive and time-consuming. Furthermore, maintenance of these identifiers is not centrally managed, so they may be out of date or ambiguous.

The NLM developed RxNorm, a drug coding system, specifically for clinical use, and has promoted its use in SCRIPT and other clinical applications. To date, however, NDC has the momentum, and the business case for moving to RxNorm has proven only partly successful (Dhavle et al. 2016).

SCRIPT is a content standard defined as an XML document; channels for exchanging these documents are defined by the communities exchanging them. As the web has displaced EDI, web services tend to be the most common channel. IHE profiles in this domain tend to use HL7 CDA, V2, and FHIR content specifications: these profiles are needed in the international space, but SCRIPT, supporting the US realm, is tightly defined, and it does not require additional profiling.

Use Case Two: Patient Summary Information—Content

A provider has a new patient and wishes to view existing documents about the patient (content layer).

At least four content standards could support this use case. The HL7 Version 2 Medical Document Management (MDM) message was designed to exchange documents of any format between healthcare information systems. The HL7 CDA Release 2.0 standard, and its accompanying implementation guide defining a Care Record Summary, was designed to be an electronic exchange format that supported semantic interchange. The ASTM Continuity of Care Record (CCR) was an evolving draft that was designed to provide a simple XML representation. And FHIR supports bundling of resources to support requirements defined by any document specification.

In 2009, when the ONC was working on specifying a standard for Meaningful Use, FHIR did not yet exist. The HL7 Version 2 standard was capable of solving the transport problem, but it did not address the requirements of the stakeholders for semantically rich content. Attention was focused on the two competing XML standards. CDA Release 2.0 had been out for less than a year, and it was not widely adopted. The ASTM CCR standard, while receiving broad industry attention because of its simple XML representation, was not completed.

In the end, the ONC selected the more fully featured HL7 CDA Release 2.0 standard over the more easily implemented CCR. This was largely influenced by the experience of the group working on the use case, many of whom had been frustrated by lack of progress in the development of CCR.

While CDA Release 2.0 resolved the issue of how to convey the clinical data, questions remained as to what standards would be used to encode key clinical information, including the type of document, types of sections within the document, and the problems, medications, and allergies information in the structured form. In this example, the work group selected LOINC for the document type and deferred specification of vocabularies to use for problems, medications, and allergies. No single terminology standard met the needs of all of the stakeholders, and choosing any single standard would have prevented others from using the resulting solution. This is a common case when standards must support the requirements of different regulatory jurisdictions and clinical domains.

Since its selection, the CCD has been harmonized with several other documents in the "Consolidated CDA" (C-CDA) specification, which lists a dozen document types that share many section definitions. Each document type specifies required and optional sections, but since each definition is "open"—that is, the document may contain additional sections not identified in the specification—it is technically possible to put any section in any document, as long as the required sections for the document type are included.

The CCD document will provide the requesting clinician with six required document sections: allergies, medications, problems, test results, social history, and vitals. The profile refines these sections to provide semantics as predictably as possible. Medications, for instance, requires RxNorm clinical drug codes, though it also supports translations from any number of other code systems that may have been used in the ordering and dispensing systems. The specification also refines 11 optional document sections; a client requesting a CCD might reasonably be expected to understand these. But all C-CDA document templates, and most other CDA document templates, are "open," meaning that while they specify required contents, they don't prohibit additional content. There are many other sections available; the C-CDA specification alone lists 70.

This variety presents a challenge, as it means that a document recipient may receive unexpected content. If that content is for human consumption, most authors would be comfortable that a receiving physician will understand those other sections. If the recipient is a computer, unpredictable data is worse than no data at all, as it can cause processing with incomplete understanding.

One final problem faces automated document exchange. When a clinician writes a note, a great deal of implicit judgment, developed over years of practice, shapes the scope and detail of the document. When a system automatically generates a summary document, it does not have access to that judgment. As a result, a document for a patient with multiple problems or hospital stays can run to scores of pages. The HL7 Relevant and Pertinent project aimed to produce guidelines for controlling this problem, and the IHE DSS project produced guidance for generating relevant text, but the difference between the needs of human and automated consumers remains wide, and strategies for dealing with this difference are still evolving.

Use Case Three: Patient Summary Information—Transport

A provider has a new patient and wishes to view existing documents about the patient (transport layer; that is, find and acquire the documents).

This is the same use case, but in addition to a standard for how to present the content that the provider seeks, the tactics the provider uses to find the content and to retrieve it also need to be agreed on. There may not be any documents about the patient in question, and if there are, the provider has no idea where to get them.

The framework for this process was put together by developers solving a tactical problem at an industry event. One of the public-sector participants in the demonstration was working with technology using metadata registries. The vendor connected that technology with the intranet-based web access via a simple HTTP POST message (as if a web form had been submitted). That message was processed by the metadata registry, and because all the vendors were connected to the same network, the system demonstrating the metadata registry was able to list all of the documents from all vendors on one screen and to display each document in response to a simple click. The casualties in this accident were the vendors whose audiences quickly migrated to the government employee's workstation to see the greatest new product on the demonstration floor. Some vendors quickly modified their software to display that same web page on the panel of their own systems, and the IHE Cross-Enterprise Document Sharing profile was demonstrated three months before the first draft text was even published.

The use case involves two contrary requirements: enable providers to access patient documents created by other providers outside their network and keep the documents secure. This use case was quickly split into two use cases, one to address the sharing network and a second one to address the secured communication channels.

The secured communication channel was addressed by adopting four common industry standards and developing one new standard. The Transport Layer Security (TLS) Protocol and X.509 certificate standards were adopted to enable system-to-system authentication and encryption. These are the same standards underlying the https protocol. The specification required that the TLS socket be encrypted using the Advanced Encryption Standard (AES), and that nodes be authenticated using digital signatures. In addition to encryption, audit trails were needed to ensure that appropriate information was captured when healthcare information was exchanged across organizational boundaries. This was a gap, and several members of the workgroup developed a draft specification via the Internet Engineering Task Force (IETF), which was then standardized in DICOM due to difficulties with the changing IETF standards development policies. The audit messages were communicated via the IETF Syslog protocol, which was itself enhanced for more reliable security.

There were several iterations and evolutions of the IHE XDS profile after some implementation experience was developed. A new use case was created to support more efficient query execution. The original ebXML specifications allowed for embedded SQL calls. This had to be modified, as a poorly formed query could negatively impact the server during testing. Other performance enhancements included the ability to bundle GET requests, so that transactions would not require too many request cycles. Additional metadata allowing the designated receiver to be identified and enabling messages to be routed through a network gave rise to the IHE

FIGURE 15.13. XDS environment

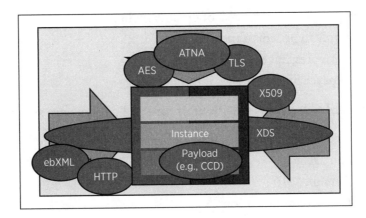

XDR profile, which is one of the foundation specifications of the HealtheWay (formerly NwHIN Exchange), supporting routable, point-to-point document exchange.

The IHE Cross-Community Access profile enhanced the Document Query and Retrieval transactions to support bridging and exchange between registries (for example, in health information exchanges). The IHE XCA profile is another of the foundation specifications found in HealtheWay. Another extension addressed manual and LAN-based exchanges, giving birth to the IHE Cross-Enterprise Document Sharing over Media profile. A third path involved using secure email to exchange documents, an effort that became the Direct Protocol. The Direct Protocol and the IHE XDR Protocol are now recognized in the Meaningful Use regulations for certified EHR systems as **transport standards**. Transport standards are data exchange standards which support connectivity between systems, allowing them to communicate using standards for discovery, enabling connections, and specifying communication protocols.

Figure 15.13 hints at the complexity of the environment where a content standard is supported by a transmission standard which itself incorporates a zoo of standards from the lower technical layers. It is important to be able to address issues at one level without being unnecessarily distracted by details that are competently addressed by other communities.

CHECK YOUR UNDERSTANDING

1. Which of the following is *not* an SDO?

   a. ASC X12N

   b. HL7

   c. IEEE-SA

   d. ONC

2. Healthcare data standardization has lagged behind other industries because

   a. It is more complex and the risk of error is higher
   b. It is too simple to be worth the effort
   c. It is more complex but the risk of error is lower
   d. The single-payer market makes it unnecessary

3. ___ is a standard to support transitions of care and patient care summaries

   a. Consolidated Clinical Document Architecture
   b. HL7 Version 2.6
   c. ASC X12 Version 5010
   d. Point-of-Care Communication

4. Health data interchange standards can be divided into:

   a. Content standards and normative standards
   b. Content standards and behavioral standards
   c. Normative standards and behavioral standards
   d. Normative standards and meaningful use

5. True or false? Healthcare organizations that use HIPAA-defined transactions must use the HL7 standard formats.

   a. True
   b. False

REVIEW

1. The X12N messaging standard is the accepted messaging standard for communicating:

   a. Clinical data
   b. Medical device data
   c. Administrative data
   d. Medical imaging data

2. ___ is a standard for the interchange of computerized biomedical images and image-related information within and between healthcare providers.

   a. DICOM
   b. NCPDP
   c. IEEE
   d. X12N 270

3. Which of the following developed a data interchange standard for reimbursement and insurance-related messaging?

   a. HIPAA
   b. IEEE-SA
   c. ASC X12N
   d. ANSI

4. ____ produces standards, implementation guides, and a data dictionary for data interchange and processing standards for pharmacy transactions.

   a. HL7
   b. NCPDP
   c. IEEE-SA
   d. NDC

5. The _____ describes how to report a quality measure.

   a. Quality Reporting Document Architecture
   b. Health Quality Measure Format
   c. Clinical Document Architecture
   d. None of the above

6. Match the three types of standards below to the correct description

   __ Transport   a. Standards for workflows, algorithms, or messaging protocols

   __ Content   b. Standards describing the syntax, semantics, data models, or vocabulary

   __ Behavior   c. Standards describing how to find, connect, or communicate to another system

7. Match the standards listed below to the correct type.

   __ HL7 Clinical Document Architecture   a. Transport

   __ SNOMED CT, LOINC, and RxNorm   b. Content

   __ The Direct Protocol   c. Behavioral

   __ Cross-Enterprise Document Sharing

8. Governments are typically:

   a. Standards developers
   b. Standards advocates
   c. Market stakeholders
   d. None of the above

9. FHIR was developed to be more _____ than existing standards.

    a. Implementable

    b. Abstract

    c. Secure

    d. Holistic

10. Which of the following organizations developed Point-of-care medical device communication standards?

    a. DICOM

    b. IEEE-SA

    c. ASC X12N

    d. NCPDP

References

Accredited Standards Committee (ASC) X12. 2018. http://www.x12.org.

Accredited Standards Committee (ASC) X12. 2017a. "X12C Purpose and scope." http://members.x12.org/policies-procedures/asc40v1-x12c-p-and-s.pdf.

Accredited Standards Committee (ASC) X12. 2017b. "X12J Purpose and scope." http://members.x12.org/policies-procedures/asc70v1-x12j-p-and-s.pdf.

Accredited Standards Committee (ASC) X12, Insurance Subcommittee, X12N. 2010. Common content. "Fig. 2.5 Segment Key – Element Summary." http://www.wpc-edi.com/reference/repository/006010CC.PDF.

Biomedical Research Integrated Domain Group (BRIDG). 2018. https://bridgmodel.nci.nih.gov/.

Bloom, B. S. 1998. Cost of treating arthritis and NSAID-related gastrointestinal side-effects. *Alimentary Pharmacology & Therapeutics* 1(Suppl 2):131–138.

Clinical Data Interchange Standards Consortium (CDISC). 2018. Expert CDISC group. https://www.cdisc.org/news/expert-cdisc-group.

Dhavle, A. A., S. Ward-Charlerie, M. T. Rupp, J. Kilbourne, V. P. Amin, and J Ruiz. 2016. Evaluating the implementation of RxNorm in ambulatory electronic prescriptions. *JAMIA* 23(e1):e99–e107. doi:10.1093/jamia/ocv131.

eCFR.gov. 2015. Electronic Code of Federal Regulations, Title 45 Subtitle A Subchapter D Part 170. https://www.ecfr.gov/cgi-bin/text-idx?tpl=/ecfrbrowse/Title45/45cfr170_main_02.tpl.

Fielding, R. "Chapter 5: Representational State Transfer (REST)." *Architectural Styles and the Design of Network-based Software Architectures* [doctoral dissertation]. 2000. https://www.ics.uci.edu/~fielding/pubs/dissertation/rest_arch_style.htm.

Grieve, G. 2011 (August, 15). HL7 needs a fresh look because V3 has failed. *Health Intersections*. http://www.healthintersections.com.au/?p=476.

Health Level Seven International (HL7). 2018. "About HL7." http://www.hl7.org/about/index.cfm?ref=nav.

Healthcare Information and Management Systems Society (HIMSS). 2018. What is Interoperability? https://www.himss.org/library/interoperability-standards/what-is.

Institute of Electrical and Electronics Engineers Standards Association (IEEE-SA). 2019a. Develop Standards: Who Oversees the Process? https://standards.ieee.org/develop/govern.html.

Institute of Electrical and Electronics Engineers Standards Association (IEEE-SA). 2019b. Develop Standards: How are Standards Made? https://standards.ieee.org/develop/govern.html.

Institute of Electrical and Electronics Engineers Standards Association (IEEE-SA). 2013. Standards Board Operations Manual. http://standards.ieee.org/develop/policies/opman/index.html.

Institute of Medicine (IOM). 2000. The Institute of Medicine Reports in 2000, "To Err is Human." https://www.ncbi.nlm.nih.gov/pubmed/25077248.

Integrating the Healthcare Enterprise (IHE). 2018. https://www.ihe.net/.

Morning, A. 2008. Ethnic classification in global perspective: A cross-national survey of the 2000 census round. *Population Research and Policy Review* 27:239. https://doi.org/10.1007/s11113-007-9062-5.

National Council for Prescription Drug Programs (NCPDP). 2009. Pharmacy: A Prescription for Improving the Healthcare System. https://www.ncpdp.org/NCPDP/media/pdf/wp/RxforImprovingHealthcare.pdf.

National Electrical Manufacturers Association (NEMA) 2018. Digital Imaging and Communications in Medicine (DICOM) current edition. https://www.dicomstandard.org/current/.

Office of Management and Budget (OMB). 1998. Circular No. A-119 – *Federal Register* (Federal Participation in the Development and Use of Voluntary Consensus Standards and in Conformity Assessment Activities). https://www.nist.gov/sites/default/files/revised_circular_a-119_as_of_01-22-2016.pdf.

Office of the National Coordinator for Health Information Technology (ONC). 2018a. Interoperability Standards Advisory, 2018. https://www.healthit.gov/isa/.

Office of the National Coordinator for Health Information Technology (ONC). 2018b. Draft U.S. Core Data for Interoperability (USCDI) and Proposed Expansion Process. https://www.healthit.gov/sites/default/files/draft-uscdi.pdf.

Office of the National Coordinator for Health Information Technology (ONC). 2015. 2015 Edition Health Information Technology (Health IT) Certification Criteria, 2015 Edition Base Electronic Health Record (EHR) Definition, and ONC Health IT Certification Program Modifications. https://www.federalregister.gov/documents/2015/10/16/2015-25597/2015-edition-health-information-technology-health-it-certification-criteria-2015-edition-base.

Patient Protection and Affordable Care Act (PPACA). 2010. Public Law 111-148.

Workgroup for Electronic Data Interchange (WEDI). 2018. About Us. http://www.wedi.org/about-us.

Resources

Boone, K. Healthcare Standards. http://motorcycleguy.blogspot.com/.

Centers for Medicare and Medicaid Services. 2014. Quality Reporting Document Architecture., Version 2.0. http://cms.gov/Regulations-and-Guidance/Legislation/EHRIncentive Programs/Downloads/Guide_QRDA_2014eCQM.pdf.

Clinical Data Interchange Standards Consortium (CDISC). 2018. BRIDG Model. https://bridgmodel.nci.nih.gov/.

Department of Health and Human Services. 2003 (February 20). Final Rule on health insurance reform: Modifications to electronic data transaction standards and code sets. *Federal Register*. http://www.aspe.hhs.gov/admnsimp/FINAL/FR03-8381.pdf.

Grieve, G. Health Intersections. http://www.healthintersections.com.au/.

Halamka, J. D. Life as a Healthcare CIO. http://geekdoctor.blogspot.com/.

HL7. http://hl7.org/.

HL7 FHIR standard. http://hl7.org/implement/standards/fhir/.

IHE. https://www.ihe.net/.

IHE wiki. https://wiki.ihe.net/.

National Committee on Vital and Health Statistics. 2007 (September 26). Letter to the Secretary, U.S. Department of Health and Human Services. http://www.ncvhs.hhs.gov/070926lt.pdf.

Office of the National Coordinator for Health Information Technology (ONC). https://www.healthit.gov/.

Office of the National Coordinator for Health Information Technology (ONC). Standards. https://www.healthit.gov/isa/.

Part IV

Application of Terminologies and Classification Systems in Healthcare

16

Centralized Locations and Tools for Multiple Terminologies: Servers, Services, Databases, and Registries

Susan A. Matney, PhD, RNC-OB, FAAN, FACMI

LEARNING OBJECTIVES

- Examine the component parts of a sample of vocabulary servers in use today
- Evaluate a standard process of accessing terminologies using common terminology services
- Explain the Unified Medical Language System (UMLS)
- Differentiate the contents of two Enterprise Specific Databases: the National Cancer Institute Enterprise Vocabulary Services (EVS) and the Public Health Information Network Vocabulary Access and Distribution System (PHIN VADS)
- Compare the names, development, and purpose of metadata registries in use within the US, including:
  - National Library of Medicine Value Set Authority Center
  - United States Health Information Knowledgebase (USHIK)

KEY TERMS

- Application Programming Interface (API)
- Common Terminology Services (CTS2)
- Metadata
- Metadata Registry (MDR)
- Metathesaurus
- NCI Metathesaurus (NCIm)
- NCI Thesaurus (NCIt)
- UMLS Terminology Services (UTS)
- Unified Medical Language System (UMLS)
- US Health Information Knowledgebase (USHIK)
- Vocabulary server

Introduction

As the emphasis on shareable and comparable healthcare data grows, the need for structured coded data also increases. As a result, the number of vocabulary, terminology, and classification systems (collectively referred to as terminologies) in healthcare has grown substantially. Additionally, terminologies are constantly developing and expanding their number of codes. At this time, multiple terminologies are required for interoperable healthcare data. The Office of the National Coordinator (ONC) as well as the Centers for Medicare and Medicaid Services (CMS) *Blueprint for the CMS Measures Management System* and *Promoting Interoperability Program* support this (CMS 2018; CMS 2019). The adoption of electronic health records (EHRs), the increase in devices connected via the Internet of Things along with the transition to a pay-for-performance model imply that structured data capture requirements will continue to increase with time.

To support the number of terminologies and the large quantity of codes, a centralized location is needed to maintain consistent terminology for implementation and use. This chapter explains the concept of databases that host multiple terminologies (known as a vocabulary server) and examines a few of the publicly available databases existing for use today.

Vocabulary Servers and Services

As mentioned previously, there is no single standard terminology that contains all the encoded concepts required for documenting care within the electronic health record (EHR). Therefore, multiple standard terminologies are required. Standard terminologies are used to collect coded patient data so that it can be stored within the EHR for longitudinal use, exchanged across systems, and aggregated for outcomes, quality measures, and research. Standards are developed by different organizations, cover different domains of healthcare data, are structured in multiple formats, and meet a variety of use cases. Vocabulary servers and services are key to working with multiple terminologies in an electronic environment.

Vocabulary Servers

Concepts from each terminology need to be integrated within one database or application for ease of use as well as convergence of multiple code systems across the enterprise and between care settings. A **vocabulary server** allows organizations to implement multiple standard terminologies. It provides the ability to house multiple standard terminologies as well as local extensions in one location, improving operational efficiency, and effective terminology management. An example of a local extension is the US Extension to SNOMED CT. This terminology is a formal extension to the International Release containing US-specific content.

Developers

Groups within both the private and public sector develop, maintain, and distribute vocabulary servers. Entities may have different use cases for the vocabulary server, contain variable standard and local terminologies, and have variable structures.

Purpose

Vocabulary servers contain variable clinical and billing concepts and cover different domains of healthcare data. Terminologies may be available for public use, require a user's license, or be proprietary. Depending on the terms of use, each terminology may require registration or royalty payment prior to download and use. Details regarding the use and distribution of each terminology should be covered in the affiliate license of each vocabulary server.

Some standard terminologies that may be included within a vocabulary server are:

- SNOMED Clinical Terms (SNOMED CT)
- Logical Observation Identifiers, Names and Codes (LOINC)
- RxNorm
- Current Procedural Terminology (CPT)
- International Classification of Diseases, Tenth Revision, Clinical Modification (ICD-10-CM)
- ICD-10 Procedure Coding System (ICD-10-PCS)
- National Drug Codes (NDC)
- Ambulatory Payment Classifications (APCs)
- Healthcare Common Procedure Coding System (HCPCS)

- Provider Taxonomy
- US Licensed Vaccine Codes (CVX)
- Health Level 7 International (HL7) Standard Code Sets (such as Drug Route, Race and Ethnicity)
- International Organization for Standardization (ISO) Terminologies
- International Classification of Functioning, Disability and Health (ICF)

Principles and Guidelines

Vocabulary servers should follow a set of basic conventions. A vocabulary server must be:

- Robust: able to incorporate and maintain multiple terminologies to be shared across systems
- Organized: able to support the nomenclatures of multiple code systems
- Functional: able to transition between identical and similar concepts present within code systems
- Usable: accessible by multiple clinical applications

Adoption and Use

Vocabulary servers are used by many different entities, including hospital systems, EHRs, software vendors and developers, informaticists, clinicians, researchers, and patients. Anyone that encounters healthcare data may access a vocabulary server without realizing it.

Vocabulary servers are important in both primary and secondary data use. Primary data use occurs at the point of care, such as documenting and reviewing data on a specific patient. Primary data capture is leveraged in the diagnosis and treatment of a unique patient by a clinician. Vocabulary servers can be helpful in primary data capture by aiding structured coded data at the point of care on assessment forms and within pick lists. Secondary data use is everything that data is used for after the point-of-care encounter. For example, providing patients access to their healthcare data, facilitating electronic health data exchange, and managing population health, analytics, or documentation to support standard of care in medical liability claims are all examples of secondary data use.

Vocabulary servers are used when clinical technologies such as clinical decision support modules, EHRs, research, and analytics systems need to incorporate medical terminologies or integrate terminologies into applications. They are also utilized to share concepts among terminologies or when there is a need to share terminologies between applications.

Process for Revision and Updates

Each vocabulary server has a different process for revisions and release of updates. Some vocabulary servers release on a calendar basis, others with standard terminology updates, still others release on an ad hoc basis. Some vocabulary servers use automated processes for updates; others require manual updates of software or content.

Terminology Services

As demonstrated by the multiple terminologies discussed in this book, terminologies vary in their structure, content, and purpose; hence there is a need for standard terminology services. Terminology services define and describe how a vocabulary server should perform instead of focusing on how the vocabulary server is organized or what type of content is present within the vocabulary server. Terminology service requirements exist for sharing and exchanging data from within an EHR, which facilitates interoperability within and between systems. These requirements have been developed within standard development organizations (SDOs) to ensure data exchange between systems and across settings. Two sets of terminology services will be described in the section Common Terminology Services Version 2 (CTS2) and the HL7 Fast Healthcare Interoperability Resources (FHIR) terminology services.

Developers

CTS2 and FHIR terminology services are HL7 Standards. FHIR terminology services was developed exclusively by HL7, and CTS2 was developed jointly between HL7 and Object Management Group (OMG). OMG is an international computer industry standard consortium that produces and maintains specifications for interoperable, portable, and reusable enterprise applications for a number of technologies and industries including healthcare (OMG 2015).

Purpose

Terminology services perform important functions in health IT. They provide specifications to assist terminology implementers in sending and receiving terminology regardless of the structure, content, and purpose of the vocabulary server. They also support applications, such as clinical decision support systems, and perform terminology lookups, translations, subsumption checks, or value set membership checks when executing logic. CTS2 and FHIR terminology services provide a standardized interface for the use and management of terminologies with the goal of enhancing the semantic interoperability of healthcare data. This means that the services designate the functions that a terminology must be able to meet without necessitating a common data structure. The terminology services are the principle functions a vocabulary server should perform in order to share the structured encoded data within standard terminologies.

Content

Terminology service specifications are designed to provide a list of the interface functions for a vocabulary server. Each specification outlines standard processes for accessing terminologies using services (HL7 2015; HL7 2018). The services describe **Application Programming Interfaces (APIs)** that can be used in procuring desired terminologies and are beneficial to both terminology suppliers and users. APIs enumerate allowed operations, how to invoke these operations, as well as their input and output requirements. An example of the CTS2 and FHIR APIs can be found on the HL7 website. The APIs between CTS2 and FHIR function similarly but differ in their underlying specifications and are programmed for HL7 different structures. Therefore, each will be further described separately.

Common Terminology Services (CTS2)

Common Terminology Services (CTS2) are rendered as Simple Object Access Protocol (SOAP) or Representational State Transfer (REST) APIs and are intended to be used with HL7 V2.x, HL7 CDA, and HL7 V3. The goals of CTS2 are defined by the following criteria:

- Ease of implementation
- Ability to act as a baseline of terminology services (not comprehensive)
- Direct and to the point
- Utilization of XML
- Compatible with the HL7 Version 3 Reference Information Model (RIM)
- Subset of the OMG terminology quality services (TQS)
- Assurance that the suppositions of terminology content and structure are limited by relevance for HL7 services

Operations addressed by the CTS2 terminology service specifications (HL7 2015) include:

- Administration: the ability to load, export, activate, or retire terminologies.
- Search Query: the ability to find concepts or value sets based on search criteria.
- Authoring/Maintenance: the ability to create and maintain content. This includes APIs for adding, changing, or deleting terminology content. This would also include the processing of change events from various terminology providers.

HL7 CTS defines runtime APIs and browsing APIs. Runtime services exist to define functions that are used within applications for accessing terminologies. Browsing APIs allow users to explore terminology content. Additionally, APIs are classified as Message or Vocabulary APIs. Message APIs interact with the messaging software while Vocabulary APIs interact with the vocabulary server itself. Vocabulary APIs access different terminologies in a standardized way. Message APIs apply only to HL7 messages. Messaging APIs make calls to Vocabulary APIs to provide the details of the code set.

- Message Runtime: construction and manipulation of content into HL7 message.
- Vocabulary Runtime: defines capabilities needed by the message runtime services.
- Message Browsing: provides details in the vocabulary domains and attributes that are recognized by the browser.
- Vocabulary Browsing: designed to be used in authoring content.
- Vocabulary Code Mapping: performs mutually exclusive one-directional mapping of concepts between different code systems.

ADOPTION AND USE

CTS2 terminology services are widely used by software developers, messaging software, and vocabulary servers. Users may implement one or many of the CTS2 APIs to meet their terminology needs. FHIR is an emerging standard and the terminology services are being gradually adopted nationwide.

PROCESS FOR REVISION AND UPDATES

CTS is a specification document which does not have routine releases. CTS2 became an OMG functional standard in July of 2011. In 2015, CTS became an ANSI-approved standard and was incorporated into the HL7 Version 3 Standard. Updates to the standard would be created collaboratively between the two organizations.

FHIR Terminology Module

FHIR terminology services are implemented using the FHIR specification which describes both the FHIR REST operations and the FHIR resource payloads needed or produced by such operations. Both terminology service specifications are designed to provide a list of the interface functions for a vocabulary server. Each specification outlines standard processes for accessing terminologies using services (HL7 2018).

HL7 FHIR terminology services were created to facilitate the use of terminology codes and value sets within FHIR resources and profiles. The goal is to facilitate ease of use by healthcare applications. FHIR terminology services are contained in the FHIR terminology module which also contains terminology resources, operations, coded data types and documentation. Figure 16.1 defines the FHIR terminology resources.

FHIR Terminology Resources

- CodeSystem: identified by a Uniform Resource Identifier (URI) and version. Properties include code, URI, description, and data type. All code systems used in FHIR have URI Identifiers.
- ConceptMap: used to define mapping from a set of concepts defined in a code system to one or more concepts defined in other code systems.
- TerminologyCapabilities: describes how the underlying terminology service works.
- ValueSet: comes from one or more code systems and has three identifiers: ValueSet. ID, the logical id; ValueSet.URL; and ValueSet.Identifier, a system value pair that identifies the value set and their contexts.
- NamingSystem: defines the extension of a code system such as the US extension of SNOMED CT.

FIGURE 16.1. FHIR terminology service needs example

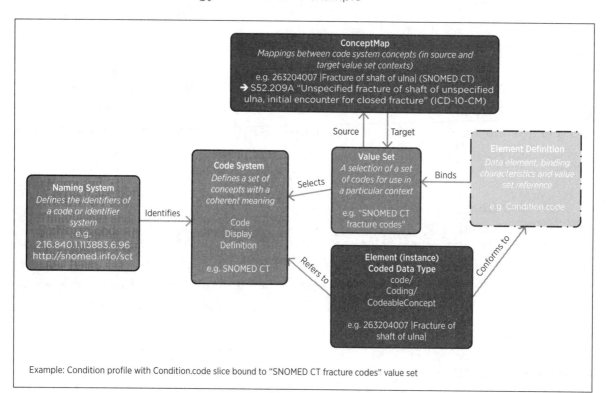

Example: Condition profile with Condition.code slice bound to "SNOMED CT fracture codes" value set

Source: HL7 2018.

FHIR Terminology Operations

Terminology operations are rules for terminology and value set processing. The rules are broken into three categories:

- CodeSystem: rules include looking up the code system by identifier; validating a code within the code system, such as the SNOMED CT ID; subsumption (is-a relationship) testing; and find-matches, which identifies complete, partial, or possible matches based on the properties in the rule.
- ValueSet: two rules for looking at or creating a collection of codes. Valueset expand is used to retrieve all value set members and validate code checks that the code is within a specific value set.
- ConceptMap: two operations used to translate one concept to another: translate used to translate a code from one value set to another and closure, which identifies new entries for the Closure table (a table built on-the-fly as new codes are seen).

ADOPTION AND USE

FHIR terminology services are being adopted and used as the FHIR resources are implemented. EHR vendors have developed APIs for the common resources such as Patient, Organization, Condition, Observation, and the like.

PROCESS FOR REVISION AND UPDATES

Revisions and updates to the FHIR terminology module are the same as all FHIR resources. The FHIR terminology resources go through the ballot process which includes a "Trial Use" period. During this time, requests for change may be submitted via the HL7 FHIR issue tracker. Implementers should understand that during this period, changes will still be occurring. The standard is considered "Normative" after the "Trial Use" period and the content will be "locked" with infrequent changes.

Unified Medical Language System (UMLS)

A **metathesaurus** is a very large, multipurpose vocabulary database that contains information about patient care, health services billing, public health statistics, indexing, and cataloging biomedical literature, or basic, clinical, and health services research. This information is obtained from source vocabularies. A methathesaurus is organized by concept or meaning, links synonymous names to the concept, and identifies semantic relationships between different concepts. The UMLS Metathesaurus is described below.

The **Unified Medical Language System (UMLS)** is a tool that aggregates, links, and packages existing computer-based clinical terminologies along with biomedical literature and knowledge bases (NLM 2017a).

Developer

The National Library of Medicine (NLM), with responsibility for coordinating terminology standards, and the Department of Health and Human Services (HHS) developed the UMLS in 1986. The UMLS provides a wide variety of applications to overcome retrieval problems caused by differences in terminology and the scattering of relevant information across many databases. It assimilates and provides terminologies to end users and houses a set of Knowledge Resources and tools that include:

- Metathesaurus: a collection of coded terms from terminologies (more than 3.6 million concepts from more than 200 terminologies and 25 languages) (NLM 2018a).
- Semantic Network: labels for organizing the concepts into domains (133 categories and 54 relationships between categories).
- SPECIALIST Lexicon and Lexical Tools: word usage information for the development of language processing tools.

Although the UMLS Knowledge Sources are provided by the NLM free of charge, a license agreement must be signed prior to download. Additional terms of use are required for the Semantic Network and Lexicon Tools. The Metathesaurus requires a license agreement because of the different restrictions placed on each vocabulary or terminology by the terminology developer. Each Metathesaurus licensee must submit a brief annual report describing how it is being used.

UMLS is directed by a multidisciplinary team of NLM staff and maintained by public funding.

Purpose

UMLS was built to be an intelligent, automated system that can understand biomedical concepts, words, and expressions and their interrelationships. The purpose of UMLS is to make it simple for health professionals and researchers to retrieve and integrate information from a variety of sources and for users to link disparate information systems, including EHRs, bibliographic databases, factual databases, and expert systems. The NLM website lists the following applications in which the UMLS could be used:

- Information retrieval
- Creation of patient and research data
- Natural language processing
- Automated indexing
- Development of enterprise-wide vocabulary services

Content

UMLS is a multipurpose resource that includes concepts and terms from many different source vocabularies developed for very different purposes. Many segments and disciplines of the healthcare process are covered in UMLS, but the total scope is controlled by the combined scope of its source vocabularies. The Metathesaurus, a very large, multipurpose, and multilingual vocabulary database, is the central vocabulary component of UMLS. The Metathesaurus is concept-oriented. The source vocabularies found in the Metathesaurus include terminologies designed for use in patient-record systems. Although the Metathesaurus does not supply a universal hierarchy, it does contain the individual hierarchies of the source vocabularies. When the same concept appears in different hierarchical contexts in different source vocabularies, the Metathesaurus includes all the hierarchies.

UMLS organizes the Metathesaurus content into categories. Major categories or categories with the largest amount of content and examples of vocabularies include:

- Clinical and Laboratory Observations
    - Logical Observation Identifier Names and Codes (LOINC)
- Procedures and Supplies
    - Current Procedural Terminology (CPT)
- Diseases and Diagnosis
    - International Classification of Diseases and Related Health Problems (ICD-10)
- Comprehensive Vocabularies and Thesauri
    - SNOMED CT

Other categories such as anatomy, drugs, genetics, nursing, and miscellaneous also exist in the Metathesaurus.

SPECIALIST Lexicon and Lexical Tools supply the lexical information and programs needed for the development of a natural language processing system. It contains words that are frequently used within the English language and medical terms. The tools assist users in the management and indexing of these words for programmers.

UMLS terminology services (UTS) is the web interface for browser downloads and to access the APIs provided by the UMLS. It was implemented in 2010 as a substitution to the

UMLS knowledge source server. Through the UTS, users with a UMLS license create an account and register for internet access to all the UMLS Knowledge sources.

Principles and Guidelines

The Metathesaurus preserves the meanings, concept names, and relationships from its source vocabularies, but additional synonymous relationships, concept attributes, and some concept names have been added (NLM 2017a). The UMLS has multiple identifiers for its content. These identifiers include:

- Concept Unique Identifier (CUI): Each concept has a permanent CUI. The CUI is a meaningless primary key, has no intrinsic meaning, and never changes. However, a CUI is removed from the Metathesaurus when it is discovered that two CUIs name the same concept. In such cases, the process is to retain one of the two CUIs, link all relevant information in the Metathesaurus to it, and retire the other CUI. Retired CUIs are never reused. "CUIs also serve as permanent, publicly available identifiers for biomedical concepts or meanings to which many individual source vocabularies are linked" (NLM 2018b).
- Lexical Unique Identifier (LUI): LUIs link lexical variants (different word types for equivalent phrases). Each LUI begins with the letter *L* and is followed by seven numbers.
- String Unique Identifier (SUI): Each unique concept representation has an SUI. If there is variation in the case, punctuation, or character, a unique SUI is assigned to the concept representation. Each SUI begins with an *S* and is followed by seven numbers.
- Atom Unique Identifiers (AUIs): The concept representation (string) from each source vocabulary has its own unique identifier. Multiple source vocabularies may have the same character representation of the concept and the AUIs uniquely identify the occurrence of each string in the source vocabulary and are the building blocks of all UMLS metathesaurus concepts. An AUI contains the letter *A* and is followed by seven numbers.

The Metathesaurus includes many relationships among different concepts in addition to the synonymous relationships, most of which come from the individual source vocabularies. The Semantic Network includes data on the categories to which all Metathesaurus concepts have been assigned and the permissible relationships among these types.

Metathesaurus construction involves understanding the intended meaning of each name in each source vocabulary and linking all the names from all the source vocabularies that mean the same thing (the synonyms). The editors determine what view of synonymy to represent in the

Metathesaurus concept structure, and each source vocabulary's view of synonymy is also present (whether or not it agrees with the Metathesaurus view).

Adoption and Use

The number of UMLS licenses has continued to increase. UMLS distributed 10,095 licenses in fiscal year 2015 (NLM 2015). This was more than 1,000 new licenses compared to fiscal year 2013. There has also been a steady increase in the use of the UMLS APIs. In 2016 users queried the APIs over 29 million times.

Results from an analysis of the 2004 UMLS user annual report show the main activities to be research, software development, healthcare provision, and education (Fung et al. 2006). This same study reported the UMLS uses were terminology research, mapping between terminologies, the creation of a local terminology, information indexing and retrieval, and natural language processing. In addition, a survey distributed to the UMLS user mailing list reported 119 uses with the top three being terminology research, information retrieval, and terminology translation (Chen et al. 2007).

Tools

The UTS provides the access point for the UMLS tools (NLM 2016). There are tools that are available online or available for download. Some of the tools include:

- UMLS browsers:
  - Metathesaurus searching—allows users to browse UML's content by text, CUI, or source terminology code. Content can be browsed by semantic or relationship type.
  - Semantic network browsing—allows users to browse by semantic types and relationships.
  - SNOMED CT Searching—searches SNOMED CT hierarchy alone or as it is included in the UMLS Metathesaurus.
- Specialist Lexicon and Lexical Tools: programs for language processing and managing lexical variations. Lexical tools include:
  - Norm Program—used to find similar terms, map terms to UMLS concepts, and find lexical variants. Example processes include removing stop words, lowercase, and sort words.
  - Word index generator—breaks strings into a unique list of lowercased "words" to produce the Metathesaurus word index.

- Lexical variant generator—a tool that combines lexical variants such as conjugations, word order, and possessiveness, and transforms them to text.
- Specialist NLP Tools
  - LexAccess—provides lookup capabilities into the SPECIALIST lexicon through queries and as a result returns lexical records.
  - Text categorization tools—provide high-level categorization of text based on Journal Description Imaging (JDI).
  - GSpell—suggests the proper spellings of misspelled words.
  - dTagger—assigns parts of speech to sentences.
  - Visual Tagging tool—provides text annotation and tagging.
  - Sub-Term mapping—identifies sub-term patterns.
- MetaMap Portal: identifies and maps biomedical texts to concepts that exist in the Metathesaurus.
- UMLS free tools available for download and personal use via UMLS Terminology Services (UTS):
  - Sample Load Scripts and Data Model: example code that supports loading Metathesaurus content into Access, MySQL, and Oracle databases.
  - MetamorphoSys: the installation wizard and customization program included in each release of UMLS. Each installation of Metathesaurus content can be customized by limiting the downloaded source vocabularies to a specific subset distributed by the UMLS. MetamorphoSys contains the rich release format (RRF) subset browser and allows users to search locally created subsets.

Process for Revision and Updates

UMLS continues to evolve through the inclusion of new vocabulary, terminology, and classification systems, and redesigns of its resources and tools based on available information technology. The Knowledge Sources are iteratively refined and expanded based on feedback from those applying each successive version. Each edition of the Metathesaurus includes files that detail any changes from the previous edition.

A formal method for expanding content involves four major steps:

1. Analysis and inversion. The semantics and structure of the vocabulary are analyzed and then "inverted" into a standard Metathesaurus input format.
2. Insertion. The terminology is inserted into the Metathesaurus maintenance system.
3. Human editing. Experts with the requisite expertise review and edit the Metathesaurus entries affected by the automated insertion routines.
4. Quality assurance (QA). QA queries are run before version releases to identify potential errors of commission and omission (NLM 2017b).

Part of the procedure includes evaluation criteria that must be addressed with all requests for a source vocabulary addition to the UMLS (NLM 2018c). This includes:

- Value to UMLS with justification for inclusion in the UMLS, interoperability benefits and documented use cases
- Description of the source vocabulary content including thesaurus characteristics, concept meanings, and associated vocabulary principles
- Technical process and development such as whether the content is available in a well-structured electronic format
- Background questions regarding terminology maintenance process, updates, authors, owner, and vocabulary integrity checking
- Terms of agreement according to the UMLS Metathesaurus License Agreement

There are no restrictions about who can suggest a vocabulary for inclusion in the UMLS Metathesaurus. However, NLM may not be able to include additions that would consume large amounts of effort in analysis, processing, or editing. NLM encourages broad use of the UMLS products by distributing semiannual updates in May (ULMS [year]AA) and November (UMLS [year]AB) free of charge.

Enterprise Terminology Systems

Some healthcare disciplines have developed terminology systems to house and centralize terminology content used within their discipline. Two examples of this are the National Cancer Institute (NCI) Enterprise Vocabulary Services and the Public Health Information Network Vocabulary Access and Distribution System (PHIN VADS) developed by the Centers for Disease Control (CDC).

National Cancer Institute Enterprise Vocabulary Services

The NCI Enterprise Vocabulary Services (EVS) is a suite of terminology tools, content, and services, which are used to code and leverage biomedical research, clinical, and public health data (NCI n.d.a).

Developer

EVS is developed by the NCI and was initiated in 1997 (NCI n.d.a). EVS forms the semantic foundation of NCI's informatics infrastructure by organizing and mapping terminologies in a consistent way to provide a rich framework for coding and retrieval.

Purpose

The core mission of EVS is to provide terminology content that cancer researchers need for data exchange and interoperability in clinical trial, research, and other activities both nationally and internationally (de Coronado et al. 2004). EVS is used to create, extend, subset, map, access, and publish biomedical terminology and ontology and for basic, translational, and clinical research; clinical care; epidemiology; public health; administration; and public information.

Content

The EVS creates two main terminology resources: the **NCI Thesaurus (NCIt)** and the **NCI Metathesaurus (NCIm)** (see figures 16.2 and 16.3). In addition, it provides a broad collection of individual terminologies, cross mappings, and value sets. The subject domain encompasses various basic and clinical research areas as well as public health and administrative content. Each reference resource contains concepts with associated codes, synonyms, definitions, and inter-concept relationships. EVS users can map to concepts in either reference resources or other EVS content as needed to support interoperability and crosswalks.

FIGURE 16.2. NCI thesaurus arrhythmia search results

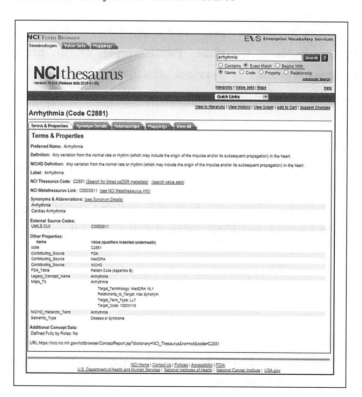

Source: NCI 2019.

FIGURE 16.3. NCI metathesaurus results

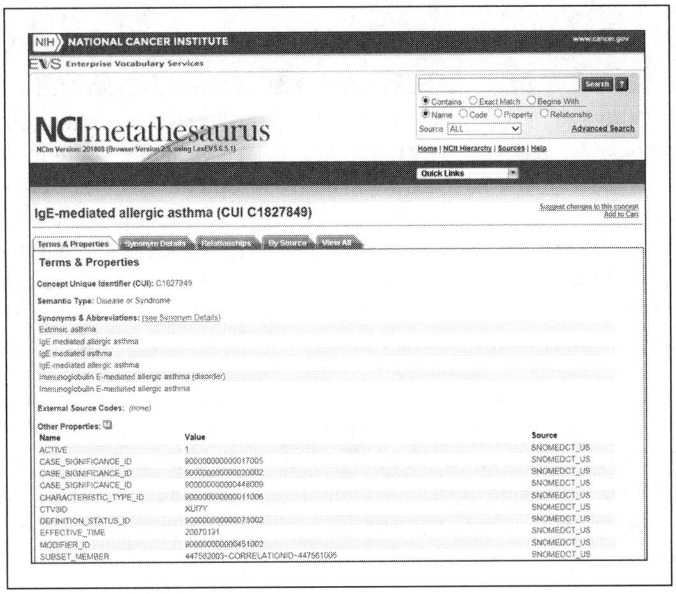

Source: NCI 2018a.

NCIt is a description logic terminology based on current science that helps individuals and software applications connect and organize biomedical information, for example, by disease and underlying biology. NCIt is developed as a web ontology language (OWL). NCIt provides textual and ontologic descriptions of key biomedical concepts. Content is generated both internally at NCI and by EVS partners and users. Content covers chemicals, drugs and other therapies, diseases, genes and gene products, anatomy, organisms, animal models, techniques, biological processes, and administrative categories. NCIt provides definitions, synonyms, and other information on cancers and related diseases, drug therapies, and a wide range of other topics related to cancer and biomedical research. It is maintained by a team of editors from multiple disciplines. NCIt serves several functions, including annotation of data in NCI's repositories and search and retrieval operations applied to these repositories. The formal structure of the thesaurus facilitates automatic reasoning.

NCIm is a comprehensive collection of biomedical vocabularies and concept-based mappings from more than 75 different terminologies. NCIm combines most public domain vocabularies from the UMLS Metathesaurus with many other vocabularies, and cross-links meanings in all of them using concept-based representations and inter-concept relationships. Table 16.1 illustrates the similarities and differences between NCIt and NCIm.

EVS supports the development and use of collections of concepts in the form of value sets or subsets. A value set is a collection of concepts from one or more standard terminology grouped together for a specific purpose (Grannis and Vreeman 2010). These collections provide a pre-curated standard set of meanings for use in coding data, metadata, and models. Organizations

TABLE 16.1. Comparison between NCI Thesaurus and Metathesaurus

Point of Comparison	NCI Thesaurus (NCIt)	NCI Metathesaurus (NCI)
Description	The NCI Thesaurus is a standard reference terminology/ontology used by the NCI to support cancer research. It is curated and maintained by NCI staff and contractors. It contains concepts and relationships needed to support NCI business and scientific programs, as well as other users and collaborators such as the FDA and CDISC.	The NCI Metathesaurus is a synthesis of many different terminologies. It is based on the National Library of Medicine's UMLS Metathesaurus, removing some proprietary and out of scope terminologies and inserting additional terminologies of interest to the NCI research community. It integrates terms and definitions from different terminologies.
Origins	The original intent was to create a stand-alone, controlled terminology in support of the NCI's software systems used for annotating, database search, data mining, text indexing, and natural language processing.	The original intent was to create a comprehensive repository as a dictionary and thesaurus containing most of the terminologies from the UMLS Metathesaurus, as well as many other biomedical terminologies created by or of interest to NCI and its partners.
Release Format	OWL	RRF - Modeled after the UMLS Metathesaurus
License	Open content license	Users may encounter each sub-terminology license separately. Some proprietary terminologies are included, with permission, and have restrictions on their use.
Subsets	Concepts in Subsets are identified within NCI Thesaurus by associations and properties, but also published separately for a number of users who require them in this format. In the future many of these will also be converted and published as value sets.	Subsets are not made available by NCI; however, individual sources can be extracted from the NCI Metathesaurus build using publicly available UMLS tools.
Updates	Monthly	Bi-annually and as needed

Source: NCI 2018b.

such as the US Food and Drug Administration (FDA), the Clinical Data Interchange Standards Consortium (CDISC), and the National Council for Prescription Drug Programs (NCPDP) have chosen to develop and integrate many of their value sets within EVS, including 500 defined subsets in NCIt.

Principles and Guidelines

NCIt is authored as a concept-based ontology called LexGrid within an open-source tool called Protégé. It is then linked to the NCIm (Ethier et al. 2013). NCIt is developed and released in the OWL format (NCI 2018c).

The structure of the NCIm is based on the UMLS Metathesaurus and complies with the structure described above in the UMLS section. Where a UMLS CUI exists, it remains the same and is used to identify concepts; otherwise, a new NCIm CUI is created. Most nonproprietary contents of the UMLS Metathesaurus are included in NCIm. In addition, the NCIm has been extended to include many other terminologies used by cancer and biomedical researchers. NCIm is released in RRF, as is UMLS Metathesaurus.

Tools

Terminologies, value sets, and cross-terminology mappings are housed in a central terminology server called LexEVS (NCI 2018d). EVS develops software to create, manage, and update terminology data within LexEVS. Tools and services to access, load, and publish vocabulary and ontology terminology resources from Lex EVS are available (NCI n.d.b). Available software for users includes the NCI Term Browser (see figure 16.4) and the NCI Metathesaurus Browser. The browser provides access to many terminologies and ontologies used by NCI and its partners such as ICD-10-CM, the Common Terminology Criteria for Adverse Events (CTCAE), the Medical Dictionary for Regulatory Activities (MedDRA), and SNOMED CT. It is linked to other information resources, including both internal NCI systems and external systems, such as the Gene Ontology and SNOMED CT. Users select the terminologies they want to search. Concepts and terms can be searched by entering a string or code. There are different types of searches such as "exact match" or "contains." Results contain matching concept records with terms and properties, synonym details such as source, relationships, and mappings.

Adoption and Use

NCI needs for terminology content, standards, and systems are often shared with the NIH and federal agencies, and by the broader cancer research and biomedical community. EVS works with many partners to build shared content and services so that information can be exchanged, interpreted, and analyzed. EVS is widely used by NCI, NIH, federal agencies, and other US and international biomedical, academic, standards, and research organizations. CDISC terminology, coded in NCIt, is required for regulatory reporting of human clinical trial data as well as preclinical data by the FDA and Japan Pharmaceuticals and Medical Devices Agency (PMDA). It is therefore deployed in clinical trial systems globally.

Process for Revision and Updates

NCIt is published monthly, and NCIm is published biannually and as needed to support a broad community of users. Below is a brief synopsis of the EVS content revision and update process.

FIGURE 16.4. NCI term browser

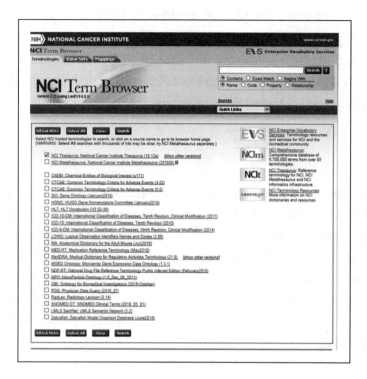

Source: NCI n.d.c.

EVS also has a published development path outlining future plans for content and software updates (NCI 2016).

New concept and term requests come from NCI as well as EVS customers. Many requests come from the term suggestion software linked to the browsers. In addition, they receive requirements and data submissions via email and other channels. NCI has a staff of curators who curate the content into the NCIt and other EVS resources.

There is a well-established QA process that occurs throughout the editing and publication cycle (de Coronado et al. 2009). QA includes both automated and manual techniques and occurs from request to publication. EVS publishes frequent updates to its documents and standards.

Public Health Information Network Vocabulary Access and Distribution System (PHIN VADS)

The Public Health Information Network Vocabulary Access and Distribution System (PHIN VADS) provides standard vocabularies to the CDC and its public health partners in one place. PHIN VADS is used in public health and clinical care practice. It promotes the use of standards-based vocabulary to support the exchange of consistent information among public health partners.

Developer

In 2004, the Centers for Disease Control and Prevention (CDC) developed a web-based enterprise vocabulary system called the Public Health Information Network Vocabulary Access and Distribution System (PHIN VADS) for accessing, searching, and distributing value sets used within the PHIN (CDC 2018a). The CDC Vocabulary and Messaging team manages the PHIN VADS application and content.

Purpose

PHIN promotes the use of a standards-based vocabulary within CDC information systems and among other SDOs. PHIN VADS was established to support shared policies, standards, practices, and services that facilitate efficient public health information access, exchange, use, and collaboration among public health agencies and with their clinical and other partners. The main purpose of PHIN VADS is to distribute the value sets associated with HL7 message implementation guides; for example, value sets associated with Arboviral v1.3 Case Notification Message Mapping Guide (CDC 2018b).

Content

PHIN VADS provides quick access to commonly and frequently used value sets by supplying all the vocabulary metadata needed for HL7 Messaging or Clinical Document Architecture (CDA) in one format at one location. Currently, PHIN VADS contains 206 code systems, over 1,500 value sets, and more than five million concepts. VADS is based on the code system or domain recommendations and value set recommendations from HITSP C80 specification. Examples of commonly used content are:

- Reportable Condition Mapping Table (RCMT): provides mapping between conditions and their associated lab tests and results.
- Public Health vocabulary (electronic lab reporting (ELR), Immunization and Syndromic Surveillance): includes value sets associated with Electronic Laboratory Reporting Implementation Guide, Immunization, and Syndromic Surveillance for Emergency Department and Urgent Care.
- Healthcare Associated Infections: all value sets associated with the National Health Safety Network.
- Flu Lab Report Vocabulary: data elements specific to influenza used for messaging public health laboratory tests and results.

Value sets are assigned a value set code, value set name, and value set Object Identifier (OID).

Principles and Guidelines

The VADS search "All Vocabularies" navigation menu includes options for searching:

- Views messaging guides
- Value sets
- Value set concepts
- Code systems
- Code system concepts
- Vocabulary groups

Hovering over any of the options reveals a pop-up window with additional information. For example, the pop-up window for value set concepts states, "A value set concept is the code and name for a concept as used in a value set (for example, Arm, Leg)" (CDC 2018c). In addition, some options provide the ability to refine the search. PHIN VADS expects users to download the code systems from the SDO or official distribution source such as the UMLS or VSAC.

Users can access and view vocabularies created in PHIN VADS for public health use, with file download options for Value Sets, Value Set Concepts, Views, and Groups, available in a tab-delimited text format or in Microsoft Excel format. Figure 16.5 illustrates the "Problem Value Set"

FIGURE 16.5. PHIN VADS Problem Value Set

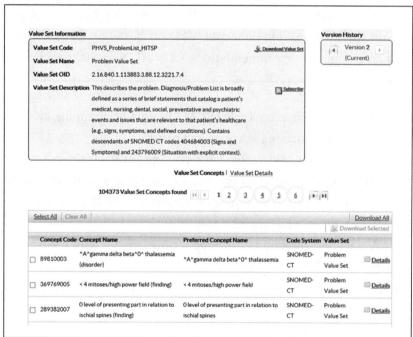

Source: CDC 2018d.

with three of the value set members and each concept's associated metadata (Concept Code, Concept Name, Preferred Name, Code System, and Value Set).

The CDC has a Meaningful Use Community of Practice (CoP) where documents and presentations are posted (CDC 2017). The members of the CoP include representatives from public health agencies, state Medicaid offices, and national public health associations.

Tools

PHIN VADS tooling is an open web service that can be directly consumed by third-party applications (CDC 2018c). These web services are built upon open standards such as HL7 CTS discussed earlier in this chapter. The web service consists of an interface, the domain objects that represent vocabulary information, and data transfer objects (DTOs) to transfer data to and from the web service. Custom programs, applications, or data extraction scripts can be written to directly use PHIN VADS Web Services.

Adoption and Use

As seen in the Problem List value set example, PHIN VADS provides the coded vocabulary within value sets that is used by the CDC and Public Health. Users access and view the files as well as download them for use in their systems. PHIN VADS users include the following:

- CDC programs
- State and local health departments
- Healthcare providers including labs
- Value set developers
- Value set implementers
- SDOs
- Standard harmonization workgroups
- EMR and public health application vendors
- Researchers

Process for Revision and Updates

PHIN VADS identifies value sets required for messaging within standards such as the HL7 Public Health Case Reports structured document or meaningful use value sets. When these are identified, the value sets are created within the PHIN VADS database. PHIN VADS uses the Universal Authoring Framework to manage the vocabulary present in PHIN VADS. The updates are based upon LOINC and SNOMED CT releases (twice a year) and to support the Reportable Condition Mapping Table (such as Dwyer Tables). In addition to this schedule, they also update

VADS when there is a new Message Mapping Guide. A notice is sent to PHIN VADS users prior to the update.

Metadata Registries

Metadata is data that defines and describes other data, such as concepts and data elements (ISO/IEC 11179 2013). A **metadata registry (MDR)** is a database that houses metadata through the use of a model (metamodel). Many MDRs exist in the US and are used for the following purposes:

- Formatting and identifying value domains
- Identifying data elements from standard information models, such as HL7 or the NCI

The two MDRs are the Value Set Authority Center (VSAC) and the US Health Information Knowledgebase (USHIK). These MDRs are described below.

Value Set Authority Center (VSAC)

VSAC provides coordination, knowledge engineering, and management for value set curation and retrieval. Prior to VSAC, value sets for Clinical Quality Measures (CQMs) and Consolidated Clinical Document Architecture (C-CDA) were not easily accessible to measure developers and implementers. Additionally, as the use of enumerated lists and codes from multiple code systems increased, the alignment, validity, and reliability of the codes needed to be assessed.

Developers

The NLM, ONC, and CMS collaborated to create the Value Set Authority Center (VSAC) as a single source host of all official versions of value sets specified by the CMS electronic Clinical Quality Measures (eCQMs). The first export of value sets to the NLM in October 2012 marked the initial curation of VSAC (NLM 2017a).

Purpose

VSAC consists of tooling that is designed to:

- Provide a centralized location for measure implementers to obtain value sets for clinical quality measures
- Confirm the validity of the codes within their code system
- Prevent the use of expired codes within value sets

- Avoid duplication of value sets (although value sets imported from PHIN VADS and SNOMED CT Reference Sets are duplicative)
- Provide value set authoring and distribution

Content

Value Sets located on VSAC contain the lists and codes required for eCQM reporting within HL7 messages. The value sets are lists of codes and descriptions that group together to define and represent clinical concepts intended for use in a specific context. Figure 16.6 illustrates the Obstetrics VTE value set. This is a value set the Joint Commission created to identify patients who have a pregnancy-related venous thromboembolism (VTE). The value set is used within the "Intensive Care Unit Venous Thromboembolism Prophylaxis" to query for every type of pregnant or obstetrics patient with a VTE diagnosis.

The VSAC provides users with a web interface for browsing the content, search, and filter constraints, APIs for recovery, and download of the value sets. The VSAC organizes its content by tabs:

- Welcome: provides a brief overview of the VSAC and hyperlinks to other sites (UMLS, NLM, and the like) that are helpful to value set users.

FIGURE 16.6. The Joint Commission obstetrics VTE value set

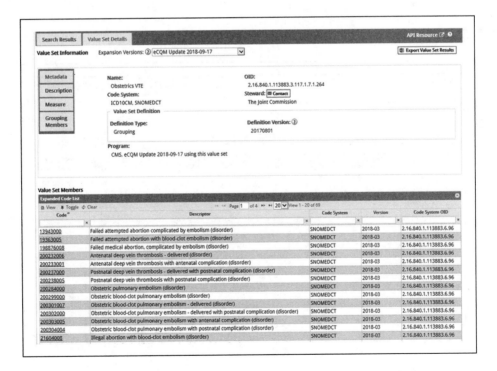

Source: NLM 2019.

- Search Value Sets: allows users to filter value sets on basic keyword search or advanced criteria (CQM number, Quality Data Model [QDM] data category, CQM developer, eligibility, code, and code system). The results of the search criteria can be downloaded in Excel and XML file types.
- Download: sorts value sets for download by publication date and then by CMS ID, Value Set Name, or QDM category. Files are provided in Excel and XML file types.
- Browse Code Systems: allows users to scan all code systems or filter by code system and code system version.
- Help: supplies a hyperlink to the NLM customer support page, instructions on how to use APIs to obtain value sets, and tips on using the filter and search criteria.

After a user logs into VSAC, the welcome screen allows the user to select the programs he or she would like to search within the NLM value set repository. The choices are: All Value Sets, CMS eCQM Value Sets, HL7 C-CDA Value Sets, or CMS Hybrid Value Sets. See figure 16.7 showing the Search All Value Sets screen for the NLM value set repository. Search constraints include Value Set Name, Code System, Definition Type, Steward, and OID. Each column in the search results can be clicked for sorting.

VSAC also allows users to obtain permissions for authoring or stewarding of value sets. This allows individual authors to curate value sets that are maintained by value set stewards. VSAC provides value set authoring guidelines in order to support best practices. Authoring can be done as an enumerated list by importing a list of codes from a code system or as rule-based

FIGURE 16.7. Search screen for NLM value set repository

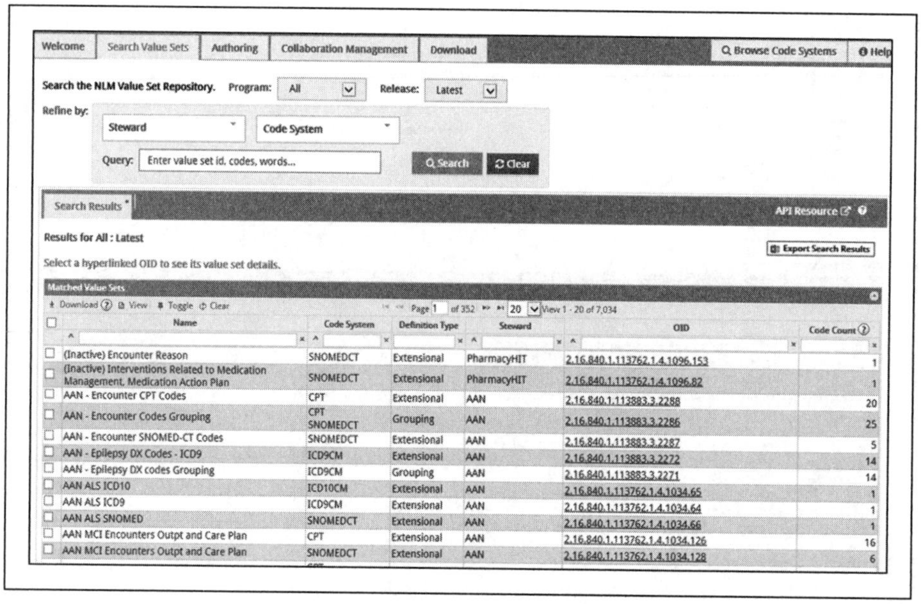

Source: NLM 2019.

(intensional) value set created by query. Additionally, the VSAC allows collaboration between authors and stewards by supporting groups to work collaboratively to publish value set content.

Principles and Guidelines

VSAC follows the Sharing Value Sets (SVS) technical framework and Common Terminology Services 2 (CTS 2) specifications. Both the SVS and CTS 2 act as means to standardize the way value sets are accessed from VSAC. VSAC also offers a FHIR terminology API. These allow users to authenticate and retrieve value set and code system content for each of the supported programs.

Adoption and Use

VSAC is the official source of value sets that appear in eCQMs required from CMS and the HL7 C-CDA value sets. A UMLS license is required to browse or download VSAC value sets.

There are eight PHIN VADS value sets used in HL7 C-CDA Implementation Guides. These value sets have been uploaded into VSAC using the code system "CDCREC." Figure 16.8 shows a screenshot of the CDC PHIN VADs value sets contained in VSAC.

FIGURE 16.8. PHIN VADs value sets

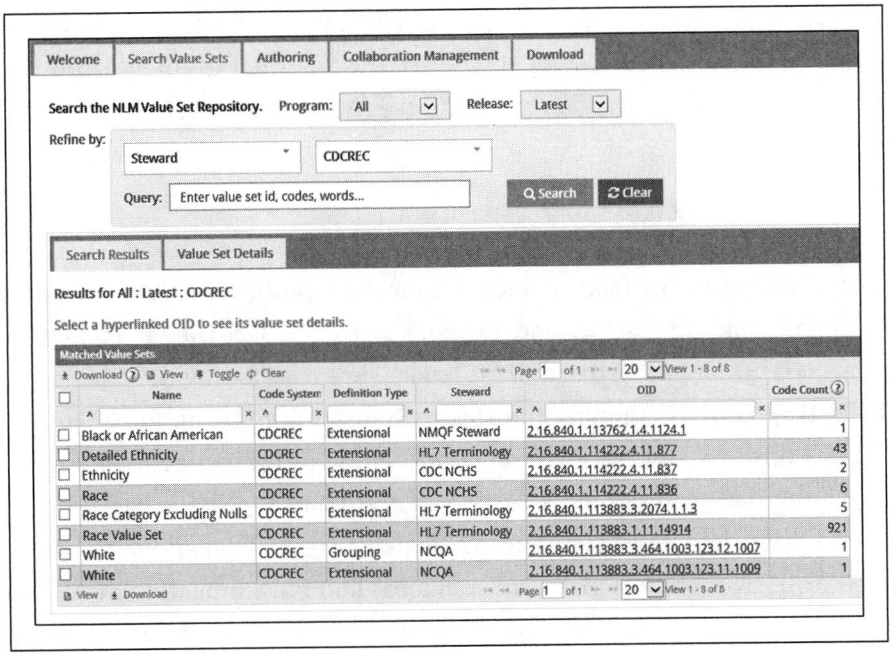

Source: NLM 2018a.

Users are prompted to provide their UMLS login information prior to accessing the value sets. VSAC offers a user's forum that targets authors, stewards, and consumers of value sets.

Process for Revision and Updates

Value set stewards are responsible for reviewing, editing, approving, and maintaining their value sets. For eCQMs, the measure contractor must re-evaluate the measure annually (Healthit.gov 2019). VSAC publishes releases as needed and users can subscribe to updates from VSAC through an NLM Listserv. The hyperlink is available via the VSAC welcome page. VSAC has published eCQM value sets starting with the 2013 reporting and performance period. In 2016 VSAC began publishing the C-CDA value sets as well as the CDC race and ethnicity roll-up codes in order to support the 2015 common clinical data set.

The US Health Information Knowledgebase (USHIK)

The **US Health Information Knowledgebase (USHIK)** is a publicly available registry and repository of specifications, standards, and metadata funded by the Agency for Healthcare Research and Quality (AHRQ) in HHS (AHRQ n.d.).

Developer

USHIK was initiated by a consortium of federal agencies and directed and funded by AHRQ beginning in 1994. The following SDOs have shared their intellectual property with AHRQ-USHIK to improve the consistent use of standards: the National Council of Prescription Data Programs (NCPDP) Accredited Standards Committee (ASC) X12 and HL7.

Purpose

The mission of AHRQ is to "produce evidence to make healthcare safer, higher quality, more accessible, equitable, and affordable, and to work with the U.S. Department of Health and Human Services (HHS) and other partners to make sure that the evidence is understood and used" (AHRQ 2017a). USHIK supports the Health Information Technology (Health IT) initiatives of the AHRQ director and the HHS secretary. These initiatives promote improved health research by creating and maintaining a system of metadata registries based on the ISO/IEC 11179 Standard for Metadata Registries (Part 3 - Registry metamodel and basic attributes) (ISO/IEC 11179 2013). USHIK promotes metadata standards and harmonization of vocabulary across standards. USHIK provides a well-organized and structured view of data elements and their specifications (attributes or metadata) for the technical and casual user. The metadata registries,

USHIK's portals, are created to provide understanding, promote interoperability, and encourage reuse of uniformly defined data. Within USHIK's portals, information models provide a means of drilling down from the overall context in which the data elements are used to the technical specifications of the data elements.

Content

USHIK contains data elements adopted by HHS as National Interoperability Standards and is divided into different portals which are accessed through tabs on its website landing page:

- USHIK – contains USHIK information, draft items, and news.
- Standards – contains healthcare IT metadata registered from SDOs that have been accredited by the American National Standards Institute (ANSI) such as ASC X12 and NCPDP.
- Health Information Technology Standards Panel (HITSP) – includes the HITSP data elements linked to all HITSP use cases, interoperability specifications, and other documents.
- Common Formats – contains the specifications for electronically reporting patient safety events that occur in hospitals to AHRQ-designated Patient Safety Organizations.
- Quality Reporting – contains eCQM data elements (names, definitions, vocabularies, and codes) associated with the quality measures' numerators, denominators, inclusions, and exclusions as well as their value sets from VSAC for CMS quality reporting programs.
- APCD (All-Payer Claims Databases) – Data element specifications from all-payer databases of multiple states, plus the ASC X12 data dictionary (of HIPAA data elements for claims transactions) and the All-Payer Claims Database Council's Core Set of payer-reported data elements for comparison purposes.
- Draft Measures – allows the browsing and comparison of measures that are currently in draft form. This page allows users to submit feedback to CMS prior to the publishing of the measure.
- Child EHR Format – outlines functional requirements and guidance on contents and standards necessary to capture and format data related to children.

Figure 16.9 is an example of the USHIK data element Healthcare-associated infection (HAI) with the associated answer codes.

FIGURE 16.9. USHIK HAI data element

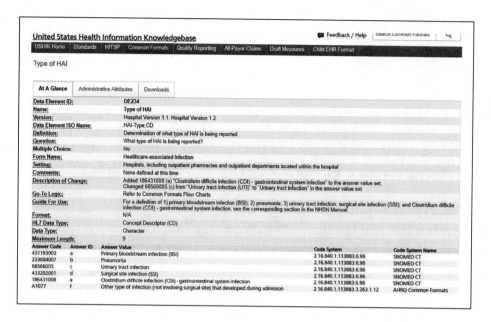

Source: AHRQ n.d.

Principles and Guidelines

USHIK houses information models and metadata in its different portals. Each information model is a map that permits the user to drill down into the portal's core components and data elements, which are the smallest unit of data pertinent to an electronic exchange of information as defined by a particular use case, standard, collection, or initiative. The ISO Standard for Metadata Registries discusses the semantics of data, including how metadata should be structured, and considers data elements' foundational concepts (ISO/IEC 11179 2013). Examples of data elements include race, gender, and laboratory test result. If the data element contains an enumerated value set for the answers (or values) from a vocabulary, the Value Domain is listed as the source of the associated values. If the value domain includes definitions for the concept, they are considered Conceptual Domains and are a collection of value meanings.

Figure 16.10 is an example of the USHIK data element Neonate Gender with the associated answer codes. The answer codes come from the Value Domain Administrative Gender Value Set (figure 16.11).

Tools

USHIK includes an All-Payer Claims Database (APCD), which contains healthcare claims from a variety of payer sources (AHRQ 2017b). The database houses claims metadata such as admission date, discharge date, charge amount, and demographics. Each state has hundreds of metadata

FIGURE 16.10. USHIK Neonate Gender data element

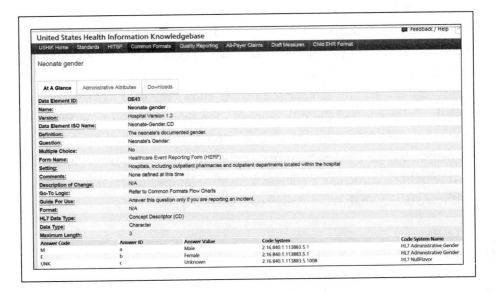

Source: AHRQ n.d.

FIGURE 16.11. USHIK Administrative Gender Value Set

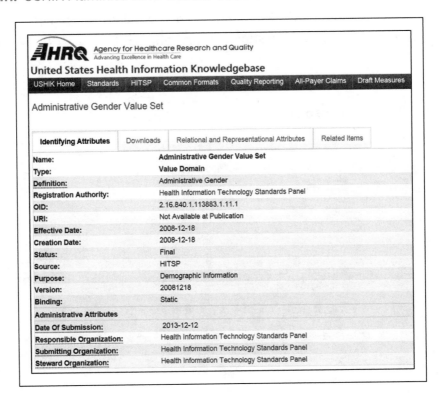

Source: AHRQ n.d.

types; for example, Utah has 578 types of metadata. Users can view metadata by state or compare metadata between states.

A USHIK comparison matrix is a tool that aids in comparing data elements' metadata across multiple standards and portals. For example, "gender" is a data element that exists in many data standards. The data elements may have different definitions or value sets in different uses (portals, or standards). The comparison matrix allows the user to see the metadata about each "gender" data element and the differences in the metadata and to evaluate the effect of these differences on the user's purpose (see figure 16.12). USHIK also offers the comparison of quality measures under the Quality Reporting tab across value sets or versions. USHIK users may include researchers, clinicians, policy makers, developers, information technology system vendors, healthcare policy analysts, and metadata users in general.

Adoption and Use

Participating SDOs include the National Council of Prescription Data Programs (NCPDP) and Accredited Standards Committee (ASC) X12. USHIK is open to anyone and provides a user-friendly metadata download format. Therefore, users who access the system are those interested in implementing the SDO data structures with the associated, or linked, standard terminologies. USHIK notifies users of updates via email. USHIK provides resources to assist users in consuming the Quality Reporting Programs eCQMs published by CMS and the Value Sets published by the NLM's Value Set Authority Center (VSAC) in support of the Quality Reporting Programs incentive payment programs. The source of truth for these artifacts is CMS and NLM VSAC; users of

FIGURE 16.12. USHIK comparison matrix

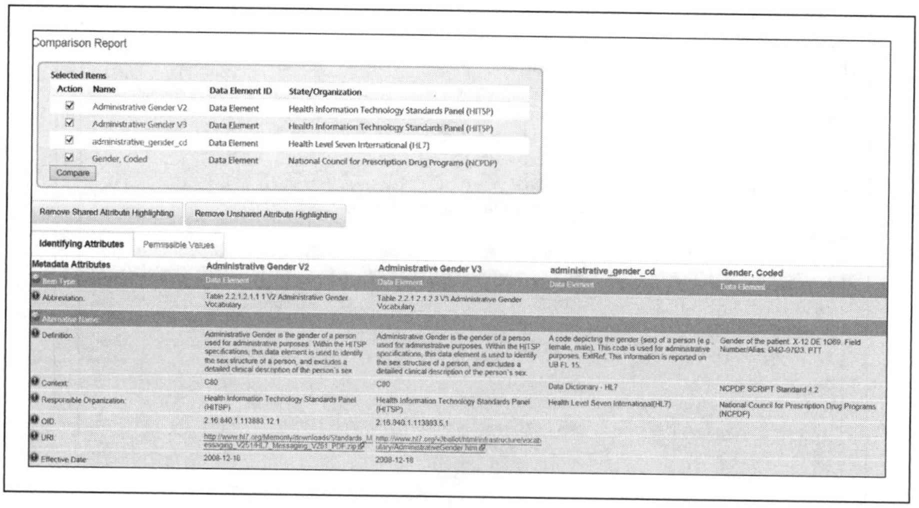

Source: AHRQ n.d.

USHIK are encouraged to consult these resources in conjunction with USHIK. Access to eCQM value sets via the UMLS requires a license to access.

Process for Revision and Updates

The data element information in each USHIK portal comes from a USHIK-registered authority, such as an SDO, a state, a federal agency, or other authority. This authority is the owner of its own intellectual property in USHIK and carries the responsibility for assuring accuracy and maintaining updated information in USHIK. Data element information may be versioned in USHIK and compared across versions.

Use Cases

Centralized vocabulary servers with associated tools and services are needed to address the increase in structured data capture requirements. The following are two examples of how a vocabulary server and a metadata registry assist with maintaining consistent terminology for implementation and use.

Use Case One: Implementing Multiple Standard Terminologies

Good Health Hospital is a healthcare organization embarking on creating encoded point-of-care assessment forms with pick lists. It is using a vocabulary server to facilitate the implementation and use of multiple standard terminologies. Because LOINC and SNOMED CT are the two standard terminologies mandated for documenting clinical assessments by the National Committee on Vital and Health Statistics (NCVHS), it has elected to use these terminologies. The requirements for documenting assessments are that the question (observation) is encoded using LOINC and the answer lists (values) are encoded using SNOMED CT. It accessed a metadata registry and located the skin assessment which describes the assessment of skin moisture, color, and turgor. The coding of the skin color observation and coded answers from both terminologies were present. The question "What is the skin color?" is the LOINC concept "Color of skin" (39107-8). The LOINC code would be the identifier for the question that is stored in the patient record and used for messaging observation data. The pick list answers are selected from a skin color value set of SNOMED CT concepts from the Clinical Findings hierarchy. Values include "skin normal color (finding)" (297952003), "yellow or jaundiced color (finding)" (267030001), or "dusky discoloration of skin (finding)" (445394005). The concept that correctly depicts the skin color observed can now be stored in the documentation system linked to the question and correctly encoded on the point-of-care assessment form using a pick list.

Use Case Two: Developing a Clinical Quality Measure

CMS contracts CQM developers to identify and create specifications that can be used to assess quality healthcare processes and outcomes. A key initiative in CQM development is harmonization across measures. Specifically, the measure developers must use the same criteria in the calculation of the numerator, denominator, and exclusion criteria of data elements. CQM developers use the VSAC to search existing value sets for data elements such as a diagnosis of "myocardial infarction" or medication lists such as "Angiotensin Converting Enzyme (ACE) Inhibitors." The VSAC browsing features allow measure developers to improve the harmonization across measures by encouraging the reuse of value sets across measures. Additionally, the VSAC allows measure developers to identify gaps in existing value sets and create a more robust repository of value sets for use across measures. Using the same value sets to define data elements across care settings provides comparable quality measures and offers a platform to provide improved quality care.

In this case, the CQM developer decided to access the VSAC for a measure it was developing for management of low blood pressure. The selection of the cohort is done by querying for all

FIGURE 16.13. eCQM value set for Hypotension

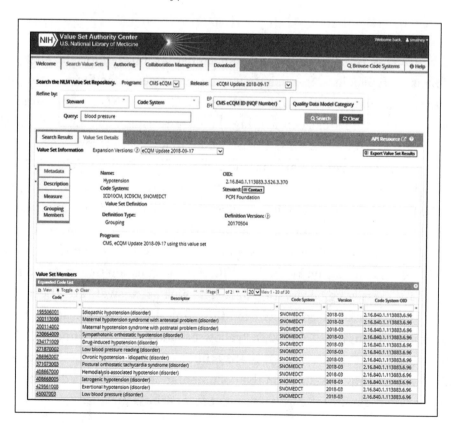

Source: NLM 2019.

patients that had a diagnosis of hypotension. From the VSAC welcome page, the CME eCQM Value Sets tab was selected. The search term "blood pressure" was entered and the value set in figure 16.13 was found and selected for inclusion in the new eCQM.

CHECK YOUR UNDERSTANDING

1. Which of the following is *not* one of the steps in NLM's methodology for expanding UMLS content?

    a. Quality assurance
    b. Analysis and inversion
    c. Human editing
    d. Public hearings

2. True or false? MetamorphoSys is a very large, multipurpose, and multilingual vocabulary database found in UMLS.

    a. True
    b. False

3. The Metathesaurus is organized by:

    a. Concept
    b. Relationships
    c. Diagnosis
    d. Disease

4. A _____ provides the ability to house multiple standard terminologies as well as local extensions in one location, improving operational efficiency, and effective terminology management.

5. Which one of the following is *not* one of the UMLS's Knowledge Resources?

    a. SPECIALIST Lexicon
    b. Semantic Network
    c. MetamorphoSys
    d. Metathesaurus

REVIEW

1. Which of the following is *not* a standard for defining how terminologies and value sets should be sent and translated? (Select all that apply.)

   a. PHIN VADS

   b. UMLS

   c. CTS2

   d. SVS

2. Which metadata repository provides content for public health reporting?

   a. PHIN VADS

   b. UMLS

   c. CTS2

   d. NCIt

3. In what terminology can cancer-specific terminology created by the NCI be found?

   a. PHIN VADS

   b. UMLS

   c. CTS2

   d. NCIt

4. Which terminology is derived from the UMLS and extended?

   a. PHIN VADS

   b. UMLS

   c. NCIm

   d. NCIt

5. What is used to hold multiple terminologies for use within EHRs?

   a. Terminology services

   b. Vocabulary servers

   c. EVS

   d. PHIN VADs

6. Which of the following content is *not* distributed from VSAC?

   a. CDC Race and Ethnicity

   b. eCQM value sets

   c. C-CDA

   d. eCQM draft measures

7. What national organization is USHIK developed under?

    a. CDC
    b. ONC
    c. ANSI
    d. AHRQ

8. What metadata repository houses standard information models?

    a. PHIN VADS
    b. ONC
    c. EVS
    d. USHIK

9. Which terminology is being curated by the National Library of Medicine?

    a. NCIt
    b. CTS2
    c. PHIN VADS
    d. UMLS

10. True or false? ISO 11179 is an international standard describing how metadata should be structured.

    a. True
    b. False

References

Agency for Healthcare Research and Quality (AHRQ). 2017a. AHRQ at a Glance. http://www.ahrq.gov/about/index.html.

Agency for Healthcare Research and Quality (AHRQ). 2017b. *All Payer Claims Databases.* http://www.ahrq.gov/about/index.html.

Agency for Healthcare Research (AHRQ). n.d. *United States Health Information Knowledgebase.* http://ushik.ahrq.gov/index.jsp?enableAsynchronousLoading=true.

Centers for Disease Control and Prevention (CDC). 2018a. *PHIN Vocabulary Access and Distribution System.* http://www.cdc.gov/phin/tools/PHINvads/index.html.

Centers for Disease Control and Prevention (CDC). 2018b. *PHIN Vocabulary Access and Distribution System: Arboviral Case Notification.* https://phinvads.cdc.gov/vads/ViewView.action?id=43AABFA7-CA19-E911-8174-005056ABE2F0.

Centers for Disease Control and Prevention (CDC). 2018c. *PHIN Vocabulary Access and Distribution System: Tools and Resources.* https://www.cdc.gov/phin/index.html.

Centers for Disease Control and Prevention (CDC). 2018d. *PHIN Vocabulary Access and Distribution System: Problem List Value Set.* https://phinvads.cdc.gov/vads/ViewValueSet. action?id=CD437C35-B979-41BD-BAD7-75810595764B.

Centers for Disease Control and Prevention (CDC). 2017. *Meaningful Use Community of Practice.* https://www. cdc.gov/ehrmeaningfuluse/cop.html.

Centers for Medicare and Medicaid Services (CMS). 2019. *Promoting Interoperability (PI).* https://www. cms.gov/Regulations-and-Guidance/Legislation/EHRIncentivePrograms/.

Centers for Medicare and Medicaid Services (CMS). 2018. *CMS Measures Management System Blueprint (Blueprint v 14.0).* https://www.cms.gov/Medicare/Quality-Initiatives-Patient-Assessment-Instruments/MMS/MMS-Blueprint.html.

Chen, Y., Y. Perl, J. Geller, and J. J. Cimino. 2007. Analysis of a study of the users, uses, and future agenda of the UMLS. *JAMIA* 14(2):221–231.

de Coronado, S., M. W. Haber, N. Sioutos, M. S. Tuttle, and L. W. Wright. 2004. NCI Thesaurus: Using science-based terminology to integrate cancer research results. *Studies in Health Technology and Informatics* 107(Pt 1):33–37.

de Coronado, S., L. W. Wright, G. Fragoso, M. W. Haber, E. A. Hahn-Dantona, F. W. Hartel, S. L. Quan, et al. 2009. The NCI Thesaurus quality assurance life cycle. *Journal of Biomedical Informatics* 42(3):530–539.

Ethier, J. F., O. Dameron, V. Curcin, M. M. McGilchrist, R. A. Verheij, T. N. Arvanitis, A. Taweel, et al. 2013. A unified structural/terminological interoperability framework based on LexEVS: application to TRANSFoRm. *JAMIA* 20(5):986-994.

Fung, K. W., W. T. Hole, and S. Srinivasan. 2006. Who is using the UMLS and how - insights from the UMLS user annual reports. *AMIA Annual Symposium Proceedings*:274–278.

Grannis, S., and D. Vreeman. 2010. "A Vision of the Journey Ahead: Using Public Health Notifiable Condition Mapping to Illustrate the Need to Maintain Value Sets." Paper read at AMIA Annual Symposium Proceedings.

Healthit.gov. 2019. eCQI Resource Center. https://ecqi.healthit.gov/ecqms#quicktabs-tabs_ecqm2.

Health Level Seven (HL7). 2018. FHIR R4 Terminology Module. https://www.hl7.org/fhir/terminology-module.html.

Health Level Seven (HL7). 2015. HL7 Version 3 Standard: Common Terminology Services (CTS), Release 2. http://www.hl7.org/implement/standards/product_brief.cfm?product_id=384.

ISO/IEC 11179. 2013. *Information technology — Metadata registries (MDR) -Part 3: Registry metamodel and basic attributes.* Geneva, Switzerland: International Organization for Standardization.

National Cancer Institute (NCI). 2019. NCI Thesaurus Arrhythmia (Code C2881). https://ncithesaurus-stage. nci.nih.gov/ncitbrowser/pages/home.jsf;jsessionid=C892C5A25E720D8626D24A5EBFB516DA.

National Cancer Institute (NCI). 2018a. NCI metathesaurus Ig-E-mediated allergic asthma (CUI C1827849). https://ncim.nci.nih.gov/ncimbrowser/pages/home.jsf.

National Cancer Institute (NCI). 2018b. NCI Thesaurus versus NCI Metathesaurus. https://wiki.nci.nih.gov/display/EVS/NCI+Thesaurus+versus+NCI+Metathesaurus.

National Cancer Institute (NCI). 2018c. NCI Thesaurus Downloads. https://cbiit.cancer.gov/evs-download/thesaurus-downloads.

National Cancer Institute (NCI). 2018d. LexEVS. https://wiki.nci.nih.gov/display/LexEVS/LexEVS.

National Cancer Institute (NCI). 2016. EVS Development Path. https://wiki.nci.nih.gov/display/EVS/EVS+Development+Path.

National Cancer Institute (NCI). n.d.a. Enterprise Vocabulary Services. https://evs.nci.nih.gov/.

National Cancer Institute (NCI). n.d.b. EVS Tools. https://evs.nci.nih.gov/tools.

National Cancer Institute (NCI). n.d.c. NCI Term Browser. https://nciterms.nci.nih.gov/ncitbrowser/pages/multiple_search.jsf.

National Library of Medicine (NLM). 2019. VSAC. https://vsac.nlm.nih.gov/.

National Library of Medicine (NLM). 2018a. Statistics - 2018AB Release. https://www.nlm.nih.gov/research/umls/knowledge_sources/metathesaurus/release/statistics.html.

National Library of Medicine (NLM). 2018b. UMLS Reference Manual. https://www.ncbi.nlm.nih.gov/books/NBK9684/.

National Library of Medicine (NLM). 2018c. UMLS Source Inclusion Evaluation Criteria and Background Questions. https://www.nlm.nih.gov/research/umls/knowledge_sources/metathesaurus/source_evaluation.html.

National Library of Medicine (NLM). 2017a. Unified Medical Language System. https://www.nlm.nih.gov/research/umls/about_umls.html.

National Library of Medicine (NLM). 2017b. UMLS Metathesaurus Source Vocabularies FAQs. https://www.nlm.nih.gov/research/umls/knowledge_sources/metathesaurus/source_faq.html.

National Library of Medicine (NLM). 2016. UMLS Basics Overview. https://www.nlm.nih.gov/research/umls/new_users/online_learning/OVR_001.html

National Library of Medicine (NLM). 2015. Programs and Services Fiscal Year 2015. https://www.nlm.nih.gov/ocpl/anreports/fy2015.pdf.

Object Management Group (OMG). 2015. Common Terminology Services 2 (CTS2) Version 1.2. https://www.omg.org/spec/CTS2/About-CTS2/.

17

Data Mapping of Clinical Terminologies, Classifications, and Ontologies

James R. Campbell, MD

LEARNING OBJECTIVES

- Explain the concept Learning Healthcare System and how it relates to the creation and use of data maps
- Describe data mapping principles and best practices for development of maps
- Compare developers of maps for US healthcare and their purposes for mapping
- Differentiate among the different types of data maps and their uses within US healthcare
- Identify the process for creating, testing, validating, and maintaining data maps for one or more use cases

KEY TERMS

- Cardinality
- Concept model
- Concordance
- Context
- Data map

- Discordance
- Fit for purpose
- Heuristics
- Learning Healthcare System
- Lexical mapping
- Semantic mapping
- Source
- Target
- Use case

Introduction

In 2007, the Institute of Medicine (IOM) set a vision for the evolution of the healthcare record in the digital age (IOM 2007). Named the **Learning Healthcare System**, the vision described a future state when data recorded in an electronic health record (EHR) would support clinical care and decision-making and then be reused securely and privately to improve the process of healthcare delivery and support clinical research and the needs of public health for population health management in a continuous cycle of process improvement. To achieve that vision, data in the EHR should be managed to support semantic interoperability, expecting that a data item can be transmitted to a different computer system, recognized for its meaning or semantics, and reused by that computer system without human intervention. Although the Office of the National Coordinator for Healthcare Information Technology (ONC) has specified a plan for achieving interoperability in the US, data reuse still faces major challenges due to inconsistent and incomplete terminologies, fragmented information architectures, and proprietary information management schemes (ONC 2017).

Data Maps

One common approach to the reuse of data from one computer system to another is to employ a **data map**, sometimes called a cross map. The International Standards Organization (ISO) defines a data map as the creation of links from concepts or terms in one classification, terminology, or ontology to another for some purpose of data reuse (ISO 2014). Maps are built to meet specific business requirements and serve one or more **use cases**, or activities or step-wise descriptions of events that describe the real-world employment and expected outcomes resulting from a piece of software or data map, for reuse. The links used to construct the map are driven by the use case and the editorial features of the two terminologies. For semantic (that is, the meaning of a concept) interoperation, an equivalence between the two concepts would be desirable, but this is not always achievable. Theoretically, identifying computable semantic equivalence is only reliable between two well-constructed ontologies with overlapping semantic domains. That is, they both apply to the same types of concepts, such as diagnoses, and they share a **concept model**, or "set of rules that determines the permitted sets of relationships between particular types of concept" (SNOMED International 2019). Since this is seldom true, the majority of maps have a directionality to the link, mapping from a concept usually in the **source** terminology, the terminology from which the data originates, to a concept in the **target** terminology, the terminology to which the concept links, and employing a type of link or relationship that serves the pragmatic purpose of the use case. Maps can be developed, published, and shared as simple tables identifying pairs of concepts from source and target, "triples" in Resource Description Framework (RDF) format constructed as records linking source, relationship (link type) and target, or as a knowledge resource which might consist of a network of IF-THEN rules supporting context-based mapping.

Mapping Purposes

Maps may be employed throughout the healthcare domain for a variety of purposes and to meet many different use cases. ISO suggests that there are three general goals or purposes for data mapping: converting legacy data to newer coding schemes, reusing data for purposes other than originally intended, and semantic interoperation of data where computer systems are using different coding schemes. Some examples of use cases targeting these goals are summarized in table 17.1 and discussed in Data Maps Use Cases and Innovation, which follows.

Types of Maps

Historically, data maps have been constructed employing a variety of approaches and serving many different use cases. There is no standard for classifying data maps although the ISO technical document does specify a set of quality indicators as noted in the following section. A data

TABLE 17.1. Purposes of data map creation and interoperation of clinical terms

Goal	Use Case	Example
Data conversion	Map EHR data from a legacy coding system to new standards	Convert coded diagnosis records from ICD-9-CM to ICD-10-CM: General Equivalence Mappings (GEMs)
Reuse	Choose medication records from the EHR corresponding to orders with a specific treatment reason	RXCLASS mapping of RxNorm medications to VA drug classes to identify cancer therapies
Reuse	Map SNOMED CT conditions to ICD-10-CM for reporting morbidity and mortality	NLM release of SNOMED CT–ICD-10-CM rules-based map
Interoperability	Extend and integrate terminology standards across domains for interoperation	The SOLOR project

map may be described minimally based upon the protocols involved in creating map records, the nature of the link used in the map, or by the characteristics of the terminology resources that are linked. Therefore, a descriptive map type may be assigned as a list of one of each of the following descriptive sets.

Mapping protocol:

- **Lexical mapping** identifies sets of terms to be linked by comparing words or character strings and is very dependent upon the language and dialect employed. The National Library of Medicine's (NLM) MetaMap program supports mapping of biomedical text to concepts in the Unified Medical Language System (UMLS) and is an example of a lexical approach.
- **Semantic mapping** employs the full definition of a concept in a source reference terminology, or ontology, to identify equivalent or related concepts in the target. A reference terminology is a controlled terminology employing a set of terms and relationships that capture and define the meaning of each concept. The map of SNOMED CT to ICD-10-CM discussed in the use cases later in the chapter is an example of a map that was constructed semantically.

Nature of the link relationship:

- Equivalence maps are designed to identify pairs of identical concepts between the source and target. Semantic equivalence and lexical equivalence can lead to very different types of map sets that may not serve the same use cases well.
- Hierarchical (taxonomic) maps order sets of concepts as having more or less specificity when traversing from source to target. They employ link relationships such as "less-than," "child-of," "more-specific than," or "is-a." A classification such as ICD-10-CM includes such implicit relationships, which specifies its hierarchical structure.
- Knowledge-based (rules-based) maps employ features of coding **context**, business case, and workflow assumptions which apply to the interpretation and application of map records, in order to create maps for terminologies where the standards developer imposes constraints on the use of the terminology scheme. The best example of a knowledge-based map is the map of SNOMED CT to ICD-10-CM where World Health Organization (WHO) classification guidelines and additional context from the patient demographics and problem list are employed by a set of rules to map each SNOMED CT concept recorded as a problem (condition) in the EHR.

Characteristics of the source and target:

- Maps may be typed based upon the nature of the terminologies involved in the map records, which may include classifications, controlled terminologies, reference terminologies, or ontologies. Hence a map such as the SNOMED CT to ICD-10-CM map may be described as a "reference terminology to classification."

Key Features of Map Quality and Documentation

In 2014 the ISO published technical report 12300, which is the most in-depth study of data mapping that has been published to date (ISO 2014). ISO defined a set of quality indicators by which to judge both a data mapping project and the resulting data map structures. Important features to consider relative to the conduct of the mapping project should:

- Include goals: "Every mapping project should explicitly state what the map is intended to achieve."
- Include use cases and scenarios: "[data maps]...should have articulated scenarios or use cases that originate from the business case" and explain how the map is intended to be used. The use case should clearly articulate any assumptions of context that may affect mapping deployment and implementation.
- Involve project team members possessing domain knowledge of the source and target terminologies to be mapped in the map development.
- Document all conventions and rules followed in the mapping, including guidance from the terminology developers.
- Explicitly define mapping guidelines and heuristics developed for the mapping project.
- Employ custodians and users of the terminologies in the mapping project.
- Document protocols for map development including manual and computational procedures.
- Clearly state the process for consensus management when employed.
- Specify a plan for quality assurance including validation of the map data and testing in the targeted use case environment.
- Employ a plan for maintenance and updating.

Applying Principles and Guidance for Map Development

Upon determining that there is a need for map development, the map developer must first clearly define the business case for the map. The business case addresses the reason for the project and expected risks and benefits associated with the mapping project, including the expected cost.

The next step is to translate the business case into a purpose and expected use for the map. The use case describes the utility of the map by identifying various scenarios wherein users will interact with and employ the map in their normal workflow. The use case essentially outlines the solution to the problem that the map is trying to address. Development of a clear set of goals, use cases, and scenarios is mandatory before undertaking any mapping project.

A governing principle of map development is that the project develops a map that is understandable, reproducible, and useful. These principles specify that the relationship between the mapped elements should be easily understood and not require a complicated user manual to deploy. In addition, the process that was used to develop the mapping relationship is straightforward, meaning that the same results can be derived by another human reviewer or machine process. The map must always support achievement of the goals of the use case it was designed to serve.

The decision to develop a data map requires careful consideration of the resources required for map development, validation, and maintenance. These resources include people, time, finances, and map tooling. The cost of mapping is influenced by the degree of variability between the source and target systems and how closely their editorial models align.

Detailed documentation is essential to the map development process. Heuristics are the set of procedures for mapping that are developed by the mapping team to achieve a useful and reproducible application of terminological constraints and Standards Development Organization (SDO) editorial guidelines. These protocols identify how differences between the source and target set, such as content or level of detail, are managed in the mapping process (Foley et al. 2007). Heuristics and guidelines are protocols for assuring reproducibility, ensuring usefulness, and specifying the use of tools used to develop and maintain the map.

As part of map development, a pilot phase to test and validate the established process is desirable. During this phase, two or more specialists independently produce the map in order to assess concordance, or agreement, and to ensure the map is reproducible. If there is discordance, or disagreement, in the map results, further refinement of procedures is necessary and may require additional pilot phases. This step is important in assessing that the map meets the objectives for which it was created.

Following successful completion of the pilot phase, map development can move into full content development. Testing should continue at regular intervals. Quality assurance is a critical component of this phase and includes review of any items that cannot be mapped.

Throughout the map creation process, communication and documentation are key components. Map development may result in the identification of discrepancies in documentation and content within the source or target systems. These issues should be communicated to the appropriate owner of the source or target systems. Documentation is critical for ensuring that the map is useful and understandable. Thorough documentation and adequate communication help to ensure transparency in the map and avoid assumptions regarding bias in map development.

Data Map Structures

Features of the data map structures that are important to the utility of the data map were also specified in the ISO technical document (ISO 2014). The data map:

- Should be well documented.
- Should be available in a "machine processable format" that is understandable and useful. Ideally, a software tool kit should support browsing and evaluation of the data map as well as use of the map in service of the use case.
- Should employ version control in a scheduled cycle of maintenance and publication.
- Should document the nature of the relationship and the degree of equivalence supported by the link in a map record. Since "equivalence" is infrequently achieved, this may include a set of relationship descriptors such as "exact match," "approximate," "no match," or "combination match" such as employed by the General Equivalence Mappings (GEMs) discussed below.
- Should explicitly document the direction of the map relationship. Most often this is from source to target.
- Should specify the cardinality of the map record set. **Cardinality** is the number of elements appropriate in the set of records for a map set and is always 1:1 for a map with semantic equivalence but is more often 1:* (one-to-many); *:* (many-to-many); or *:1 (many-to-one).
- Must clearly define the data map structures, distribution formats, and licensing requirements.

Map Tooling

An important consideration in map project planning is the map tooling software that will be utilized to create, maintain, validate, and sometimes deploy the map. Map tooling can be a simple spreadsheet or a sophisticated software application. Open source mapping tools are available to the public to utilize in mapping projects. An example of an open source mapping tool useful for browsing and validation studies is the Interactive Map-Assisted Generation of ICD codes (I-MAGIC) Mapping Tool, developed by the NLM. This tool allows users to enter a set of diagnoses or conditions as well as facts about the patient and the episode of care, and provides mapping results from SNOMED CT to ICD-10-CM. The tool is useful to familiarize the user with the map function and supports assessment of fitness for purpose.

The Regenstrief Institute provides a mapping tool for browsing and mapping from local code sets to Logical Observation Identifiers Names and Codes (LOINC). This tool, which is called the Regenstrief LOINC Mapping Assistant (RELMA), is a Windows program for searching the LOINC database and helping to map local laboratory data dictionaries to LOINC codes. It is available free from the LOINC website along with the LOINC release files (see [LOINC 2018] in the resources section at the end of the chapter).

Other organizations, such as EHR vendors, terminology developers, and distributors often develop their own mapping tools. Maps developed by some companies are proprietary mapping tools, meaning these tools are owned by the entity that created them and may require licensing. As with many other products, users must assess functionality and features of mapping tools relative to their data mapping requirements and goals.

Validation for Mapping Projects

After the map is developed, the final step before deployment should be an independent validation process. In order to avoid bias and confirm reproducibility, validation should be performed by an entity not involved in the map development process or with special interest in the use of the map. The entity should not include personnel involved in the map development or with a financial or political interest in the map's development or use. Map validation is necessary to ensure credibility that a data map is useful, reproducible, and achieves its goals. Those validating the map must have experience in both the source and target systems and confirmed experience in map development and quality control. The map validation process requires addressing the following questions:

- Is the map easy to understand? Does it solve the problem outlined in the use case requirements?
- Can the results be reproduced? Do independent users employing the map achieve a high rate of concordance in mapping identical source code sets?
- Is it evident that the map supports the use case and can be useful in the scenario proposed?

The use case should be compared to the map results to ensure the map is consistent (Maimone 2011). General validation reviews should be completed. These reviews should optimally include the following features:

- Use of authoritative sources from standards development organizations as reference
- Development of a statistically appropriate sample of the map records to validate the map results in the environment in which the maps are going to be deployed
- Review and confirmation of compliance with map heuristics and guidelines
- Use of a blinded comparison by independent mapping specialists in order to assess statistical concordance
- Evaluation of the results, accounting for any discordance and employing feedback for map quality improvement

- Execution of an "in use" validation study in the scenario proposed by the project comparing map target assignment to a reference "gold standard" from the standards development organizations

The map can be implemented following satisfactory testing by these processes.

Maintenance of Maps

If classifications and terminologies are being mapped, they typically are updated at different times of the year, adding to the challenge for maintaining a current map. Data maps require maintenance to remain current. Maintenance is needed when any update is made to either the source or target terminology systems including any new, revised, or retired data elements in either terminological resource. Map maintenance must also occur if there are changes in the data reporting requirements, standards, or databases. These updates may include revised guidelines that must be communicated to those in the organization that use systems or reports derived from the maps. Maps that are not properly maintained are likely to introduce errors.

In most cases involving data maps, a designated time for sunsetting the map is appropriate when it is no longer needed. This will always be important in the case of using a map for legacy data conversion. Once the migration has been accomplished, there is no longer a need to maintain the map. Any maps used for migration should be properly archived to provide for audit should any question arise in the future concerning the migration project.

Exploring the Management and Use of Data Maps

A use for data maps can arise in any field of human endeavor employing pencil and paper or a computer. Information management in healthcare is no exception. The US information architecture of the Learning Healthcare System must deal with many valid requirements for reuse of data originating within the EHR or other healthcare information systems. Following are some exemplars of information reuse in US healthcare systems and how organizations have employed data maps to manage those challenges.

Data Reuse within the EHR

Clinical information is documented as part of patient care during a healthcare encounter primarily to support clinical decision-making and also to record information necessary for reimbursement. Middleware vendors of terminology services employed by EHR vendors supply data maps that link from clinical term sets used in the clinical user interface to ICD-10-CM classification and SNOMED CT reference terminology for reporting encounter diagnoses and supporting clinical decision-making. Maps from laboratory data dictionaries to LOINC and locally coded procedure data to CPT-4 are common data map use cases for compliance with interoperability reporting requirements specified by ONC.

Interoperation—Health Information Exchange

Sharing of clinical information between two EHRs in support of a lifetime electronic patient record requires exchanging standard code sets specified by ONC. These consist of RxNorm for medications, LOINC for lab results and clinical observations, SNOMED CT for problem lists, and ICD-10-CM and ICD-10-PCS for encounter diagnoses and procedures. EHR site managers create data maps from internal data dictionaries employing local terms and codes to the relevant terminology standards in order to populate HL7 Clinical Document Architecture (CDA) record summaries which support healthcare quality and safety for the patient who is in the process of transition of care. Data maps usually include lab master to LOINC, problem list to SNOMED CT, and medications to RxNorm and National Drug Code (NDC) codes.

Interoperation—Value Set Authority Center (NLM)

In order to support uniformity of data gathered from patient interviews, it is necessary to have a standard question and standard set of answers. The NLM maintains the Value Set Authority Center (VSAC 2019) as a clearinghouse for value sets, which are code lists corresponding to standard "answer lists." For meaningful use stage 2 compliance, ONC identified a core set of social history data that all EHRs are required to maintain for their patients. One such data element is: "What is the patient tobacco smoking status?" This was specified as LOINC 72166-2 for storage

TABLE 17.2. VSAC value set map for smoking status

Data Element	Value Set	Code System	Code	Descriptor
LOINC:72166-2	Tobacco smoking status	SNOMED CT	266919005	Never smoked tobacco
LOINC:72166-2	Tobacco smoking status	SNOMED CT	266927001	Tobacco smoking consumption unknown
LOINC:72166-2	Tobacco smoking status	SNOMED CT	428041000124106	Occasional tobacco smoker
LOINC:72166-2	Tobacco smoking status	SNOMED CT	428061000124105	Light tobacco smoker
LOINC:72166-2	Tobacco smoking status	SNOMED CT	428071000124103	Heavy tobacco smoker
LOINC:72166-2	Tobacco smoking status	SNOMED CT	449868002	Smokes tobacco daily
LOINC:72166-2	Tobacco smoking status	SNOMED CT	77176002	Smoker
LOINC:72166-2	Tobacco smoking status	SNOMED CT	8517006	Ex-smoker

and representation in the EHR. NLM VSAC publishes the value set of SNOMED CT "answers" for that question as shown in table 17.2. VSAC maintains these data maps linking standard data elements specified by HL7, LOINC, and others to the approved lists of values in ONC standard code sets, supporting interoperability of EHR data.

Data Reuse—Public Health Reporting

The Centers for Disease Control and Prevention (CDC) maintains a network for clinical enterprises to submit statistics for reportable diseases such as Zika virus and syndromic surveillance for conditions such as "flu-like illnesses." The Public Health Information Network Vocabulary Access and Distribution System (PHIN VADS) maintained by CDC publishes numerous data maps, which are also called value sets, identifying ICD-10-CM, ICD-10-PCS, LOINC, and SNOMED CT code sets which are to be employed in these reporting use cases. These data maps are one-to-many links from CDC reportable conditions to codes occurring in laboratory and clinical systems that are expected to trigger a report to the CDC.

Data Reuse—Supporting Healthcare Research

A number of healthcare research data networks have emerged in the US in recent years, including the Patient-Centered Outcomes Research Institute network (PCORI) and the Observational Health Data Sciences and Informatics (OHDSI). (See [PCORI 2018] and [OHDSI 2018] in the resource list at the end of the chapter.) These networks support free communication of research data queries between their participating datamarts, allowing clinical researchers to query EHR, billing, claims, and other data sets for millions of patients. An example of a network research query recently circulated was: "How many children age 12 and under had lead levels drawn in the past year? How many were at toxic levels?" In constructing the programs that site managers use to retrieve the data from these sources, data maps are employed to translate the information from the information models employed by the feeder systems to interoperable coding standards specified by ONC. These coding standards are a critical common language used by researchers in constructing their queries.

Legacy Data Conversion—Terminology Version Control

Terminologies and classifications evolve over time, creating requirements for updating data coding between versions. On October 1, 2015, US healthcare systems transitioned from ICD-9-CM to ICD-10-CM for encounter diagnosis reporting. In order to support the necessary changes to healthcare software and coding tables, the Centers for Medicare and Medicaid Services (CMS) developed General Equivalence Maps (GEMs) to support those modifications (CMS 2018).

These maps will be discussed in a use case that follows. Another code transition is anticipated after WHO releases ICD-11.

Data Reuse Supported by Standards Development Organizations

Standards development organizations (SDOs) frequently develop data maps to support interoperation use cases faced by their community of users. The International Health Terminology Standards Development Organisation (IHTSDO), now called SNOMED International, provides a mapping service that is responsible for linking SNOMED CT to other important classifications, including ICD-10 (not ICD-10-CM) and ICD-O-3. Although not an SDO, the NLM has developed and maintains maps including SNOMED CT to ICD-10-CM, LOINC to CPT-4, and SNOMED CT to ICD-9-CM. The Unified Medical Language System (UMLS) Metathesaurus was developed as a semantically based concept equivalence map meant to link identical concepts in many classifications, code sets, and reference terminologies.

When Is a Data Map Fit for Purpose?

For use in scenarios that affect patient care, it is critical for data maps to be understandable, reproducible, and useful. These three principles underlie quality data map development. Data integrity problems originating in poorly designed maps may cause harm if applied without validation and testing. The coding specialist should carefully evaluate maps and a decision should be made whether the map is **fit for purpose**. From the discussion above, it should be understandable that determining a data map to be fit for purpose requires minimally that:

- The goals of the proposed use for the map align reasonably with the goals set for the mapping project that developed it.
- The use case scenarios align with the intended real-world deployment scenario for the map data set.
- There is software or tools available to support assessment of the map and to employ the data map in real-world scenarios. The tools must employ the data map in a manner consistent with the design of the map link, the direction, and cardinality.
- The map and map data structures are well documented and understandable in terms of its intended use.
- The map has been validated to reproducibly meet use case requirements and accomplish stated goals.
- Map maintenance is current and the maintenance cycle is appropriate to the publication schedule of the source and target terminologies.

Data Map Use Cases and Innovation

There are a number of use cases for data maps, some of which are described below. Investigation into an innovative method of developing terminology extensions for interoperable information exchange is also explained.

Use Case One: Legacy Diagnosis Code Conversion Using General Equivalence Mappings (GEMs)

Table 17.3 details an ICD-9-CM to ICD-10-CM GEMs use case.

When CMS mandated US conversion from ICD-9-CM (Volumes 1 and 2) to ICD-10-CM on October 1, 2015, the National Center for Health Statistics (NCHS) created the GEMs to support conversion of legacy ICD-9-CM data so that healthcare systems could analyze longitudinal trends in patterns of care. CMS published bidirectional maps supporting retrospective use cases as well as GEMs for ICD-10-PCS. A sample of map records for ICD-10-CM is included in table 17.4. CMS published yearly updates for three years ending in 2018 (CMS 2018) anticipating that legacy conversion requirements would be completed.

TABLE 17.3. ICD-9-CM (ICD-9-CM volumes 1 and 2) to ICD-10-CM General Equivalence Mappings (GEMs) use case

Goal	Conversion of ICD-9 to ICD-10 data for longitudinal analysis
Use case/Scenario	A coding specialist must report trends in the occurrence of infectious disease incidence in the hospital from 2008 to 2018. GEMs are used to convert legacy diagnosis reports from 2008 through 2015 to ICD-10-CM and then compute yearly incidence by ICD-10-CM code.
Map type	Classification to classification
Source	ICD-9-CM volumes 1 and 2
Target	ICD-10-CM
Relationship/Link	Multifactorial – approximate, no map, combination, scenario, choice list
Direction	Bidirectional, published as two sets of links
Cardinality	One-to-many
Map data structures	Tabular with source, target, and relationship codes
Documentation	https://www.cms.gov/Medicare/Coding/ICD10/2017-ICD-10-CM-and-GEMs.html
Guidelines and heuristics	https://www.cms.gov/Medicare/Coding/ICD10/2017-ICD-10-CM-and-GEMs.html
Maintenance plan	Yearly updates

TABLE 17.4. Examples of General Equivalence Maps (GEMs)

Source	Target	GEM Equivalence	
ICD-9-CM	**ICD-10-CM**	Relationship	Meaning
042	B20	00000	Exact match
59972	R311	10000	Approximate match
59972	R3121	10000	Approximate match
59972	R3129	10000	Approximate match
ICD-10-CM	**ICD-9-CM**		
Z3A00	NoDx	11000	No match
Z3A01	NoDx	11000	No match
T422X1A	9662	10111	Combination map
T422X1A	E8558	10112	Combination map
T422X1A	9660	10121	Combination map
T422X1A	E8558	10122	Combination map

Source: CMS 2018.

Use Case Two: Reuse of RxNorm Coded Data for Clinical Research Using RXCLASS Data Map

Table 17.5 details a Veterans Administration (VA) National Drug File - Reference Terminology (NDF-RT) to RxNorm map use case.

The RXCLASS website and API supported by the NLM support data maps from a set of medication classifications including the a) VA drug classifications, b) Anatomic and Therapeutic Classification (WHO 2018), c) Established Pharmacologic Classes from Daily Med, and d) the FDA Structured Product Labelling to RxNorm codes of term type ingredient. RxNorm codes are sometimes called RXCUIs. This map is supplemented by the additional data maps between different RxNorm term types found on the RXNAV website. RxNorm term types are abbreviated as TTY in the RxNorm semantic network. NLM supports these mappings with each monthly update of RxNorm. The purpose of the mappings is to support the deployment and use of RxNorm codes (RXCUIs) in applications supporting US healthcare. The RXCLASS website provides a browser that allows the user to explore each of the data maps (NLM 2018a). The maps are also accessible from NLM using the RXCLASS API and retrievable by web service call. The API is useful for retrieving data maps in machine-readable form.

TABLE 17.5. VA medication classes (NDF-RT) to RxNorm

Goal	Support access to subsets of medication events coded with RXCUI by classification of therapeutic intent
Use case/Scenario	A research data warehouse manager downloads the map of VA drug classifications to RxNorm and installs the classification in the data warehouse browser in order to provide support for the researcher who wants to retrieve medication orders coded in RxNorm indexed by therapeutic class such as "Antineoplastics."
Map type	Terminology to classification
Source	VA drug classification code
Target	RxNorm ingredients (TTY = IN)
Relationship/Link	has_RXCUI
Direction	Source to target
Cardinality	One-to-many (1:*)
Map data structures	RESTful or SOAP web services as structured text or XML
Documentation	https://rxnav.nlm.nih.gov/RxClassIntro.html https://rxnav.nlm.nih.gov/RxClassAPIs.html#
Guidelines and heuristics	Not documented
Maintenance plan	Monthly updates available by RXCLASS API

RxNorm term types IN, MIN, and PIN listed in table 17.6 are types of medicinal ingredients found in drug products and are all summarized on the RXNAV website for a particular drug ingredient. Type BN contains brand names of products assigned by drug manufacturers. Types SCDC and SBDC are generic and branded drug components that are not orderable because they do not include a formulation. Types SCD, GPCK, SBD, and BPCK are manufactured drug products of a specific formulation, available for use in the US pharmacopoeia, and orderable drugs that are valid for use in an inpatient medication order or an outpatient prescription. Type DFG is a drug formulation group. SCDG and SBDG are generic and branded drug groups, respectively.

The VA drug classification, for example, is used as a therapeutic classification browser in the RXCLASS map for identifying a set of medications used for a specific purpose. Table 17.7 lists samples of the data maps from RXCLASS and RXNAV websites for types of anticancer drugs (antineoplastics) that are mapped from the VA classification. The map links the VA drug classification therapeutic concept to the set of medication ingredients that are useful for that objective. Links from the RXCLASS ingredient directly to the RXNAV map allow browsing of the various term types of medications for that ingredient including the orderable drug term types (SCD, SBD, GPCK, BPCK) that can be used to issue electronic orders in the EHR.

TABLE 17.6. RxNorm term types

TTY	Term Type
IN	Ingredient (generic)
MIN	Multiple ingredients
PIN	Precise ingredient (salt or specific molecular formula)
BN	Brand name
SCDC	Semantic clinical drug component
SBDC	Semantic branded drug component
SCD	Semantic clinical drug (orderable)
GPCK	Generic drug pack (orderable)
SBD	Semantic branded drug (orderable)
BPCK	Branded drug pack (orderable)
SCDG	Semantic clinical drug group
DFG	Drug formulation group
SBDG	Semantic branded drug group

Source: NLM 2018b.

TABLE 17.7. RXCLASS-RXNAV medication classification map

Source	RXCLASS Target		RXNAV Target	
VA Drug Class	TTY	RXCUI	TTY	RXCUI
AN000 Antineoplastic	IN	301739 Abarelix	SCD	402100 Abarelix 50mg/ml injectable
AN000 Antineoplastic	IN	1946825 Ademaciclib	SCD	1946838 Ademaciclib 100mg oral tablet
AN000 Antineoplastic	IN	1946825 Ademaciclib	SCD	1946842 Ademaciclib 150mg oral tablet
AN000 Antineoplastic	IN	1946825 Ademaciclib	SCD	1946846 Ademaciclib 200mg oral tablet
AN000 Antineoplastic	IN	1946825 Ademaciclib	SCD	1946830 Ademaciclib 50mg oral tablet

Source: NLM 2018a; NLM 2018b.

Use Case Three: Reuse of SNOMED CT Problem List as ICD-10-CM Billing Codes

Table 17.8 details a SNOMED CT problem list to ICD-10-CM map use case.

SNOMED CT is a reference terminology designed to record clinical data with a high degree of precision and to support retrieval and clinical decision support. The International Classification

TABLE 17.8. SNOMED CT conditions (clinical findings, events, and situations) to ICD-10-CM

Goal	Convert SNOMED CT problem list to ICD-10-CM
Use case/Scenario	A coding specialist wishes to translate SNOMED CT problem records reported by the clinician to ICD-10-CM codes that may be used as candidate billing codes.
Map type	Knowledge-based map; Reference terminology to Classification
Source	SNOMED CT Clinical findings, Events and Situations with explicit context
Target	ICD-10-CM
Relationship/Link	IF-THEN rule sets
Direction	SNOMED CT to ICD-10-CM
Cardinality	One-to-many (1:*)
Map data structures	Reference set of ordered rules linking source to target(s)
Documentation	https://download.nlm.nih.gov/mlb/utsauth/ICD10CM/doc_Icd10cmMapTechnicalSpecifications_Current-en-US_US1000124_20180301.pdf
Guidelines and heuristics	https://download.nlm.nih.gov/mlb/utsauth/ICD10CM/doc_Icd10cmMapTechnicalSpecifications_Current-en-US_US1000124_20180301.pdf
Maintenance plan	Yearly updates

of Diseases published by the WHO is designed to provide statistical reporting of morbidity and mortality and is employed across the world serving use cases of reimbursement, resource planning, and population health. Clinical care data recorded in the US EHR must first support clinical decision-making, but the NCHS architecture for information management expects that data to be reused for other purposes best served by ICD-10-CM. SNOMED CT is mandated by ONC for encoding of clinical problem lists and the use case supported by this data map repurposes that problem list data for use in encounter diagnosis reporting.

Recognizing that ICD-10-CM employs many inclusion and exclusion rules, the data map employs a rule-based structure which assumes access to basic information a) about the patient—age and gender; b) about the episode of care; and c) about comorbidities identified as other conditions in the patient problem list. For each source concept, the map has one group of ordered map rules for each target code to be produced. Since the map has cardinality of one-to-many, multiple groups of map rules support the need for the number of ICD-10-CM target codes required for proper classification of some events.

In the example shown in table 17.9 for mapping of the SNOMED CT concept 10050004|Contusion of chest(disorder)|, guidelines call for assignment of two ICD-10-CM codes for proper classification. The mapGroup (GRP) identifies the set of rules for each target code and the mapPriority (PRTY) specifies the sequence in which the rules are to be evaluated. The first rule testing true when evaluated by order of mapPriority assigns the target code linked to that rule. So if the patient problem list includes 80907003|Contusion of scapular region|, but

TABLE 17.9. Sample map records from SNOMED CT to ICD-10-CM map

SOURCE	G R P	P R T Y	RULE	TARGET
10050004|Contusion of chest|	1	1	IFA 428016006 | Contusion of rib |	S20.20X?|Contusion of thorax, unspecified|
10050004|Contusion of chest|	1	2	IFA 448321000124104 | Sternal fracture with retrosternal contusion |	S22.20X?|Unspecified fracture of sternum|
10050004|Contusion of chest|	1	3	IFA 80907003 | Contusion of scapular region |	S40.019?|Contusion of unspecified shoulder|
10050004|Contusion of chest|	1	4	OTHERWISE TRUE	S20.019?|Contusion of unspecified front wall of thorax|
10050004|Contusion of chest|	2	1	IFA 448321000124104 | Sternal fracture with retrosternal contusion |	S20.2019?|Contusion of unspecified front wall of thorax|
10050004|Contusion of chest|	2	2	OTHERWISE TRUE	CANNOT BE CLASSIFIED AS SPECIFIED

Source: NLM 2018c.

no other code in the rule list, the first code assigned by the rule scheme for mapGroup one will be S40.019?|Contusion of unspecified shoulder|. If a problem of sternal fracture is on the problem list as comorbidity, the second group rule will test true and assign the second ICD-10-CM code to the classification. Otherwise, there is insufficient information to fully classify the source concept and assign a second code.

The NLM publishes and updates the map annually and supports a tool for browsing called I-MAGIC (I-MAGIC 2018), which employs the map to produce a candidate ICD-10-CM code list once the user has entered birth date and gender and recorded the SNOMED CT problem list. Reports from NLM in 2017 indicated that there were more than 2,300 licensed users of the data map across the US and that the Indian Health Service was employing the map in their EHR application (Fung 2017).

Use Case Four: Interoperation of Clinical Terms; the SOLOR Project

Table 17.10 details an innovative method of developing a terminology-extensions use case.

SOLOR stands for System Of Logical Representation and employs only terminology standards identified by ONC as central aspects of the interoperability road map. The VA initiated the project to promote semantic interoperability of EHR data within the VA and Department of Defense.

TABLE 17.10. Developing an interoperation framework for the EHR: SOLOR

Goal	Semantic interoperation of EHR clinical data
Use case/Scenario	An EHR terminology manager uses the SOLOR tool kit to semantically model and define concepts that cannot be accurately represented with existing SNOMED CT, LOINC, or RxNorm concept codes. This supports interoperation of EHR data for clinical, research, and public health purposes.
Map type	Not a data map; a framework and tools for interoperable semantic modelling of EHR concepts
Source	SNOMED CT, LOINC, RxNorm
Target	N/A; SOLOR is **NOT** a data map
Relationship/Link	Semantic equivalence (EQUALS) and subsumption (IS_A) will be supported for queries across cooperating EHRs
Direction	N/A
Cardinality	N/A
Map data structures	SOLOR tools for semantic modelling of EHR concepts
Documentation	http://solor.io
Guidelines and heuristics	Not documented
Maintenance plan	Not developed

Planning is predicated on the observations that data maps always involve loss of meaning when reusing clinical data and that the only opportunity for complete semantic interoperability occurs between ontologies with a well-defined and shared concept model. Of ONC data standards, only SNOMED CT supports a concept model that supports logical definition of concepts. The SOLOR project is developing tools that will allow modelling and definition of local enterprise terminology requirements using just the SOLOR standards set and the SNOMED CT concept model. The expectation is that these terminology extensions can be exchanged and reused with full semantic interoperation. The SOLOR project team is cooperating with the Clinical Information Modeling Initiative to develop the tools and protocols necessary for interoperable information exchange (HL7 2018).

CHECK YOUR UNDERSTANDING

1. True or false? The goal of data mapping is always to identify items that are semantically equivalent within two terminologies.

   a. True
   b. False

2. The General Equivalence Mappings use terms such as "no match," "exact match," and "approximate match" to specify which of the following:

    a. Source
    b. Target
    c. Degree of equivalence
    d. Use case

3. Which is the target system for a data map from SNOMED CT to ICD-10-CM?

    a. SNOMED CT
    b. ICD-10-CM
    c. None of the above
    d. All of the above

4. A map that fulfills the use case requirements, is well documented, and generates valid and reproducible results may be considered to be:

    a. Fit for purpose
    b. Semantically interoperable
    c. Concordant
    d. None of the above

5. A data map from SNOMED CT conditions to ICD-10-CM classification links a single source concept to one, two, or three target records (1:*). This characteristic of the data map is called:

    a. Map purpose
    b. Semantic equivalence
    c. Cardinality
    d. Multiplicity

REVIEW

1. The goals and purpose of the map should be found in the:

    a. Map tooling
    b. Source
    c. Target
    d. Use case

2. The guideline rules created by and for map developers are known as:

    a. Heuristics
    b. Requirements

c. Business case

d. Mapping advice

3. To ensure the map is consistent, map results should be compared to and consistent with the:

a. Lexicon

b. Heuristics

c. Use case

d. Target

4. The map life cycle includes:

a. Use case specification

b. Development

c. Maintenance

d. All of the above

5. Semantic interoperation of data means that:

a. The data can be transmitted from computer A to computer B

b. Computer B recognizes the meaning of the data

c. Computer B can employ the data in a meaningful way

d. All of the above

6. True or false? A single definition for data mapping exists.

a. True

b. False

7. Vendor A provides data maps to developer B of an EHR, which maps the procedure data dictionary of system B to CPT-4 codes. The billing module uses the CPT-4 codes for documentation and reporting of professional services. This is an exemplar use case of a map supporting:

a. Legacy data recoding

b. Data reuse

c. Semantic interoperation

d. Heuristics

8. True or false? Data maps may only involve classifications and terminologies as source and target.

a. True

b. False

9. A map from SNOMED CT to ICD-10-CM is an example of mapping from:

    a. Classification to terminology

    b. Terminology to classification

    c. Classification to classification

    d. Terminology to terminology

10. According to ISO's principles of mapping technical report, it is important that specialists with domain knowledge of the source and target terminologies be involved in the data mapping life cycle during:

    a. Use case development

    b. Map development

    c. Map maintenance

    d. None of the above

References

Centers for Medicare and Medicaid Services (CMS). 2018. ICD-10 PCS and GEMs. https://www.cms.gov/Medicare/Coding/ICD10/2018-ICD-10-PCS-and-GEMs.html.

Foley, M., C. Hall, K. Perron, and R. D'Andrea. 2007. Translation please: Mapping translates clinical data between the many languages that document it. *Journal of AHIMA* 78(2):34–38.

Fung, K.W. 2017. "SNOMED CT to ICD-10-CM map and the I-MAGIC tool." AMIA 2017 NLM booth presentation. https://lhncbc.nlm.nih.gov/sites/default/files/AMIA_SNOMED_CT_map_and_I-MAGIC_tool.pdf.

Health Level Seven International (HL7). 2018. Clinical Information Modeling Initiative. http://www.hl7.org/Special/Committees/cimi/index.cfm.

Institute of Medicine (IOM). 2007. *The Learning Healthcare System: Workshop Summary.* Washington, DC: National Academies Press. http://www.ncbi.nlm.nih.gov/books/NBK53494/.

Interactive Map-Assisted Generation of ICD Codes (I-MAGIC), National Library of Medicine. 2018. https://imagic.nlm.nih.gov/imagic/code/map.

International Standards Organization (ISO). 2014. ISO/TR 12300:2014 Health Informatics – Principles of Mapping between Terminological Systems. https://www.iso.org/standard/51344.html.

Maimone, C. 2011. Data mapping best practices. *Journal of AHIMA* 82(4):46–52.

National Library of Medicine (NLM). 2018a. RXCLASS. https://mor.nlm.nih.gov/RxClass/.

National Library of Medicine (NLM). 2018b. RxNav. https://mor.nlm.nih.gov/RxNav/.

National Library of Medicine (NLM). 2018c. SNOMED CT United States Edition. https://www.nlm.nih.gov/healthit/snomedct/us_edition.html.

Office of the National Coordinator for Health Information Technology (ONC). 2017. Connecting Healthcare for the Nation: A Shared Nationwide Interoperability Roadmap. https://www.healthit.gov/sites/default/files/hie-interoperability/nationwide-interoperability-roadmap-final-version-1.0.pdf.

SNOMED International. 2019. SNOMED CT Editorial Guide. https://confluence.ihtsdotools.org/display/DOCEG/SNOMED+CT+Editorial+Guide.

Value Set Authority Center (VSAC). 2019. https://vsac.nlm.nih.gov.

World Health Organization (WHO). 2018. The Anatomical Therapeutic Chemical Classification System with Defined Daily Doses. http://www.who.int/classifications/atcddd/en/?

Resources

Brewin, B. 2012. VA Launches a Data Mapping Project. http://www.nextgov.com/health/2012/05/va-launches-healthcare-data-mapping-project/55727.

Centers for Disease Control (CDC). 2018. Public Health Information Network Vocabulary Access and Distribution System (PHIN VADS). https://phinvads.cdc.gov/vads/SearchVocab.action.

Fung, K.W. 2012. How the SNOMED CT to ICD-10 Map Facilitated the Map to a National Extension of ICD-10. http://www.ihtsdo.org/fileadmin/user_upload/doc/slides/Ihtsdo_Showcase2012_MappingNationalExtensionICD10.pdf.

Fung, K.W. and J. Xu. 2012. Synergism between the mapping projects from SNOMED CT to ICD-10 and ICD-10-CM. *AMIA Annual Symposium Proceedings* 2012:218–227. http://www.ncbi.nlm.nih.gov/pmc/articles/PMC3540534/.

Fung, K., R. Schichilone, and K. Giannangelo. 2010. Benefits and use cases of a SNOMED CT to ICD-10 map. *AMIA Annual Symposium Proceedings* 2010:1049.

Giannangelo, K. and J. Millar. 2012. Mapping SNOMED CT to ICD-10. *Studies in Health Technology and Informatics* 180:83–87.

LOINC. 2018. https://loinc.org/.

McBride, S. et al. 2006. Data mapping. *Journal of AHIMA* 77(2): 44–48.

National Library of Medicine. n.d. UMLS Metathesaurus – Mapping Projects. https://www.nlm.nih.gov/research/umls/knowledge_sources/metathesaurus/mapping_projects/index.html.

Observational Health Data Sciences and Informatics (OHDSI). 2018. http://www.ohdsi.org.

Patient-Centered Outcomes Research Institute (PCORI). 2018. https://www.pcori.org/.

Regenstrief Institute. Regenstrief LOINC Mapping Assistant (RELMA). http://loinc.org.

Ross-Davis, S. 2012. Preparing for ICD-10-CM/PCS: One payer's experience with general equivalence mappings (GEMs). *Perspectives in Health Information Management.* http://perspectives.ahima.org/preparing-for-icd-10-cmpcs-one- payers-experience-with-general-equivalence-mappings-gems/#.UjHc9x8o6ig.

SNOMED International. 2019. Mapping Information. https://www.snomed.org/snomed-ct/sct-worldwide.

Wilson, P. 2007. What mapping and modeling means to the HIM professional. *Perspectives in Health Information Management* 4:2. http://library.ahima.org/xpedio/groups/public/documents/ahima/bok1_033815.pdf.

18

Use of Terminologies, Classifications, and Value Sets

Jay Lyle, PhD

LEARNING OBJECTIVES

- Review the use of terminologies and classifications in electronic health record systems
- Examine the use of classifications and value sets in administrative applications
- Explain how terminologies, classifications, and value sets work together in an electronic healthcare environment
- Identify implementation issues surrounding the use of terminologies, classifications, and value sets in healthcare
- Explain the terminology connection to semantic interoperability

KEY TERMS

- Binding strength
- Classification
- Code
- Code system
- Concept identifier
- Controlled terminology
- Description logics (DL)
- Extensional

- Intensional
- Model binding
- Model impedance
- Monohierarchy
- Nonsemantic identifier
- Ontology
- Polyhierarchy
- Term
- Terminologies
- Terminology
- Terminology binding
- Unified Code for Units of Measure (UCUM)
- Values
- Value binding
- Value set
- Value set definition
- Value set expansion

Introduction

When one fills out a form, whether on paper or on a computer screen, it is easy to infer what kinds of values should be put in the form fields. A "first name" field requires a string of letters; "age" or "temperature" a number; "birth date" a date. A more difficult challenge for the form designer arises when the form requires a value like race or gender. In these cases, the designer may use check boxes, or a drop-down selection tool for a computer form. These tools record concepts, and to record concepts in a predictable, standardized way, a controlled terminology must be implemented.

This chapter builds on the previous chapters that described the use of terminologies, classifications, and code sets in electronic health record (EHR) and administrative systems. The focus is on explaining the connection the systems have to semantic interoperability, understanding how they work together, and identifying implementation issues surrounding their use.

Several terms that have clear meanings in general conversation but that become problematic in more detailed investigations, must be clarified in this chapter. First is the distinction between "terminology" and "terminologies." **Terminology** is the domain of terms, codes, and their design and use. **Terminologies**, also known as code systems, are specific knowledge assets in a domain. The distinction between classifications and other kinds of terminologies is important enough that they are usually referred to as "terminologies and classifications."

The contents of terminologies are often referred to as concepts. However, what the terminology actually contains is codes and terms that represent the concepts. **Term** refers to the linguistic representations of a concept, such as Acute myocardial infarction. **Code** refers specifically to the coded (usually nonsemantic) identifier, such as I21, not the term or concept referenced by the code. Codes are also known, in concept-oriented terminologies, as **concept identifiers**. The abstract idea of "concept" is considered an axiom; codes and terms refer to them, but they don't have to define the idea.

Given these distinctions, **values** refer to the contents of terminologies when terms are not distinguished from codes, or when referring to both; for example, a requirement to draw "values" from LOINC.

Types of Terminologies and Classifications

A terminology is the set of terms specific to a domain. It may be a very small, informal, locally defined set, such as the set of gender concept identifiers embedded in a registration form and used only by the registration application, or it may be an extremely complex assembly of millions of concept identifiers, terms, and relationships, curated by rigorous governance processes and published to a global audience, such as SNOMED CT. The terms "lexicon" and "vocabulary" are often used to convey the more general meaning, synonymous with nomenclature. The term **controlled terminology** is often used to distinguish a specific, managed knowledge asset from these more general meanings.

A key kind of terminology is the **classification**, which uses a monohierarchical system to arrange or organize like or related entities. Classifications have many uses such as providing data that are used in monitoring public health and risks or determining the correct payment for healthcare services. These uses require that each value inhabit a single category.

Another important kind of terminology is the **ontology**. An ontology, like a classification, assigns hierarchical relationships, but it can assign other relationships as well, including additional hierarchical relationships. These additional relationships mean that an ontology cannot be used as a classification without taking this into account and designing processes for selecting unique hierarchical relationships.

Or, graphically, a terminology may simply list terms, as seen in figure 18.1.

FIGURE 18.1. Terminology

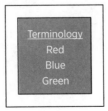

Source: © AHIMA.

A concept-oriented terminology is the specification of a set of words or phrases intended to represent the concepts required for a particular use. It is based on the idea that terms may be ambiguous, so it uses concept identifiers (codes) with at least one but potentially many associated terms. It does not, therefore, depend on terms, which may not be appropriate for certain contexts (see figure 18.2).

FIGURE 18.2. Concept-oriented terminology

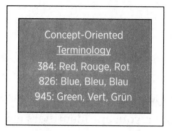

Source: © AHIMA.

FIGURE 18.3. Classification

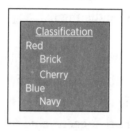

Source: © AHIMA.

FIGURE 18.4. Ontology

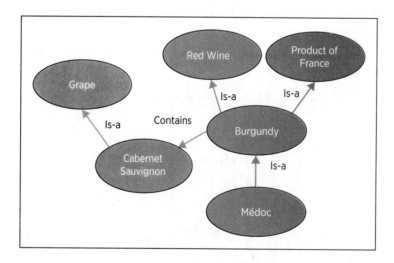

Source: © AHIMA.

A taxonomy or classification asserts hierarchical relationships, as seen in figure 18.3.

Lastly, an ontology may assert a variety of kinds of relationships, including multiple hierarchies, as seen in figure 18.4.

Several terminologies and classifications are common in health information technology. They can be used for a variety of conceptual domains and for a variety of uses. Medication substances, for instance, can be identified in a variety of ways. Orders and prescriptions may specify drugs, strengths, and forms, but not brands; dispensing and administration records will record specific products; FDA approval processes need specific chemical formulations; and allergy records may document broad classes of substances. Each of these use cases has an appropriate drug terminology. Table 18.1 summarizes some of the most common terminologies and classifications used in health records.

TABLE 18.1. Common terminologies and classification systems used in health records

Terminology/ Classification	Domain	Kind	Context
SNOMED CT	Disorders, Procedures, Substances, Observations, etc.	Terminology/Ontology	Clinical record
ICD-10-CM	Disorders	Classification	Administrative classification
ICD-10-PCS	Procedures	Classification	Administrative classification
LOINC	Observations	Terminology/Ontology	Clinical record
CPT	Procedures	Terminology	Ordering
RxNorm	Medications	Terminology/Ontology	Ordering/Billing
Med-RT	Medications	Terminology	Allergy
UNII	Medications	Terminology	Pharmacovigilance
HCPCS	Procedures	Terminology	Billing

Features of Terminologies

These terminologies and classifications exhibit a variety of design choices. Terminologists recognize a variety of best-practice design features for terminologies and classifications. A concise summary of many of these features is the landmark paper "Desiderata for Controlled Medical Vocabularies in the Twenty-First Century." Some of the author's key insights are summarized here (Cimino 1998).

A good terminology should be concept-oriented. This means that terms are not vague, ambiguous, or redundant; that is, each term has a specific meaning, each term has a single meaning, and each meaning has a single term. Since words can be ambiguous, this guideline is typically taken to apply to the code, not the term. A terminology can use the ambiguous term "cold" to mean a temperature range, an emotional affect, and a viral upper respiratory infection as long as the codes, also called "concept identifiers," are distinct.

A good terminology exhibits concept permanence. This means that, although the terminology may evolve over time, the meanings of its concepts do not. If a concept is found to be too broad, more precise concepts can be added; if it is found to be incorrect, it can be deactivated, but kept in the documentation. But the code, or concept identifier, should always refer to the concept it started with.

Those two desiderata are widely—though not universally—supported. Some are less widely supported.

A good terminology uses **nonsemantic identifiers**. This means the codes, or concept identifiers, don't mean anything; one can't infer information about what a code means without dereferencing its terms. This desideratum is not always followed, as it can be very convenient to understand that, for example, K21 in ICD-10-CM (Gastro-esophageal reflux disease with esophagitis) is a disorder of the digestive system (signified by the letter K) without having to look it up, while SNOMED CT's 235595009 would have to be looked up. But the semantic identifier binds the meaning to the form in a way that constrains the update process. When the system is revised, it is sometimes necessary to reassign concept parents. If the identifier determines the parent, this is impossible to do without creating a new concept identifier with the same meaning as the old one.

A good terminology supports a **polyhierarchy**. This means that a concept can have more than one parent. Viral pneumonia is both a viral disorder and a respiratory disorder. A **monohierarchy** has to choose which of these parents to assign, and then it must provide guidance both for the assignment of the code and for correctly conducting statistical analysis on the results.

Per Cimino (1998), a good terminology rejects "not elsewhere classified." As a terminology evolves, the meaning of such terms will change. "Hepatitis not elsewhere classified" would include Hepatitis C in 1988, and not in 1989. Instead, if new concepts cannot be authored expeditiously, more general parent concepts should be used.

Cimino's desiderata (there are seven more) focus on terminologies for accurate and reusable clinical knowledge. Terminologies designed for specific purposes, such as billing and statistical aggregation, may have different priorities and requirements. Experts from different communities disagree about the desiderata and the best ways to support them, but these are business decisions, and different terminology stewards make different decisions.

Examples of Design Features Found in Terminologies and Classifications

The following are examples of how terminologies stack up against the best-practice design features of Cimino's desiderata. In some cases, the terminology or classification meets best practice while in others, that is not the case.

UNIFIED CODE FOR UNITS OF MEASURE

One of the most basic code systems is the **Unified Code for Units of Measure (UCUM)**. UCUM was developed by the Regenstrief Institute, Inc. to define codes for units of measure. They are mostly abbreviations of words: meter is "m"; second is "s." Because of the limited number of letters available, some have longer abbreviations: "mol" for mole, "Hz" for Herz. Differences in standards make it necessary to differentiate some traditional terms with brackets; e.g., "[lb_av]" for avoirdupois pounds, "[lb-tr]" for troy.

UCUM is compositional. Millimeters of mercury, for instance, is abbreviated "mmHg"; meters per second as "m/s." Because of this compositional nature, there are infinitely many valid codes of UCUM, though only a few hundred commonly used ones. They are often found in laboratory and vitals measurements.

UCUM does not follow the principle of nonsemantic identifiers, but because unit names are not volatile, change does not cause problems for the stewards. It is concept oriented. There is an implicit hierarchy, as each unit falls into a "base unit" category (length, time, mass and so on) or some combination thereof.

UCUM does not support "not elsewhere classified" concepts.

LOGICAL OBSERVATION IDENTIFIERS NAMES AND CODES

Logical Observation Identifiers Names and Codes (LOINC), also developed by the Regenstrief Institute, started out as an effort to standardize codes for laboratory results. It has since proven its value in other areas where there is a question for which an answer is sought, whether it be "blood glucose mass concentration" (2341-6) or "did the vehicle airbag deploy?" (67500-9).

LOINC codes have nonsemantic identifiers. They are implicitly polyhierarchical, as they have definitional "axes":

- Component: the thing observed; for example, glucose
- Property: the characteristic of the thing; for example, mass concentration
- Time: the time frame of measurement; for example, 4 hour post-challenge
- System: where measured; for example, blood, serum

- Scale: what kind of answer is expected; for example, ordinal scale, or quantity
- Method: optionally, how the measurement was taken; for example, test strip

LOINC does not provide "not elsewhere classified" concepts.

INTERNATIONAL CLASSIFICATION OF DISEASES, TENTH REVISION, CLINICAL MODIFICATION

The *International Classification of Diseases, Tenth Revision, Clinical Modification* (ICD-10-CM) is the US's adaptation of the World Health Organization's *International Statistical Classification of Diseases and Related Health Problems, 10th revision* (ICD-10). It is developed by the National Center for Health Statistics. It contains a monohierarchical set of codes describing disorders. The monohierarchy is designed to support statistical aggregation. This supports use in public health statistics, billing, and a variety of management and quality control tasks. It also uses semantic identifiers; this helps human abstractors work more efficiently with the values.

For example, the code for "Acute myocardial infarction" is I21. There are several more specific codes under this code, and there are guidelines specifying which codes are valid for use and which are simply present to support the hierarchy. I21 is a semantic code because the I tells a knowledgeable coder that this is a disease of the circulatory system.

ICD-10 CM includes "not elsewhere classified" values.

RxNORM

The National Library of Medicine (NLM) designed RxNorm to provide normalized names for clinical drugs and links to many of the drug vocabularies commonly used in pharmacy management and drug interaction software. It does not assert a hierarchy, though it does define relationships between, for example, drug ingredients, the clinical drugs that contain them, and the products and packaging in which they are marketed. RxNorm uses concept unique identifiers, or CUIs, which are nonsemantic.

RxNorm codes and terms identify drug ingredients (IN), semantic clinical drug components (SCDC), clinical dose form groups (CDFG), and relationships among these values.

RxNorm also provides maps to FDA's Unique Ingredient Identifier and National Drug Codes for packaged products. RxNorm codes are used in NDF-RT (now Med-RT) classifications.

RxNorm does not provide "not elsewhere classified" values.

SNOMED CT

SNOMED CT, published by SNOMED International, is the largest and most general terminology in widespread use. It defines almost half a million unique concepts with 1.3 million descriptions (terms) and 2.7 million relationships. SNOMED CT is technically an ontology because it defines not only concepts, but their relationships. It states not only that viral pneumonia is both a viral disorder and a respiratory disorder, but that it has a causative agent of a virus, a finding site of the lungs, an associated morphology of inflammation and consolidation, and a pathological process of infection. The semantic richness of this knowledge base supports a variety of use cases, including use cases that may not yet be known.

SNOMED CT is published in a set of files that can be used to support automated inference using Description Logics. Its publication has recently been augmented with files in the Ontology Web Language (OWL), supporting these logical capabilities more fully and easily. SNOMED CT is licensed for use in the US by the NLM. In countries without national licenses, users must establish their own licenses.

SNOMED CT is very broad in content scope and can be used to standardize codes and terms for a variety of purposes. Its logical design is intended to support more sophisticated uses, such as clinical decision support.

SNOMED CT follows all of Cimino's desiderata.

Implementation Issues

Terminologies and classifications are useful outside of computer systems. Linnaeus's system of classification for organisms and its supporting nomenclature was so useful that it is still in use today, despite revolutionary changes in our understanding of underlying biological relationships. But since most medical data systems are computerized, most of the work in designing terminologies focuses on optimizing their use in computers.

The meaning of a concept in a terminology is incomplete. It is only useful when it is instantiated in a record, and the record provides half of the meaning. A code for a laparotomy refers to an abstract idea; the field it populates must be known in order to know whether it is a laparotomy order, a laparotomy that has been conducted, a prohibition, recommendation, or some other use of the concept represented by the code. And before the clinician can complete the form (to order a laparotomy, for instance), the form must be designed to associate the "procedure ordered" field with the appropriate list of orderable procedures from a terminology.

This process is called **terminology binding**: the tying-together of the data element in the information model, form, or other structured specification with the set of concepts that may appropriately complete the thought. Key sources for defining binding requirements and designs include the ISO 11179 standard for metadata registries and the HL7 Vocabulary workgroup publications, including the *Core Principles and Properties of HL7 Version 3 Models, Characteristics of a Value Set Definition*, and a work in progress entitled *Vocabulary Binding Semantics*.

In most cases, the set of appropriate values for a data element is smaller than the set of values found in a terminology. The element must be bound to a subset of the terminology. The subset is referred to as a value set. The value set designates the values (codes and terms) appropriate to the data element—for example, not all 90,000 LOINC codes, but only those selected to support a vital signs form, or a physical examination form. Figure 18.5 illustrates the use of a value set in a data element designed for a vital signs data entry form.

A value set definition may be constructed in two ways. The obvious way is by explicitly listing the required values (codes and terms)—an extensional definition. It is also possible to state some rule for inclusion such as "all the children of *disorder of the spleen*" or "all disorders with a finding site *of bone structure*"—an intensional definition. Most value set definitions are extensional.

When a value set definition is applied to the terminologies (usually referred to as a code system in this context) from which it draws its terms, the resulting list of values is called a value set expansion. The distinction is clearer for intensionally defined value sets than for extensionally defined value sets, but it's applicable for both: if a code system inactivates a code, then an expansion may differ from its extensional definition by excluding that code.

Value sets may change over time, so they support versioning. This volatility, combined with the fact that a value set may be defined intensionally, and may contain references to multiple code

FIGURE 18.5. Binding a data element in a form to a value set

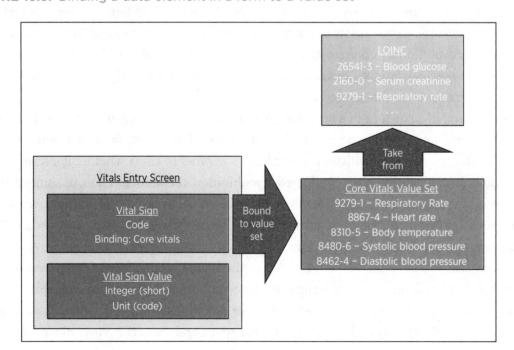

Source: © AHIMA.

systems and other value sets, means that understanding the current valid contents of a value set at a point in time can be challenging. When discussing value set maintenance, it's important to be clear about the distinction between the value set definition and the value set expansion. Using the unspecified term "value set" may lead to confusion.

When a data element is bound to a value set, the designer will also specify a **binding strength**. Strength refers to the level of rigor with which the constraint should be enforced. In some cases, the value set is absolute: the only valid way to complete the element is to choose from the value set. But in medicine, information may change more quickly than the technology that supports it, so allowances must be made for users to choose values not specified in the value set. For instance, there was no code for exposure to the Zika virus in ICD-10-CM in 2017, so public health agencies wishing to record such exposure had to use interim values. Any system with too strong a binding, that prevented the use of codes other than those specified, would make life difficult in these cases. Strength is a property of the data element, not the value set.

Coded data elements may require other qualifications in binding than strength. Examples include the ability to record source text, or to record multiple codes, possibly with some metadata indicating which code was chosen by a human user or was the result of translation.

Binding is a semantic task: it involves the designer joining the semantics defined by an information model to the semantics defined by the value set. Sometimes, the join will be imperfect. An allergy form, for instance, may have a data element to represent the substance to which the patient is allergic. If the same form is used to record the fact that the patient has no allergies, it might seem convenient to capture the "no known allergies" in the same field where one might otherwise capture "penicillin." This is an example of **model impedance**, the phenomenon where the semantics of the model and the terminology don't quite fit. Other examples include a vitals screen where one might record that the patient was seated for a blood pressure reading in a "patient body position" field, or one might use a more specific "seated blood pressure" question code. Either way works, but they differ, and subsequent consumers of the data have to anticipate both paths in order to understand the data correctly.

Model impedance is a key impediment for attempts to construct standards specifications that support semantic interoperability. More constrained specifications are one way to avoid impedance. A vitals observation implementation guide, for instance, might constrain the observation codes to those that already include position, and prohibit use of a patient position field, or vice versa. This is the approach of HL7 Fast Healthcare Interoperability Resources (FHIR), but there is no capability to harmonize these approaches across implementation communities.

Another approach to resolving model impedance is the use of ontologies to model both scenarios consistently, and to use **model binding** to ensure they can be understood. In the body position example, the body position element of the information model would have a **value binding** to a value set of body positions, but it would also have a model binding to a single value specifying "this is the body position of the patient for which this measurement is being taken." This requires the use of a foundational terminology that includes these relationship values. SNOMED CT includes a set of relationship concepts with defined domains and ranges that form an implicit information model within the terminology. An "observable entity" like blood pressure may have an attribute of "precondition," which might have a value such as "patient sitting." If the position element had a model binding to the "precondition" value, then an intelligent system would be able to determine that the "blood pressure" value combined with the "patient sitting" precondition is equivalent to a "seated blood pressure" value, as long as that value is so defined in the terminology.

Another example would be that a clinical finding can have a causative agent as a defining attribute, and viral pneumonia, as mentioned previously, has "virus" as such an attribute. However, one might record pneumonia as a finding and associate it with a cause (virus) captured in another element of the information model. The existence of the causative agent value allows an intelligent system to discover that the viral pneumonia value in one field is synonymous with a pneumonia finding with a cause of virus.

Maps

When clinical systems need to produce interoperable messages using standard terminologies, they have two options: they can implement those terminologies natively, or they can map.

Most systems are not designed around standards; code values are defined to meet the needs of the implementing provider team. Once the system is functional, attention turns to secondary uses of data, including analysis, quality measures, and interoperability—the kinds of uses for which standards are necessary. The obvious solution is to provide a map: a set of assertions that a code in the local system is equivalent to and can be expressed by a code in the appropriate standard. For example, code XYZ in the local system is equivalent to and can be expressed by code ABC in the appropriate standard. The use of a map introduces overhead to the process of generating standards-compliant content and the separation of concerns prevents either endeavor from interfering with the other.

However, mapping presents a critical problem: the content of the local system may not map cleanly to the standard. One solution is to use the next-best broader term in the standard. It is semantically sound to assert that a patient with "Hepatitis A" has "Hepatitis," even though the assertion is lossy, meaning it loses a bit of the precision of the original. This approach is sufficient for statistical purposes, but it fails to provide information that may be necessary for patient care. The use of "original text" fields in association with coded data ameliorates the problem for human recipients, who can read the text, but not for computer systems. A further issue is that the author of the data and the author of the map may not have perfectly aligned assumptions about the meaning of the codes, and a local identifier for "pre-cancerous dysplasia" might not be classified in the target system as a critical risk factor. Mapping is an unavoidable task in many environments, but it does present costs and risks.

A more elegant solution is native standardization. This approach involves implementing standard codes directly in the operational system. This way, a user selecting a value ("sitting") from a drop-down box on a screen has already identified the SNOMED CT code, and no translation is necessary. This approach minimizes the extra work involved in maintaining a local set of codes and makes it unnecessary to translate them to produce standards-compliant communications. However, systems sometimes need to record information for which no code yet exists. A new code can be requested, but even the most responsive code system maintainers can't provide such a thing the instant a need is identified. For these cases, even systems that commit to native standardization must create their own "local" codes. In the Zika example, a local code might have been stored at the point of care, and the ICD-10-CM code added in later, when it became available. Medico-legal requirements around recordkeeping usually mean that, even if a standard code is requested and provided, the original record cannot be modified. At this point, a system striving to use native standards now has both a native code and a local code.

One option is to record a local value in every instance, but to also record a standard code when one is available, or to add such a code after the fact, when necessary. This design supports flexibility and standardization. It does create a correspondence that looks a lot like a map: the governance of such a system must strive to defend the position that the standard system is the system of record, and that the local codes must not extend or enhance the semantics so provided.

Terminology and Semantic Interoperability

The semantics supported by terminologies can extend beyond the uses cases in which the data is captured and can support intelligent use of information for clinical decision support, quality measures, and research. The complex relationships captured by some terminologies qualify them as ontologies. Ontologies are characterized as terminologies that specify a variety of relationships, but they are designed to provide a comprehensive framework for knowledge representation. In philosophy, ontology is the science of what exists; in knowledge management, it has come to denote a kind of representation of what exists, and it is defined as "a formal, explicit specification of a shared conceptualization" (Studer et al. 1998).

The result of this formal rigor is that a properly constructed ontology will support automated logical inference using a class of tools known as **description logics (DL)**. DL supports the inference of new facts from previously asserted facts. Some logical inferences can be made with relatively simple applications of rules, such as clinical decision support rules that encode guidelines to propose administration of aspirin to patients who present at the emergency department with chest pain. Sometimes the rule author may not know all the coded values that might be considered chest pain. If all the values ("radiating chest pain," for example) are modeled in the ontology as kinds of chest pain, then the rule will be able to infer that this patient's symptom is a kind of chest pain and make the appropriate recommendation. No extra effort is required to maintain the list of values that are kinds of chest pain for use in the rule; they are already classified in the terminology.

Other common cases of this sort of rule include drug checks. A drug order is recorded to support administration, but the system happens to know that the drug interacts with another drug the patient is taking. The clinical decision support system can use record data to perform additional safety checks. For instance, nonsteroidal anti-inflammatory drugs (NSAIDs) may be contraindicated for a patient on warfarin. Most providers will know this and avoid acetaminophen, ibuprofen, and the like. But if a provider at a different facility prescribes a less well-known NSAID, such as piroxicam, the applicability of the rule may not be clear. A rule written against the category of NSAIDs, rather than against a list, will be more likely to stay up to date.

This principle, that the data can be looked at from different perspectives, can support more complicated inferences. A provider may record that a patient has "bacterial pneumonia" purely for the purpose of supporting the orders for treatment. The concept identifier attached to the diagnosis will also support billing, in concert with the orders for procedures and medications. However, the diagnosis concept identifier has, in SNOMED CT, definitional relationships that may support automated inference. It has a "finding site" of "lung structure," making it possible for the system to put together the fact that the patient had been intubated and suggest investigation of a ventilator-associated infection. Normally, a clinician would recognize such a detail, but in cases where a patient may have been transferred, or staff changes obscured the record, or there is a time lag, the ability to make such connections systematically may be important.

Recognition of clinically significant relationships in situations where humans may not have sufficient perspective is a key value proposition for ontologies. But there are limits to the promise. Each of the millions of relationships in SNOMED CT is authored by a person, and the authors do not all share the same assumptions. SNOMED International spends significant resources on assuring the quality of the terminology, but quality sufficient to support actionable clinical recommendations remains in the future. One effort, the Federal Health Information Model, has authored over 200 value sets, but has yet to identify a case where an intensional definition (for example, a SNOMED concept and its descendants) can be used to define a value set for a specific use case. Whether this limit results from human engineering and our ability to communicate clearly across organizations or from inherent messiness in the underlying information remains to be seen.

CHECK YOUR UNDERSTANDING

1. Terminology is the domain of:
   a. Codes and concept identifiers
   b. Terms

   c. Terms, codes, and their design and use

   d. Terms, codes, and translation

2. Concept permanence:

   a. Refers to the Platonic essence of a concept

   b. Means that meaning of a concept will not change

   c. Refers to medical recordkeeping

   d. Means that the clinical concept will not evolve

3. A value set expansion is:

   a. An intensional definition of a value set

   b. A method for extending a value set across terminologies

   c. The result of applying a value set definition

   d. A value added to a value set

4. The practice of using standard terminologies in a software system is known as:

   a. Taxonomy

   b. Binding

   c. Native standardization

   d. None of the above

5. A value set is:

   a. A terminology

   b. Used to select appropriate subsets of a terminology

   c. Used to assert relationships in a terminology

   d. Used to modify a terminology

REVIEW

1. True or false? The meaning of a concept in a terminology is incomplete because it needs to be tied together with a data element in the information model, form, or other structured specification.

   a. True

   b. False

2. A nonsemantic identifier

   a. Refers to a syntactic rather than a semantic code

   b. Does not embed meaning in the code

    c.   Refers to a term rather than a concept

    d.   Does not refer to a concept with relationships

3.   Which way(s) may a value set definition be constructed?

    a.   Extensional

    b.   Binding and expansion

    c.   Intensional and binding

    d.   Extensional and intensional

4.   Which of the following demonstrates model impedance?

    a.   A system needs to record a value not yet provided by the specified terminology.

    b.   A system requires a body position when capturing blood pressure.

    c.   A system does not require a body position when capturing blood pressure.

    d.   A test code supports glucose measurement with a test strip method, and the information model also has a dedicated test method field.

5.   A terminology in which a value can have more than one parent is a

    a.   Classification

    b.   Controlled terminology

    c.   Polyhierarchy

    d.   Concept-oriented terminology

6.   The use of "not elsewhere classified" prevents a terminology from achieving

    a.   Nonsemantic identifiers

    b.   Polyhierarchy

    c.   Taxonomy

    d.   Concept permanence

7.   Which of the following is a concept-oriented terminology?

    a.   LOINC

    b.   UCUM

    c.   SNOMED CT

    d.   RxNorm

8.   The need for a data element to support new and unanticipated values implies a need for

    a.   A more rigorous binding strength

    b.   A less rigorous binding strength

    c.   A more extensional binding strength

    d.   A more intensional binding strength

9. Which of the following is a classification?

    a. LOINC

    b. CPT

    c. SNOMED CT

    d. ICD-10-CM

10. When discussing value set definition and maintenance, it is important to distinguish

    a. Value set definition from value set expansion

    b. Value set intension from value set expansion

    c. Value set definition from value set extension

    d. Value set version from value set extension

References

Cimino, J. 1998. Desiderata for controlled medical vocabularies in the twenty-first century. *Methods of Information in Medicine* 37(4-5):394-403.

Studer, R., R. Benjamins, and D. Fensel. 1998. Knowledge engineering: Principles and methods. *Data & Knowledge Engineering* 25(1–2):161–197.

Resources

Agency for Healthcare Research and Quality (AHRQ). n.d. United States Health Information Knowledgebase (USHIK). https://ushik.ahrq.gov/mdr/portals.

Health Level Seven International (HL7). 2012. HL7 Version 3 Standard: Core Principles and Properties of V3 Models, Release 1. http://www.hl7.org/implement/standards/product_brief.cfm?product_id=58.

Health Level Seven International (HL7). 2019. HL7 Specification: Characteristics of a Value Set Definition, Release 1. http://www.hl7.org/implement/standards/product_brief.cfm?product_id=437.

ISO/IEC 11179. 2013. Information technology – Metadata registries (MDR) -Part 3: Registry metamodel and basic attributes. Geneva, Switzerland: International Organization for Standardization.

National Cancer Institute. 2018. NCIthesaurus. https://ncit.nci.nih.gov/ncitbrowser.

National Library of Medicine. 2018. RxNorm. https://www.nlm.nih.gov/research/umls/rxnorm/.

National Library of Medicine. 2018. Unified Medical Language System (UMLS). https://www.nlm.nih.gov/research/umls/.

National Library of Medicine. 2018. Value Set Authority Center (VSAC). https://vsac.nlm.nih.gov.

Office of the National Coordinator for Health Information Technology (ONC). n.d. "Introduction to ISA." https://www.healthit.gov/isa/

Regenstrief Institute. 2018. LOINC. https://loinc.org/.

Regenstrief Institute. 2018. Unified Code for Units of Measure (UCUM). http://unitsofmeasure.org/.

SNOMED International. 2018. SNOMED CT. http://www.snomed.org/.

US Food and Drug Administration. 2018. Unique Ingredient Identifier (UNII). https://fdasis.nlm.nih.gov/srs/.

Glossary

ABC codes Five-character alphabetic codes that describe a wide assortment of procedures, treatments, and services provided during an encounter with a complementary and alternative medicine, nursing, or other integrative healthcare provider. These codes are a registered vocabulary of Health Level Seven (HL7) and were incorporated into the National Library of Medicine's Unified Medical Language System (UMLS) in 1998.

Accountability measure A measure that meets specific criteria to be used for purposes of accountability.

Accredited Standards Committee (ASC) X12N The subcommittee responsible for insurance and insurance-related business processes standards. ASC develops and maintains X12 EDI and XML standards, standards interpretations, and standards guidelines.

Activity The execution of a task or action by an individual.

Activity limitation Difficulties an individual may have in executing activities.

Alphabetical Index Section of the Current Dental Terminology (CDT) Code that provides a listing of codes by subcategory, nomenclature, or relationship along with the page(s) where the CDT code(s) are found.

American Dental Association (ADA) A professional association that provides advocacy, facilitates research, and promotes professional development to the dentistry profession throughout the US.

American Hospital Association's Central Office on HCPCS Provides coding guidance for the following Level II HCPCS codes: A codes for ambulance services and radiopharmaceuticals; C codes; G codes; J codes; and Q codes, except Q0136 through Q0181 for hospitals; physicians; and other health professionals who bill Medicare.

American Medical Association (AMA) The national professional membership organization for physicians that distributes scientific information to its members and the public, informs members of legislation related to health and medicine, and represents the medical profession's interests in national legislative matters; maintains and publishes the Current Procedural Terminology (CPT) coding system (AMA 2019).

American National Standards Institute (ANSI) The agency that coordinates the development of voluntary standards to increase global competitiveness in a variety of industries, including healthcare.

American Nurses Association (ANA) A professional organization representing the interests of nurses.

American Psychiatric Association (APA) A medical specialty society consisting of members involved in psychiatric practice, research, and academia. The APA develops and publishes the *Diagnostic and Statistical Manual of Mental Disorders* (DSM).

Application Programming Interface (API) A set of definitions of the ways in which one piece of computer software communicates with another or a programmer makes requests of the operating system or another application; operates outside the realm of the direct user interface.

Artefact In the Patient Summary Standards Set (PSSS), a named standard, profile, guide, or implementation specification used to achieve interoperability.

Atom A drug name, plus additional characteristics (NLM 2018).

Attributes Characteristics or aspects of a concept's meaning; used in SNOMED CT to characterize and define concepts.

Barrier A physical, social, or attitudinal environmental factor that hinders a person's ability to live and conduct their life.

Behavioral standards Data exchange standards that describe messaging protocols, workflows, and algorithms to be executed by communicating systems.

Binding strength When a data element is bound to a value set, a binding strength is specified. Strength refers to the level of rigor with which the constraint should be enforced.

Biopsychosocial Model A blend of the Medical Model and the Social Model that views functioning and disability as an interaction among one's biological, psychological, and social factors.

Body functions Physiological and psychological functions of the body (for example, mental functions or sensory functions).

Body structures Anatomical parts of the body including organs, limbs, and their components.

Candidate class A data class that is considered to be next in line for inclusion in the US Core Data for Interoperability.

Capacity A person's ability to do a task or action in a standardized testing environment.

Cardinality The numbers of source and target concepts that may logically participate in populating a data map record for a specific use case. Map relationships may be one-to-one (1:1) for equivalence maps but often are one-to-many (1:*) or many-to-many (*:*) for other relationship types.

CDT Coding Companion A publication of the American Dental Association (ADA) that advises on using the Current Dental Terminology (CDT) Code by providing definitions, coding scenarios, and questions and answers for each of the 12 dental service categories.

Centers for Medicare and Medicaid Services (CMS) The US Department of Health and Human Services (HHS) agency responsible for Medicare and parts of Medicaid. CMS is responsible for the oversight of Health Insurance Portability and Accountability Act (HIPAA) administrative simplification transaction and code sets, health identifiers, and security standards. CMS also maintains the Healthcare Common Procedure Coding

System (HCPCS) medical code set and the Medicare Remittance Advice Remark Codes administrative code set (CMS 2006).

Classification A key kind of terminology that uses a monohierarchical system to arrange or organize like or related entities.

Classification of diseases A "system of categories to which morbid entities are assigned according to established criteria" (WHO 2016).

Clinical Care Classification (CCC) A nursing classification designed to document the steps of the nursing process across the care continuum.

Clinical Data Abstraction Center (CDAC) Independent review firms contracted by the Centers for Medicare and Medicaid Services to perform data collection.

Clinical Data Interchange Standards Consortium (CDISC) A voluntary consensus standards development organization recognized by ISO. The organization's mission is to develop and support interoperable data standards for medical research and related areas of healthcare (CDISC 2018).

Clinical Document Architecture (CDA) An interchange standard to support electronic documentation of patient encounters and services. CDA is the basis for several widely used and internationally adopted implementation guides, including the Continuity of Care Document (CCD), the harmonized collection of 12 CDA document templates called Consolidated CDA (C-CDA), and the Quality Reporting Document Architecture (QRDA).

Clinical quality measure (CQM) A mechanism for measuring and tracking the quality of healthcare services. Measures contain defined data elements that, when reported, define the measure.

CMS HCPCS Workgroup A group that manages permanent national codes. It is comprised of public and private insurers including Medicare; Medicaid; the Department of Veterans Affairs; and Pricing, Data Analysis, and Coding contractor.

Code Refers specifically to the coded (usually nonsemantic) identifier, not the term or concept referenced by the code. Codes are also known, in concept-oriented terminologies, as concept identifiers.

Code on Dental Procedures and Nomenclature (Code) Lists the dental codes used for billing dental procedures and supplies.

Code Maintenance Committee (CMC) The committee established to maintain the Current Dental Terminology (CDT) Code. It includes representatives from third-party payers, the American Dental Association (ADA), dental specialty organizations, the Academy of General Dentistry (AGD), and the American Dental Education Association (ADEA). The delegates from these entities cast votes to accept or decline CDT code changes, additions, or deletions.

Code system When a value set definition is applied to the terminologies from which it draws its terms.

Coding Clinic A publication issued quarterly by the American Hospital Association (AHA) and approved by the Centers for Medicare and Medicaid Services (CMS) to give official coding advice and direction.

Coding string In the International Classification of Functioning, Disability and Health (ICF), a set of relevant codes used to describe an individual's health situation.

Comité Européen de Normalisation (CEN), or European Committee for Standardization Consisting of the national standards bodies in Europe as well as associates representing broad industrial sectors and social and economic partners, the association develops and defines European Standards and other formal documents for healthcare as well as other fields and sectors.

Common Ontology A prototype semantic scaffolding developed by the World Health Organization (WHO) and SNOMED International shared between ICD-11 and SNOMED CT, from which all foundation layer entities can be defined.

Common Terminology Services (CTS2) Define and describe how a terminology server should perform instead of focusing on how the server is organized or what type of content is present within it.

Complementary and alternative medicine (CAM) A group of diverse medical and healthcare systems, practices, and products that are not considered to be part of conventional medicine.

Concept A unique unit of knowledge or thought created by a unique combination of characteristics.

Concept identifier In concept-oriented terminologies, the code assigned to each concept. In SNOMED CT, the identifier is a unique number.

Concept model "The set of rules that determines the permitted sets of relationships between particular types of concept" (SNOMED International 2019a).

Concept orientation Concepts in a controlled medical terminology are based on meanings, not words.

Concept permanence A code representing a concept in a controlled clinical terminology is not reused and thus meanings do not change.

Concordance The fractional rate of agreement between two coding specialists in selecting a mapping target when creating or using a data map.

Configurable Able to address specific terminology needs as authorized organizations add concepts, descriptions, relationships, and subsets to complement the SNOMED CT International Release through the extension mechanism.

Consolidated CDA (C-CDA) The harmonized collection of 12 CDA document templates.

Content model The explicit information model for each ICD-11 rubric.

Content standards A data exchange standard that describes the information to be communicated over a connection, addressing syntax, semantics and data models, terminology, and rendering of information.

Context For data maps, this consists of business case and workflow assumptions that apply to the interpretation and application of map records. For example, in mapping classifications such as ICD-10-CM, are comorbidities to be used in assessing "excludes" guidelines. Since most data map structures are incapable of managing such complexities, simple maps should generally be explicitly "context free."

Controlled terminology A terminology whose governance processes ensure that it is structurally sound, accurate, and up to date.

Cooperating Parties A group of four organizations (the American Health Information Management Association, the American Hospital Association, the Centers for Medicare and Medicaid Services, and the National Center for Health Statistics) that collaborate in the development and maintenance of ICD coding guidelines.

Coordination and Maintenance Committee (C&M Committee) Committee composed of representatives from the National Center for Health Statistics (NCHS) and the Centers for Medicare and Medicaid Services (CMS) that is responsible for maintaining the United States' clinical modification version of the International Classification of Diseases and ICD-10 Procedure Coding System.

Core sets A guide for identifying common ICF codes that relate to a person's particular health experience. Core sets have been developed for specific conditions and populations.

Council on Dental Benefit Programs The group responsible for developing a standard set of codes describing dental procedures, which led to CDT-1.

Counseling A discussion of one or more of the following topics: diagnostic results, impressions, or recommended diagnostic studies; prognosis; risks and benefits of management; instruction for management; importance of compliance; risk factor reduction; or patient and family education.

CPT Editorial Panel A panel composed of seventeen members which is authorized to revise, update, or modify CPT codes, descriptors and the rules and guidelines.

Cross map Enables SNOMED CT to effectively reference other terminologies and classifications.

Current Dental Terminology (CDT) The code set recognized as the standard dental procedural code reference for dentists practicing in academic, clinical, and administrative settings.

Current Procedural Terminology (CPT) A comprehensive terminology published by the American Medical Association (AMA) and used for reporting diagnostic and therapeutic procedures and medical and surgical services.

Data class A high-level grouping of similar data types made up of data objects (USCDI 2018).

Data dictionary A descriptive list of names (also called representations or displays), definitions, and attributes of data elements to be collected in an information system or database.

Data element A unit of data for which the definition, identification, representation and permissible values are specified by means of a set of attributes (ISO 2013).

Data element domain A specification (list or range) of the valid, allowable values that can be assigned for each data element in a data set (Shakir 1999).

Data governance 1. The overall management of the availability, usability, integrity, and security of the data employed in an organization or enterprise (Data Governance Institute 2013) **2.** A specific enterprise information management function that supports coordination among all other EIM functions. It is the enterprise authority that ensures control and accountability for enterprise data through the establishment of decision rights and data policies and standards that are implemented and monitored through a formal structure of assigned roles, responsibilities, and accountabilities.

Data map A set of links from concepts or terms in one classification, terminology, reference terminology, or ontology to another for some purpose of reuse (ISO 2014).

Data quality management (DQM) The business processes that ensure the integrity of an organization's data (Davoudi et al. 2015). Governance functions ensure that the use and management of data and information is compliant with jurisdictional law, regulations, standards, and organizational policies.

Data set A list of recommended data elements with uniform definitions.

Department of Health and Human Services (HHS) A cabinet-level agency that oversees all the health and human services-related activities of the federal government.

Derivative work A resource, such as a subset or cross map, that consists of, includes, references, or is derived from one or more SNOMED CT components (SNOMED International 2019b).

Derived classification One based on a reference classification such as ICD or ICF by adopting the reference classification structure and categories and providing additional detail or through rearrangement or aggregation of items from one or more reference classifications (WHO 2018).

Description In SNOMED CT, the term or text for a concept.

Description logics (DL) A class of tools that support the inference of new facts from previously asserted facts.

Descriptive text A component of the DSM through which narrative content, such as diagnostic chapter introductory sections and informative material following the diagnostic criteria, helps support diagnosis.

Descriptor Descriptors assigned to codes represent the official definition of the items and services.

Designated Standards Maintenance Organization (DSMO) A category of organization established by the Health Insurance Portability and Accountability Act to maintain the electronic transaction standards mandated by HIPAA.

***Diagnostic and Statistical Manual of Mental Disorders* (DSM)** A standard classification of mental disorders developed by the American Psychiatric Association.

Diagnostic classification A listing of all the disorders, diagnostic codes, subtypes, specifiers, and notes that are unique to a system such as DSM-5.

Diagnostic criteria Content within DSM-5 that summarizes a description of each disorder.

Differentiation Histological grading or the degree to which a tumor resembles the normal tissue from which it arose.

Digital Imaging and Communications in Medicine (DICOM) A standard for the interchange of computerized biomedical images and image-related information within and between healthcare providers.

Disability An umbrella term for impairments, activity limitations, and participation restrictions that denotes the negative aspects of the interaction between the health condition and contextual factors.

Discordance The fractional rate of disagreement between two coding specialists in selecting a mapping target when creating or using a data map.

Domain A sphere or field of activity and influence.

Dose form The physical form of a dose.

Drug Listing Act 1972 In 1972, the Federal Food, Drug and Cosmetic Act (FDCA) was amended to make submission of information on all commercially marketed drugs mandatory. Under its new name, the Drug Listing Act of 1972 required all domestic and foreign firms (manufacturers, repackagers, and labelers) marketing drug products in the US to list with the FDA prescription drug products manufactured, prepared, propagated, compounded, or processed for commercial distribution in the US.

DSM-5 *See Diagnostic and Statistical Manual of Mental Disorders* (DSM).

Editorial Guide A guide for clinical personnel, business directors, software product managers, and project leaders that explains the capabilities and uses of SNOMED CT from a content perspective.

Electronic clinical quality measure (eCQM) Use data from electronic health records or health information technology systems to measure healthcare quality (eCQI 2019). eCQMs are assigned a specific, unique CMS eCQM identifier, which is a semantic identifier that includes the version number.

Electronic data interchange (EDI) A standard transmission format using strings of data for business information communicated among the computer systems of independent organizations.

Electronic dental record system (EDR) The EDRs used in dentistry generally include a database specifically for CDT that is updated by the EDR vendor to keep up with the latest CDT release.

Electronic prescribing (e-Rx) The process of entering prescription information into a computer application and securely transmitting the prescription directly to the retail pharmacy's information system.

Emerging data class The data class under evaluation for potential promotion to candidate class in the US Core Data for Interoperability.

Encoder Specialty software used to facilitate the assignment of diagnostic and procedural codes according to the rules of the coding system.

Environmental factors External influences that facilitate or hinder functioning and health (for example, accessible buildings, weather); or make up the physical, social, and attitudinal environment in which people live and conduct their lives.

Evaluation and management (E/M) codes Codes that are designed to report physician work as performed in different clinical settings. With a few exceptions, E/M codes are based on the practitioner's documentation of history, physical examination, and medical decision-making.

Exhaustive A requirement of a statistical classification wherein every condition has a place to be coded, even if that is a residual category.

Extension A structure that enables authorized organizations to add concepts, descriptions, relationships, and reference sets to complement the SNOMED CT International Release.

Extensional One of the two ways of constructing a value set definition. This method lists explicitly the required values (codes and terms).

Facilitator A physical, social, or attitudinal environmental factor that helps a person's ability to live and conduct their life.

FAIR data principles A set of guidelines to ensure that data are Findable, Accessible, Interoperable, and Reusable.

Fast Healthcare Information Resources (FHIR) A standard for health data exchange that focuses on implementation.

Federal Food, Drug and Cosmetic Act (FDCA) A federal law establishing the legal framework within which the FDA develops regulations.

Fit for purpose A map data set that aligns with the needs of the user and employs documentation and data structures that are understandable, useful, and reproducible in achieving the goals of the use case.

Food and Drug Administration (FDA) The federal agency responsible for protecting the public health by assuring certain foods are safe, wholesome, sanitary and properly labelled; ensuring human and veterinary drugs and vaccines and other biological products and medical devices are safe and effective; assuring cosmetics and dietary supplements are safe and properly labelled; protecting the public from products that emit radiation; regulating tobacco products; and advancing public health by speeding product innovations (FDA 2018a).

Foundation Component The semantic network of all terms, meanings, and practical relationships, or the core of the ICD-11.

Foundational interoperability "Allows data exchange from one information technology system to be received by another and does not require the ability for the receiving information technology system to interpret the data" (HIMSS 2018).

Fully specified name (FSN) 1. The unique text representing the meaning of a concept that is independent of the context in which it is used (SNOMED International 2019c). 2. The primary name for a LOINC term.

Functioning An umbrella term for body structures, body functions, and activities and participation. It denotes the positive or neutral aspects of the interaction between the health condition and contextual factors.

General Assembly The highest authority of SNOMED International. It "ensures that the purpose, objects and principles of the association are pursued and that the interests of the organization are safeguarded" (SNOMED International 2019d).

Granularity Consisting of small components or details.

Harmonization The process of identifying and resolving differences by coming to an agreement.

HCPCS Level I Current Procedural Terminology (CPT), maintained by the American Medical Association (AMA).

HCPCS Level II Codes not covered by Current Procedural Terminology (CPT) and modifiers that can be used with all levels of HCPCS codes, developed by the Centers for Medicare and Medicaid Services (CMS); also referred to as National codes.

Healthcare Common Procedure Coding System (HCPCS) A standardized system for healthcare providers and medical suppliers to report professional services, procedures, and supplies.

Healthcare Effectiveness Data and Information Set (HEDIS) A set of standard performance measures designed to provide healthcare purchasers and consumers with the information they need to compare the performance of managed healthcare plans.

Health condition The particular disorders/diseases/injuries of the individual.

Health Information Technology for Economic and Clinical Health (HITECH) Act Legislation created to promote the adoption and meaningful use of health information technology in the United States. Subtitle D of the Act provides for additional privacy and security requirements that will develop and support electronic health information, facilitate information exchange, and strengthen monetary penalties. Signed into law on February 17, 2009, as part of ARRA (Public Law 111-5 2009).

Health Insurance Portability and Accountability Act (HIPAA) The federal legislation enacted to provide continuity of health coverage, control fraud and abuse in healthcare, reduce healthcare costs, and guarantee the security and privacy of health information.

Health Level Seven (HL7) A voluntary consensus standards development organization recognized by the International Organization for Standardization (ISO) and accredited by the American National Standards Institute. The organization's mission is to provide standards for interoperability (HL7 2019). The number seven in the name of the organization refers to the application level (the highest level) in the ISO seven-layer communication model known as the Open Systems Interconnection model.

Heuristics Sets of pragmatic guidelines employed as rules for map developers that are developed in a mapping project to systematically manage issues of ambiguity or uncertainty when interpreting terminological editorial guidance.

Hierarchical Condition Category (HCC) risk adjustment model A statistical process designed to predict the health spending for a specific patient population using attributes such as age, demographics, and medical condition.

Hierarchy An ordered grouping of concept codes linked together through | is a | relationships (SNOMED International 2019b).

Histology The microscopic study of tissue and cells.

ICD-11 for Morbidity and Mortality Statistics (ICD-11-MMS) The classification that replaces the World Health Organization's ICD-10.

ICD-11-MMS Reference Guide A guide that provides material such as explanations of terms and rules to assist in the correct classification of its content. It contains three parts: An Introduction to ICD-11, Using ICD-11, and New in ICD-11.

ICF Model A nonlinear, systemic, biopsychosocial model consisting of multiple components.

Impairment Problems in body structures or functions such as a significant deviation or loss.

Implementation guide An artifact designed to be handed to a software developer who, ideally, does not need to know anything about the subject matter; the guide should contain all the information necessary to build the message.

Institute of Electrical and Electronics Engineers Standards Association (IEEE-SA) A standards-setting body of the IEEE that develops standards in a broad range of industries including healthcare.

Integrating the Healthcare Enterprise (IHE) An initiative by healthcare professionals and industry to improve the way computer systems in healthcare share information. The organization promotes the coordinated use of established standards such as DICOM and HL7 to address specific clinical need in support of optimal patient care.

Intensional One of the two ways of constructing a value set definition. This method states some rule for inclusion of the required values (codes and terms).

International Classification for Nursing Practice (ICNP) A unified nursing language system. It is a compositional terminology for nursing practice that facilitates cross-mapping of local terms and existing terminologies.

International Classification of Diseases (ICD) An international classification system developed by the World Health Organization to translate diagnoses of diseases and other health problems into an alphanumeric code.

International Classification of Diseases, Eleventh Revision (ICD-11) The most recent revision of the World Health Organization's disease classification system.

International Classification of Diseases for Oncology, Third Edition (ICD-O-3) A derived classification of ICD published by the World Health Organization (WHO). It is used primarily by tumor or cancer registries to code the topography (site) and morphology (histology) of neoplasms.

International Classification of Diseases, Tenth Revision, Clinical Modification (ICD-10-CM) The United States' clinical modification of the World Health Organization's ICD-10.

International Classification of Functioning, Disability, and Health (ICF) Both an international classification system and a model developed by the World Health Organization (WHO). The overall aim of the ICF is to provide a "unified and standard language and framework for the description of health and health-related states" that can be used with *all* people, not just those with disability (WHO 2007, 3).

International Classification of Primary Care, Second Edition (ICPC-2) Classification used for coding patient data related to general and family practice and primary care.

International Conference on Harmonization (ICH) of Technical Requirements for Registration of Pharmaceuticals for Human Use A joint project established in 1990 that brought together the drug regulatory authorities of the European Union, Japan, and the United States, as well as representative associations of the pharmaceutical research-based industry in the three regions.

International Council of Nurses (ICN) A federation of national nurses' associations representing millions of nurses worldwide that was instrumental in developing the International Classification for Nursing Practice.

International Organization for Standardization (ISO) A worldwide, nongovernmental, internationally recognized standards development body.

Interoperability Standards Advisory (ISA) A guide published by the Office of the National Coordinator for Health Information Technology (ONC) to help clarify the current state of standards regulation (ONC 2018).

| is a | relationship A parent-child relationship that links concepts within a hierarchy.

Labeler Any firm that manufactures, repacks, or distributes a drug product.

Labeler code The first segment of the National Drug Code (NDC); assigned by the US Food and Drug Administration (FDA) to a firm.

Learning Healthcare System The Institute of Medicine (IOM) vision for the evolution of the healthcare record in the digital age (IOM 2007).

Lexical mapping A mapping activity that identifies links between two terminologies based on the similarity of the wording or character strings they share.

Linearizations A subset of the ICD-11 Foundation Component that is fit for a particular purpose
(reporting mortality, morbidity, or other uses); jointly exhaustive of the ICD universe (Foundation Component); and composed of entities that are mutually exclusive of each other; and in which each entity is given a single parent.

Logical Observation Identifiers, Names, and Codes (LOINC) A standard of universal identifiers developed by the Regenstrief Institute that is used worldwide to facilitate the exchange and aggregation of clinical results for many purposes, including care delivery, quality assessment, public health, and research purposes.

LOINC Committee A voluntary group of interested experts organized by the Regenstrief Institute in 1994 focused on standardizing observation identifiers.

Management Board A board within SNOMED International responsible for the strategic direction of the organization.

Mapping The process of associating concepts from one coding system with concepts from another coding system and defining their equivalence in accordance with a documented rationale and a given purpose.

Meaningful Use An initiative to encourage adoption of electronic health records by specifying what it meant for such a system to "meaningfully" use data from other systems, and by tying Medicaid and Medicare payments to proof that such a system was in use.

Medical Dictionary for Regulatory Activities (MedDRA) A terminology designed to facilitate medical product regulation and related electronic data interchange.

Medical Model A model that follows the assumption that the medical problem resides within the individual (such as a problem in the immune system that causes multiple sclerosis).

Metadata Data that defines and describes other data, such as concepts and data elements (ISO 2013).

Metadata Registry (MDR) A database that houses metadata through the use of a model (metamodel).

Metathesaurus A very large, multipurpose vocabulary database that contains information about patient care, health services billing, public health statistics, indexing, and cataloging biomedical literature or basic, clinical, and health services research.

Minimum Data Set (MDS) One of the three components of the resident assessment instrument; a minimum data set of core elements for use in conducting comprehensive assessments.

Miscellaneous codes Codes that are used when a supplier submits a bill for an item or service for which no existing National code adequately describes the item or service being billed.

Model binding The assignment of meaning to a data element in a model by associating it with a semantic code (for example, "patient blood type").

Model impedance The phenomenon in which the semantics of the model and the terminology do not quite fit.

Modifiers Two-character extensions added to a Current Procedural Terminology (CPT) code to indicate that a particular event modified the service or procedure without changing its basic definition.

Monohierarchy A hierarchy in which a concept has a single parent.

Morbidity The state of being diseased (including illness, injury, or deviation from normal health); the number of sick persons or cases of disease in relation to a specific population.

Morphology The science of structure and form of organisms.

Mortality **1.** The state of being mortal (destined to die); **2.** Incidence of death in a specific population.

Mortality Reference Group (MRG) A group established by the World Health Organization (WHO) to make recommendations regarding mortality to the Update and Revision Committee (URC).

Mutually exclusive A requirement of a statistical classification wherein events cannot occur at the same time to avoid double-counting them.

NANDA-I A classification of nursing diagnoses developed by NANDA International used to describe patients' responses to actual or potential health problems and life processes responses to diseases rather than classifying the conditions of diseases and disorders.

Namespace identifier A number assigned by SNOMED International to an organization that is allowed to maintain a SNOMED CT extension (SNOMED International 2019c); the part of the SNOMED CT Identifier (SCTID) that is controlled by the organization that provides the extension identifier.

National Center for Health Statistics (NCHS) An agency within the Department of Health and Human Services (HHS) that develops and maintains ICD-10-CM and its *Official Guidelines for Coding and Reporting*.

National Council for Prescription Drug Programs (NCPDP) A not-for-profit, ANSI-accredited standards developing organization (SDO) founded in 1977 that develops standards for exchanging prescription and payment information.

National Drug Code (NDC) A product identifier maintained and approved by the US Food and Drug Administration (FDA) that uniquely identifies human drugs and biologics and veterinary drugs. The NDC system is the Health Insurance Portability and Accountability Act (HIPAA) standard medical data code set for reporting drugs and biologics for retail pharmacy transactions.

National Drug Code (NDC) Directory A public repository of NDC numbers and related drug product information populated by domestic and foreign drug labelers that are required to list drugs manufactured, prepared, propagated, compounded, or processed for commercial distribution in the US. There is a separate Electronic Animal Drug Product Listing Directory organized by NDC number.

National Release Center (NRC) Part of a network of national entities responsible for customizing, distributing, supporting, and releasing SNOMED CT for each country.

National Technology Transfer and Advancement Act (NTTAA) A law enacted in 1995 that gives the US Office of Management and Budget (OMB) the authority to direct federal agencies to use voluntary consensus standards unless inconsistent with law or impractical.

NCI Metathesaurus (NCIm) One of two main terminology resources created by the National Cancer Institute Enterprise Vocabulary Services (EVS). Each reference resource contains concepts with associated codes, synonyms, definitions, and inter-concept relationships.

NCI Thesaurus (NCIt) One of two main terminology resources created by the National Cancer Institute Enterprise Vocabulary Services (EVS). Each reference resource contains concepts with associated codes, synonyms, definitions, and inter-concept relationships.

Nonsemantic identifier The codes, or concept identifiers, do not mean anything; one cannot infer information about what a code means without dereferencing its terms.

Normalized name The ingredient, strength, and dose form (in that order) for a generic drug.

Normative standard A standard that carries the legitimacy and enforceability of the completed standards developing organization (SDO) process.

Numeric Index A complete listing of every Current Dental Terminology (CDT) code and the page where the code is found.

Nursing Interventions Classifications (NIC) A terminology that describes the treatments that nurses perform.

Nursing Outcomes Classification (NOC) A classification of patient or client outcomes developed to evaluate the effects of nursing interventions.

Office of the National Coordinator for Health Information Technology (ONC) The lead agency charged with formulating the federal government's health information technology (health IT) strategy and coordinating federal health IT policies, standards, and investments.

Ontology A controlled terminology that employs a formal, computable model of meaning that captures uniquely the defining features of a concept and supports queries of equivalence and relatedness. Well-designed and documented ontologies are generally the best terminological approach to achieving full semantic interoperability.

Open tooling framework (OTF) An open framework that provides tools for the SNOMED CT community. It includes standardized application programming interfaces (APIs) that provide fundamental software services for business applications.

Outcomes and Assessment Information Set (OASIS) A standardized data set that represents items of a comprehensive assessment designed to gather and report data about Medicare beneficiaries who are receiving services from a Medicare-certified home health agency.

Package code The part of the National Drug Code (NDC) that identifies package size and type.

Participation Involvement in a life situation.

Participation restriction Problems an individual may experience in involvement in life situations.

Patient Summary Standards Set (PSSS) A patient summary data set for health information exchange and interoperability developed by the Joint Initiative on SDO Global Health Informatics Standardization (JIC).

Performance A person's ability to do a task or action in a real-life living situation (for example, in a home, neighborhood, store, or recreation center).

Permanent national codes Maintained by the CMS HCPCS Workgroup, permanent national codes provide a standardized coding system that is managed jointly by private and public insurers.

Personal factors Internal influences that facilitate or hinder functioning and health (for example, age, gender, race, habits, upbringing, education, profession).

Polyhierarchy A hierarchy in which a concept can have more than one parent.

Post-coordination A combination of concept identifiers that are joined to convey clinical meaning (SNOMED International 2019e).

Pre-coordination A representation of a commonly used clinical term as a single concept. (6)

Preferred term (PT) In SNOMED CT, the term assigned to a concept that, according to language and dialect, is the most clinically appropriate way of describing it (SNOMED International 2019c).

Pricing, Data Analysis, and Coding (PDAC) contractor Provides coding guidance for manufacturers and suppliers on the proper use of the HCPCS codes used to describe durable medical equipment, prosthetics, orthotics, and supplies (DMEPOS) for the purpose of billing Medicare.

Product code The part of the National Drug Code that identifies a specific strength, dosage form, and formulation of a drug for a particular firm.

Product trade name Name (also referred to as proprietary name) assigned or supplied by the labelers (firms) as required under the Food, Drug, and Cosmetic Act.

Profile One of the degrees of specificity within interoperability levels that constrains any ambiguities and options left in a specification so that implementers in a particular community can communicate clearly, without irrelevant or confusing extra decisions.

Promoting Interoperability (PI) A Centers for Medicare and Medicaid Services (CMS) rebrand of Meaningful Use to indicate the focus on increasing health information exchange and patient data access.

Prospective payment system (PPS) A type of reimbursement system that is based on preset payment levels rather than actual charges billed after the service has been provided; specifically, one of several Medicare reimbursement systems based on predetermined payment rates or periods and linked to the anticipated intensity of services delivered as well as the beneficiary's condition.

Provenance The metadata, or extra information about data, that can help answer questions such as when and by whom the data was created.

Quality Reporting Document Architecture (QRDA) The data submission standard used for a variety of quality measurement and reporting initiatives. QRDA creates a standard method to report quality measure results in a structured, consistent format and can be used to exchange eCQM data between systems. (CMS 2019).

Reasons for encounter (RFE) In the International Classification of Primary Care (ICPC) system, the subjective experience of the problem by the patient, or the "reason for encounter."

Reference model General-level standards (for example, HL7's Reference Information Model [RIM] and ISO's Electronic Health Record Communication standard EN 13606).

Reference set (RefSet) Structured format for a set of references to SNOMED CT components (SNOMED International 2019c).

Reference terminology A controlled terminology employing a set of terms and relationships that capture and define the meaning of each concept.

Regenstrief Institute, Inc. The overall steward and developer of Logical Observation Identifiers, Names, and Codes (LOINC) and nonprofit medical research organization associated with Indiana University.

Regenstrief LOINC Mapping Assistant (RELMA) A desktop program for browsing the database and mapping local test codes to LOINC terms.

Related classification A term that partially refers to a reference classification or is associated with the reference classification at specific levels of structure only and describes important aspects of health or the health system not covered by reference or derived classifications (WHO 2018).

Relationships 1. A type of connection between two concepts. 2. In RxNorm, relationships link drug names to other drug names and ingredients as well as other information, such as National Drug Codes (NDCs), marketing categories, and pill imprint information from the source data (NLM 2018).

Resident assessment instrument (RAI) A federally mandated standard consisting of three components used to collect demographic and clinical data on residents in Medicare- or Medicaid-certified nursing homes and noncritical access hospitals with swing bed agreements.

Root concept A single special concept that represents the root of the entire content in SNOMED CT.

Rubrics In the context of the International Classification of Primary Care (ICPC), the second axis components of an ICPC code.

RxNorm A standardized nomenclature for clinical drugs that supports semantic interoperation between proprietary drug terminologies and pharmacy knowledge base.

RxNorm concept unique identifier (RXCUI) An identifier for the drug concept.

SCRIPT An electronic prescribing standard published by the National Council for Prescription Drug Programs (NCPDP).

Semantic Branded Drug (SBD) In RxNorm, the semantic clinical drug (SCD) with the brand name, i.e., <SCD>[Brand name]. For example, Amoxicilin 250 MG Oral Capsule [Amoxil]. Amoxil is the brand name.

Semantic Clinical Drug (SCD) Standardized names created in RxNorm for every clinical drug; consists of ingredient, strength, and dose form.

Semantic data model A modelling mechanism that describes of how vocabulary items can be combined to make a valid representation of medical information (Huff et al. 1998).

Semantic interoperability "A feature of a terminology or ontology which assures that data recorded in one computer system can be transmitted to a different computer and used with full appreciation of its meaning. This requires that both computers share a computable concept model which defines the data element and that the data are generated compliant with that model" (HIMSS 2018).

Semantic mapping A map developed by making use of the full definition of a concept in a source reference terminology, or ontology, to identify equivalent or related concepts in the target.

Semantic type A domain within a semantic network.

Semicolon Has a special meaning in Current Procedural Terminology (CPT). In order to make the format less cluttered, common information is not repeated. Within a code set, an initial code may contain a procedure description, a semicolon, and additional information. The information to the left of the semicolon applies to that code and all the codes indented under it; the information to the right of the semicolon changes.

Separate procedure Is commonly part of another, more complex procedure.

SNOMED Clinical Terms (SNOMED CT) A systematized, multiaxial, and hierarchically organized controlled terminology developed by the College of American Pathologists and currently owned by SNOMED International.

SNOMED CT Identifier (SCTID) A unique integer assigned to each SNOMED CT component (SNOMED International 2019c).

SNOMED International The organization that owns and maintains SNOMED CT.

SOAP An acronym for a component of the problem-oriented medical record that refers to how each progress note contains documentation relative to **S**ubjective observations by the patient of the problem or the reason for encounter; **O**bjective observations not classified with ICPC; **A**ssessment or diagnosis of the patient's problem; and **P**lans or process of care.

Social Model A model where disability is viewed as a social construction, where problems lie not within the person with a disability but in the environment that fails to accommodate people with disabilities and in the negative attitudes of people without disabilities (where people with disabilities are seen as a minority group).

Source The terminology, classification, or ontology from which a data map originates.

Specifications One of the degrees of specificity within interoperability levels that serve named purposes and often provide sufficient detail to implement without further guidance.

Standards development organization (SDO) An organization involved in the development of standards at a national or international level and in a variety of domains such as healthcare informatics.

Standards set A "coherent collection of standards and standards artefacts that support a specific use case" (JIC 2018).

Structural interoperability "An intermediate level that defines the structure or format of data exchange (i.e., the message format standards) where there is uniform movement of healthcare data from one system to another such that the clinical or operational purpose and meaning of the data is preserved and unaltered. Structural interoperability defines the syntax of the data exchange. It ensures that data exchanges between information technology systems can be interpreted at the data field level" (HIMSS 2018).

Structured Product Labeling A Health Level Seven (HL7) standard labeling format that provides a mechanism for exchanging product and facility information (FDA 2018b).

Surgical package A concept that is based on a single, readily identifiable procedure that may contain a number of services.

Systematized Nomenclature of Dentistry (SNODENT) An official subset of SNOMED CT, it is a terminology providing standardized terms for clinicians, academics, and researchers to record oral health data (ADA 2019).

Target The terminology, classification, or ontology to which a data map links.

Taxonomy 1. The principles of a classification system, such as data classification **2.** The study of general principles of scientific classification.

Technical Implementation Guide (TIG) Contains guidelines and advice about the design of applications using SNOMED CT and covers topics such as release file specifications, concept model, terminology services, entering and storing information, and migration of legacy information (SNOMED International 2019b).

Temporary national codes Codes that give insurers the flexibility to establish codes that are needed before the next annual update for permanent national codes or until consensus can be reached on a permanent national code.

Term The linguistic representations of a concept.

Term type (TTY) Term that indicates generic and branded names of products at different levels of specificity (NLM 2018).

Terminologies Specific knowledge assets in a domain.

Terminology The domain of terms, codes, and their design and use.

Terminology binding The tying-together of the data element in the information model, form, or other structured specification with the set of concepts that may appropriately complete the thought.

Topography The site of origin of the neoplasm. In ICD-O, the same three-character and four-character codes as in the malignant neoplasm section of the second chapter of ICD-10, except those categories that relate to secondary neoplasms and to specified morphological types of tumors.

Transport standards Data exchange standards which support connectivity between systems, allowing them to communicate using standards for discovery, enabling connections, and specifying communication protocols.

UMLS Terminology Services (UTS) The web interface for browser downloads and access to the APIs provided by the UMLS.

Understandable, Reproducible, Useful (URU) principle Three basic operational criteria followed by SNOMED CT modelers when assessing whether content is creating and sustaining semantic interoperability (SNOMED International 2019a).

Unified Code for Units of Measure (UCUM) A system that defines codes for units of measure.

Unified Medical Language System (UMLS) A tool that aggregates, links, and packages existing computer-based clinical terminologies along with biomedical literature and knowledge bases
(NLM 2017).

Uniform Hospital Discharge Data Set (UHDDS) A core set of data elements that are collected by acute care, short-term stay (usually less than 30 days) hospitals to report inpatient data elements in a standardized manner. It was developed through the National Committee on Vital and Health Statistics (NCVHS) and has been required by Department of Health and Human Services (HHS) policy since January 1, 1975.

Uniform Resource Identifiers (URIs) A unique character string for each entity in the International Classification of Diseases (ICD).

Update and Revision Committee (URC) Established by the World Health Organization (WHO) in 2000 to review the reference classifications such as the International Classification of Diseases (ICD) and recommend changes to the Heads of WHO Collaborating Centres each year.

US Core Data for Interoperability (USCDI) A standardized set of health data classes and component data elements for interoperable health information exchange.

US Health Information Knowledgebase (USHIK) A publicly available registry and repository of specifications, standards, and metadata funded by the Agency for Healthcare Research and Quality (AHRQ) in the US Department of Health and Human Services (HHS) (AHRQ n.d.).

Use case A list of activities or step-wise description of events that describe the real-world employment and expected outcomes resulting from a piece of software or data map.

Values The contents of terminologies when terms are not distinguished from codes, or when referring to both (for example, a requirement to draw "values" from LOINC).

Value binding The association of a data element with a set of valid values that may be used to populate it (for example, "A", "B", "AB", "O").

Value set The values (codes and terms) appropriate to a data element.

Value set definition A formal definition of the values in a value set, whether by enumeration ("A", "B", "AB", "O") or by rule ("ABO blood types").

Value set expansion The set of values determined by a value set definition under a certain set of circumstances (for example, a date implying a specific version of the underlying code system).

Vocabulary A list or collection of clinical words or phrases with their meanings; also, the set of words used by an individual or group within a particular subject field.

Vocabulary server A database that hosts multiple terminologies.

WHO Family of International Classifications (WHO-FIC) "A suite of integrated classification products that share similar features and can be used individually or jointly to provide information on different aspects of health and on the health care system" (WHO 2016).

Wonca International Classification Committee (WICC) The Wonca committee responsible for ICPC.

Workgroup for Electronic Data Interchange (WEDI) A cross-sectional coalition of individuals in the healthcare industry that has been involved in improving electronic data interchange standards for billing transactions.

World Health Organization (WHO) The global organization responsible for the development and publication of the reference classifications within the family of international classifications.

World Organization of Family Doctors (Wonca) An organization previously known as the World Organization of National Colleges, Academics, and Academic Associations of General Practitioners/Family Physicians. It was instrumental in the development of ICPC.

References

Agency for Healthcare Research and Quality (AHRQ). 2019. United States Health Information Knowledgebase. http://ushik.ahrq.gov/index.jsp?enableAsynchronousLoading=true.

American Dental Association (ADA). 2019. SNODENT. https://www.ada.org/en/member-center/member-benefits/practice-resources/dental-informatics/snodent.

American Medical Association (AMA). 2019. https://www.ama-assn.org/.

Centers for Medicare and Medicaid Services (CMS). 2019. Quality reporting document architecture. https://ecqi.healthit.gov/qrda-quality-reporting-document-architecture.

Centers for Medicare and Medicaid Services (CMS). 2006. Glossary. https://www.cms.gov/apps/glossary/default.asp?Letter=C&Language=English.

Clinical Data Interchange Standards Consortium (CDISC). 2018. Expert CDISC Group. https://www.cdisc.org/news/expert-cdisc-group.

Data Governance Institute. 2013. Defining Data Governance. http://www.datagovernance.com/defining-data-governance/.

Davoudi, S., J. A. Dooling, B. Glondys, T. D. Jones, L. Kadlec, S. M. Overgaard, K. Ruben, and A. Wendicke. 2015. Data Quality Management Model (2015 Update). Journal of AHIMA 86, no.10 (October 2015): expanded web version. http://bok.ahima.org/doc?oid=107773#.XDPMPlxKhaQ.

eCQI Resource Center. 2019. eCQMs. https://ecqi.healthit.gov/ecqms.

Health Level 7 (HL7). 2019. About HL7. http://www.hl7.org/about/index.cfm?ref=nav.

Healthcare Information and Management Systems Society (HIMSS). 2018. What is interoperability?" https://www.himss.org/library/interoperability-standards/what-is.

Huff, S. M., R. A. Rocha, C. J. McDonald, G. J. De Moor, T. Fiers, W. D. Bidgood, A. W. Forrey et al. 1998. Development of the Logical Observation Identifier Names and Codes (LOINC) vocabulary. JAMIA 5(3):276–292.

Institute of Medicine (IOM). 2007. The Learning Healthcare System: Workshop Summary. Washington, DC: National Academies Press. http://www.ncbi.nlm.nih.gov/books/NBK53494/.

International Standards Organization (ISO). 2014. ISO/TR 12300:2014 Health Informatics – Principles of Mapping between Terminological Systems. https://www.iso.org/standard/51344.html.

ISO/IEC 11179. 2013. Information technology — Metadata registries (MDR) -Part 3: Registry metamodel and basic attributes. Geneva, Switzerland: International Organization for Standardization.

Joint Initiative Council (JIC). 2018. Patient Summary Standards Set Guidance Document, January 2018 v1.0. http://www.jointinitiativecouncil.org/registry/Patient_Summary_Standards_JIC_Jan_2018.pdf.

National Library of Medicine. 2018. RxNorm overview. https://www.nlm.nih.gov/research/umls/rxnorm/overview.html.

National Library of Medicine (NLM). 2017. *Unified Medical Language System*. https://www.nlm.nih.gov/research/umls/about_umls.html.

Office of the National Coordinator for Health Information Technology (ONC) 2018. Interoperability Standards Advisory, 2018. https://www.healthit.gov/isa/.

Public Law 111-5. 2009. 123 Stat. 115, Short title, see 26 U.S.C. 1 note. http://uscode.house.gov/.

Shakir, A.M. 1999. Tools for defining data. Journal of AHIMA 70(8):48–53.

SNOMED International. 2019a. SNOMED CT Editorial Guide. https://confluence.ihtsdotools.org/display/DOCEG/SNOMED+CT+Editorial+Guide.

SNOMED International. 2019b. SNOMED CT Technical Implementation Guide. https://confluence.ihtsdotools.org/display/DOCTIG/Technical+Implementation+Guide.

SNOMED International. 2019c. SNOMED CT Glossary. https://confluence.ihtsdotools.org/display/DOCGLOSS/SNOMED+Glossary.

SNOMED International. 2019d. Governance and Advisory. https://www.snomed.org/our-organization/governance-and-advisory.

SNOMED International. 2019e. SNOMED CT Starter Guide. https://confluence.ihtsdotools.org/display/DOCSTART/SNOMED+CT+Starter+Guide.

U.S. Core Data for Interoperability (USCDI) Task Force. 2018. USCDI Task Force Draft Recommendations. https://www.healthit.gov/sites/default/files/facas/2018-04-18_USCDI_TF_DraftRecommendations-508.pdf.

U.S. Food and Drug Administration (FDA). 2018a. FDA Fundamentals. https://www.fda.gov/AboutFDA/Transparency/Basics/ucm192695.htm.

U.S. Food and Drug Administration (FDA). 2018b. Structured Product Labeling Resources. https://www.fda.gov/forindustry/datastandards/structuredproductlabeling/.

World Health Organization (WHO). 2018. Derived and Related Classifications in the WHO-FIC. http://www.who.int/classifications/related/en/.

World Health Organization (WHO). 2016. *International Statistical Classification of Diseases and Related Health Problems 10th Revision, Volume 2*, 5th ed. Geneva: WHO.

World Health Organization (WHO). 2007. *International Classification of Functioning, Disability, and Health: Children and Youth Version*. Switzerland: WHO.

INDEX

Trust AHIMA for Your Coding Education and Training

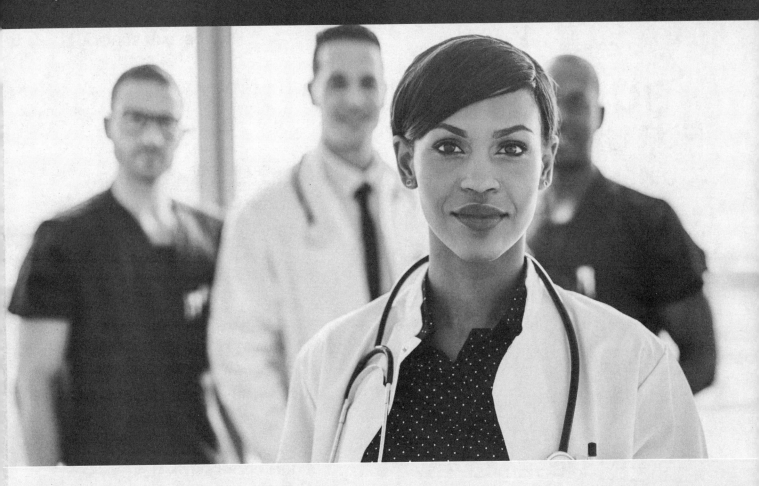

AHIMA is widely recognized and highly regarded as a leader in coding education and training. AHIMA has been at the forefront of providing coding expertise for over 85 years and served as one of four cooperating parties responsible for the ICD-10 Coding Guidelines.

AHIMA HAS A VARIETY OF CODING PRODUCTS AND RESOURCES TO ASSIST YOU AND YOUR TEAM:

- Professional Books and Textbooks
- Meetings
  - In-Person
  - Virtual
- Online Courses
- Toolkits and Practice Briefs
- Webinars

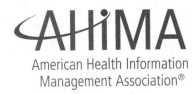

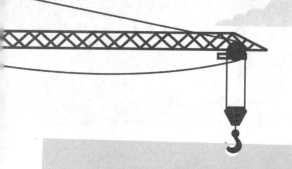

BUILDING A FUTURE CAREER?
YOU NEED THE RIGHT CREW!

You work hard to earn the skills and know-how you need for a job in health information management (HIM). Now lay a strong foundation with AHIMA membership at the affordable Student Member rate—of $49—almost 75% off active member dues!

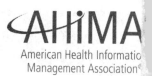